# UNDERSTANDING MOTOR DEVELOPMENT IN CHILDREN

# UNDERSTANDING MOTOR DEVELOPMENT IN CHILDREN

**DAVID L. GALLAHUE**
**Indiana University**

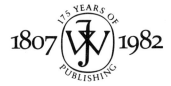

**JOHN WILEY & SONS**
New York • Chichester • Brisbane • Toronto • Singapore

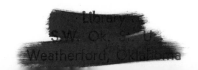

*Library of Congress Cataloging in Publication Data:*

Gallahue, David L.
    Understanding motor development in children.

    Bibliography: p.
    Includes indexes.
    1. Motor ability in children.   2. Child develop-
ment.   3. Physical education for children.
I. Title.

RJ133.G34        155.4′12        81-16279
ISBN 0-471-08779-3                AACR2

Printed in the United States of America

10 9 8 7 6 5 4 3 2 1

Gratefully dedicated to
Douglas and Loretta Gallahue and
Robert and Beatrice Bredenberg
for sharing their wisdom and love
of children throughout a productive life.

# FOREWORD

The acquisition of fine and gross motor skills has historically been regarded as a developmental process that begins during the intrauterine period and continues throughout a lifetime. Evidence accumulated during the last two decades has reinforced the concept that motor development is an orderly, sequential process under favorable conditions, but we have also learned that a variety of agents and conditions can affect the rate and degree to which motor tasks are learned. *Understanding Motor Development in Children* incorporates an impressive body of knowledge from the areas of biology, education, psychology and sociology into a volume that has practical implications for anyone who seeks a greater understanding of motor development during infancy and childhood. The author combines his knowledge of the research literature with years of experience in teaching children into a text that is permeated with practical, down-to-earth suggestions for teachers of motor skills.

Despite its prominence in the literature of child development during the 1920s and 1930s, motor development has received little more than a cursory treatment in texts of child development since then. This trend was also evident in the scientific reports and papers written by psychologists and personnel from the medical professions. Emphasis was directed at cognitive and social growth, while motor development was regarded as a natural, continuous, and unalterable process that would reach specific predictable outcomes through the passage of time. This volume counteracts that omission by identifying the numerous variables that influence motor development and by accentuating the ages and stages when specific elements and events are likely to have their greatest influence. We are reminded of the important interaction between maturation and experience that must occur if children are to reach their potential in motor skill acquisition. The confusing literature on perceptual motor programs is interpreted and summarized so that it has practical utility for educators who seek a comprehensive review, or for those who wish to acquire a base from which to initiate their own programs.

Although theory and the results of research undergird the content, it is the practical application of information that sets this volume apart from contemporary texts devoted to motor development. The acquisition of motor skills from infancy to adolescence is integrated with significant variables as they wax and wane in importance during the course of development. The interrelationship of physical, social, and cognitive development—a pervasive theme—is then carried to its culmination in the motor skills curriculum. The fragmentation of content that frequently occurs in books written by physical educators is avoided by the author's dedication to a holistic approach to motor development.

The current emphasis on learning in early childhood is also likely to bring with it significant changes in the knowledge on which courses and curricula in motor development are based. The author's emphasis on principles and themes provides for the incorporation of new information without disrupting the structure of this text. In fact, the acquisition of supplemental information by students is encouraged through use of a reading list at the end of each chapter. Although these references will soon be outdated, the format suggests that additional information is available and students of motor development are encouraged to search for it.

The ultimate utility of information lies in its ability to enhance the quality of human existence. *Understanding Motor Development in Children* enables teachers to enter a new relationship with children. Readers who have digested the contents of this book and understand the relationships of growth discussed here will be able to observe movement with greater comprehension and interpret its meaning to students with greater clarity.

**VERN SEEFELDT**
**Michigan State University**

# PREFACE

*Understanding Motor Development in Children* is designed for undergraduate and graduate students taking a first course in the growth and motor behavior of children. It is written in an easy-to-understand and easy-to-use manner in order for it to be of value to early childhood, elementary, and physical education teachers. Each chapter contains an introduction to the specific topic, followed by a research-based discussion. The summary and chapter highlights at the end of each chapter provide the reader with a condensed overview and delineation of the major points discussed earlier. A list of critical readings is presented at the end of each chapter for the student who desires further information on the particular subject. Each chapter contains tables and figures, line drawings and photographs, to provide the reader with a clearer understanding of the process of motor development.

Since development is a process that begins at conception and continues throughout life, I have chosen to discuss the prenatal period through childhood (roughly age 12), and have included those cognitive and affective factors that influence the psychomotor development of children. All that we are, or aspire to be, is rooted in the early years of life. Therefore, we will view development during the prenatal period and infancy in terms of its impact on later behavior.

The text is divided into six sections. Section One provides background on the study of motor development. Chapter 1, Understanding Motor Development: An Overview, examines the history, methods of study, research problems, and terminology used in the study of motor development. Chapter 2 provides a discussion of models of child development. Particular attention is given to the theoretical models of Jean Piaget, Erik Erikson, and Robert Havighurst and their implications for motor development. In Chapter 3, Motor Development: A Theoretical Model, a systematic approach to the study of motor development is presented. The phases and stages of this model serve as the theoretical and organizational framework for the remainder of the text; these phases and stages are discussed more fully in Section Four.

Section Two is devoted to factors affecting motor development. Chapter 4 deals with prenatal factors affecting motor development. Chapter 5 focuses on infant and childhood factors affecting motor development.

Section Three deals with the process of growth. Prenatal and infant growth are the topics of Chapter 6. Chapter 7 focuses on childhood growth. In Chapter 8 the general growth and development characteristics of childhood are discussed. A summary of the cognitive and affective characteristics of children during early and later childhood are presented here, along with implications for implementing the physical education program.

Section Four is in many ways the heart of the text. It deals with the phases and stages of motor development. Chapter 9 is devoted to the reflexive movement activity of the newborn and the young infant. Primitive and postural reflexes are discussed, with particular attention given to their role in later movement behavior. Chapter 10 is devoted to rudimentary movement during infancy. The major stability, locomotor, and object manipulation tasks of this period are discussed and summarized. Fundamental movement of preschool and primary grade children is the topic of Chapter 11. A wide variety of locomotor, manipulative, and stability movements are analyzed at their initial, elementary, and mature stages of development. Where possible, these developmental sequences are based on biomechanical research data. Where such data are not available, observational assessment data are used. Chapter 12 focuses on sport-related movement as an outgrowth of fundamental movement abilities. Sport skills as they are related to fundamental movements are presented for a variety of individual and team sports.

Section Five deals with the abilities of children. In Chapter 13 we examine the physical abilities of children. Chapters 14 and 15 focus on perceptual-motor abilities and the self-concept of children, respectively.

Section Six synthesizes information from the preceding sections and deals with programming for children. Chapter 16 examines children's play, toys, and play spaces. Chapter 17 focuses on the education of young children, with particular attention given to the motor development dilemma, educational programs for young children, and the interaction between learning to move and learning through movement. Chapter 18, Developmental Physical Education: A Curricular Model, may be the most important to the practitioner. This chapter presents a developmental approach to the physical education program during the preschool, primary, and elementary school years. Diagrams are used to synthesize the concepts presented in this chapter. Chapter 18 forms the basis for the companion text to this book: *Developmental Movement Experiences for Children,* which puts the concepts and principles dealt with here to practical use through the implementation of developmentally appropriate movement experiences. Finally, Chapter 19 takes a critical look at selected motor development assessment instruments with a view to both their strengths and weaknesses.

As with all authors, there are many people to thank for their contributions to the formulation and completion of this text. I am especially indebted to Jacqueline Herkowitz (Ohio State University), Andrew Ostrow (West Virginia University), and Vern Seefeldt (Michigan State University) for their critical review of the manuscript and their many helpful comments. Lolas Halverson and Mary Ann Roberton (University of Wisconsin), two colleagues whom I have admired from afar for many years, and who are unknowingly responsible for my initial and continuing interest in motor development, deserve special recognition. I am also grateful for the support and contributions of several of my colleagues, especially: John Haubenstricker and Crystal Branta (Michigan State University); Anthony Annarino (Purdue University); Bruce McClenaghan and Diane Ward (University of South Carolina); and Harold Morris, Tony Mobley, and Wynn Updyke (Indiana University). I wish also to thank several of my former students and colleagues from around the world for their contributions to this effort. The dissonance they created in me provided opportunities for refinement of the Phases of Motor Development. I especially wish to thank Farouk Abdulwahab (Cairo University), Mesaed Al-Haroun (University of Kuwait), Fouad Kamal (University of Ottawa), Marika Botha (Namibia), and Richard LaPage, Gordon Payne, and Lawrence Switzer (Winnipeg, Manitoba). Thanks are also due former students Steven Frederick (Wright State University), George Luedke (Southern Illinois University), Robert Koslow (Southern Methodist University), Gregory Payne (California Polytecnic University), and current students Violet Johnson, Sandra Stupiansky and Barbara Willer for their many direct and indirect contributions. The splendid cover photograph as well as the photographs in Chapters 10 and 11 are the work of Ken Gustin. The others are credited to Robert Koslow. A special thank you is extended to Wayne Anderson, Wiley editor, for his support of this project, to my secretary, Laura Shipley, for typing and retyping the manuscript and, of course, to my family (Ellie, David Lee, Jennifer, and Al) for their patience and encouragement.

**DAVID L. GALLAHUE**

## COMPANION TEXT

Gallahue, D.L.: *Developmental Movement Experiences for Children*. New York: Wiley, 1982.

This text provides practical application of the theory and research information that is presented in *Understanding Motor Development in Children*. The book is intended for teachers and students who view physical education from a developmental standpoint and use movement activities as a means of developing and refining fundamental movement abilities. It will be of value to early childhood, elementary classroom, and physical education teachers who wish to use a developmental skill theme approach to improve children's fundamental movement abilities.

The text is divided into four sections. Section I provides a brief overview of the potential outcomes of a quality movement program, a curricular model for teaching developmental physical education, and suggestions for effective teaching by skill themes. Sections II, III, and IV focus on developing and refining fundamental locomotor, manipulative and stability abilities, respectively. Section V provides numerous examples of how to integrate rhythmic, perceptual-motor, visual, auditory, and tactile experiences into the developmental movement program.

This 416-page soft-cover text is available from:

John Wiley & Sons, Inc.
605 Third Avenue
New York, New York 10016

## COMPANION FILM

### THE PROGRESSIVE DEVELOPMENT OF MOVEMENT ABILITIES IN CHILDREN

(15 minutes, sound, color)

This film, developed by the author and Marika Botha, and produced and directed by Ken Gustin, was made possible through a grant from Indiana University and John Wiley & Sons, Inc. The film depicts the development of children's movement abilities, ranging from the first reflexive movements of newborns and the rudimentary movements of infants to the fundamental and sport skill abilities of children and adolescents. Based on research information and the theoretical model presented in this text, the film is an excellent device for introducing the topic of motor development to students, parents, and professional groups.

The film is available for rental ($15.00*) or purchase ($120.00*) from:

Indiana University
Audio Visual Center
Student Services Building, Room 008
Bloomington, Indiana 47405     *Current costs; prices are subject to change.

# CONTENTS

# SECTION FOUR   PHASES AND STAGES OF MOTOR DEVELOPMENT   135

# SECTION FIVE   ABILITIES OF CHILDREN   265

# SECTION SIX    PROGRAMMING FOR CHILDREN

# SECTION ONE

# BACKGROUND

AGE PERIODS OF MOTOR DEVELOPMENT

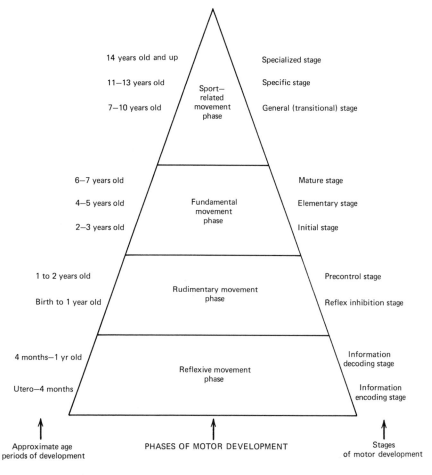

14 years old and up — Specialized stage

11–13 years old — Specific stage

7–10 years old — General (transitional) stage

Sport—related movement phase

6–7 years old — Mature stage

4–5 years old — Elementary stage

2–3 years old — Initial stage

Fundamental movement phase

1 to 2 years old — Precontrol stage

Birth to 1 year old — Reflex inhibition stage

Rudimentary movement phase

4 months–1 yr old — Information decoding stage

Utero–4 months — Information encoding stage

Reflexive movement phase

Approximate age periods of development

PHASES OF MOTOR DEVELOPMENT

Stages of motor development

# Understanding Motor Development: An Overview

The study of human growth and development has been of keen interest to scholars and educators for many years. Knowledge of the processes of development lies at the very core of education whether it be in the classroom, in the gymnasium, or on the playing field. Without a sound knowledge of the developmental aspects of child behavior, one can only guess at the appropriate educational techniques and intervention procedures to use in skill development. Considerable research has been conducted and a number of texts have been written on the processes of development. Although a fair amount of research has been conducted on the developmental aspects of movement behavior, it is of considerably less scope and magnitude in comparison with the amount that has been conducted on the cognitive and affective processes of development.

Developmental psychologists tend to be only marginally interested in motor development and then only as a visual indicator of cognitive functioning. Likewise the social psychologist is interested in affective development with only fleeting attention given to movement and its influences on the social and emotional development of the individual. Since the primary thrust of research and study has come from the many branches of psychology, it is only natural that motor development has often been viewed in terms of its potential influences on other areas of behavior, and a convenient and readily observable means of studying behavior, instead of a phenomenon worthy of study for its own sake.

The study of motor development as a specialized field is a relatively new addition to the physical education profession, although motor development is recognized by many to be at its very heart. The decade of the 1980s has given rise to the full recognition of motor development as a legitimate area of study that cuts across the fields of exercise physiology, biomechanics, motor behavior, and motor control, as well as the fields of developmental psychololgy and sociology. The early and continuous work of physical education professionals such as Helen Eckert, Anna Espenschade, Ruth Glassow, Lolas Halverson, and G. Lawrence Rarick did much to kindle interest in the study of motor development. The quest for understanding progressed at a slow but steady pace into the 1960s, and then the pace began to escalate as physical educators and psychologists alike shifted their focus away from achievement-oriented norms back to the study of underlying developmental processes. During the 1970s an ever-expanding body of research led by a new generation of scholars heightened interest in the study of motor development. Interest has continued into the 1980s, and now the study of motor development has taken its place as a legitimate area of study and research in the fields of physical education and psychology.

Unfortunately, the process of human development is often studied from a compartmentalized standpoint, which has led to a rather unbalanced view of growth and development. Development has been studied in terms of domains (cognitive, affective, psychomotor), age-related behaviors (infancy, childhood, adolescence, adulthood, middle age, old age), and from either a biological or an environmental bias (Figure 1.1). It is crucial that those interested in the study of motor development not compound the errors of compartmentalization. The study of motor development must be viewed from the perspective of the totality of humankind. It

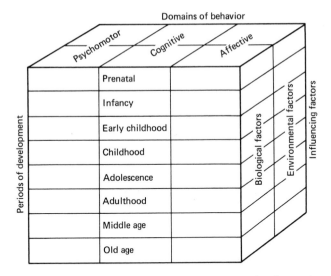

**Figure 1.1.** The compartmentalized view of human development.

must encompass both the biological and environmental aspects of cognitive and affective behavior that impact on motor development, and it must look across various age periods of development. If it is to be of any real value to the practitioner the study of motor development must not focus only on the skilled performer in a controlled environment. It must instead analyze and document what individuals of all ages can do under normal and augmented circumstances. Figure 1.2 provides a schematic representation of the interrelated nature of the study of motor development.

It is apparent that a full discussion in one text of all aspects of growth and development from conception to old age would be a monumental task. Therefore, this book will focus on physical growth and motor development during childhood (roughly ages 2 through 12). Background information from the prenatal period and infancy is provided in terms of its relationship to development in childhood. The cognitive and affective aspects of development are discussed in terms of how they impact on motor development and of how motor development impacts on each of them. Discussion, where possible, is research-based and documented. Information is, however, presented in nontechnical terms demonstrating practical application of knowledge wherever possible. The Chapter Highlights at the end of each chapter list the main concepts dealt with in that chapter.

The information contained here is not the "last word" on the physical growth and motor development of children. Research and study in this area are still in their infancy in comparison to other other areas of developmental research. Our knowledge base is constantly expanding, and even as this text is being written new

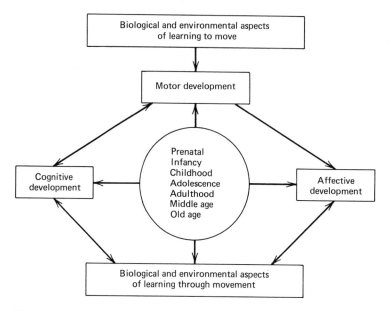

**Figure 1.2.** The interrelated nature of the study of motor development.

hypotheses are being formulated and new conclusions being drawn from the excellent research being conducted throughout North America and Europe.

## STUDY OF THE DEVELOPMENTAL PROCESS

Development is a continuous process that begins at conception and ceases at death. Development encompasses all aspects of human behavior and as a result may only be artificially separated into domains, categories, or age periods. The growing acceptance of the concept of "lifespan" development is important to keep in mind. Just as study of the skilled athlete during adolescence and adulthood is important so also is the study of movement important during infancy, childhood, and later life. There is much to be gained by learning about motor development at all ages and by viewing it as a continuous process.

Motor development is highly specific. The once accepted notion of general motor ability has been disproved to the satisfaction of most. Superior ability in one area does not guarantee similar ability in others. The outmoded concept that one either possesses or does not possess ability in movement activities has been replaced by the concept that each person has specific capabilities within each of the many performance areas.

Various factors involving movement abilities and physical abilities interact in complex ways with cognitive and affective abilities. Each of these abilities is in turn affected by a wide variety of biologically and environmentally related factors.

The process of development, and more specifically the process of motor development, should constantly remind us of the individuality of the learner. Each individual has his or her own unique timetable for the development and extent of acquisition of movement abilities. Although our "biological clock" is rather specific when it comes to the sequence of acquisition of abilities, the rate and extent of development are individually determined. Typical age periods of development are just that: typical, and no more. Age periods merely represent approximate time ranges during which certain behaviors may be observed. Overreliance on these time periods would negate the concepts of continuity, specificty, and the individuality of the developmental process.

The study of growth and motor development dates back only to the 1930s. Since then a number of methods of study have evolved, and a variety of problems have influenced both the quantity and quality of information available. The following sections briefly review the history, methods of study, and problems encountered in the study of motor development.

## History

The first serious attempts at the study of motor development in children were made in the 1930s by Bayley (1935), Gesell and Thompson (1934), McGraw (1935), Shirley (1931), and others. Since their early pioneering efforts, their names have become legend in motor development research. The surge of interest that their research brought about was motivated by interest in the relationship of the processes of maturation and learning to cognitive development. In their separate but remarkably similar research, the early researchers chronicled the well-known sequences of motor development during infancy. Their naturalistic observations of children provided a great deal of information about the sequential nature of the progression of normal development from the acquisition of early rudimentary movements to mature patterns of behavior. Although the rate at which children acquired selected movement abilities varied somewhat, the investigations revealed that the sequence of acquisition was universal and invariant.

The studies of Gesell and Thompson (1929) and McGraw (1935) are classics in the use of the co-twin control method of studying development. Their research provided considerable insight into the influence of augmented and restricted practice on the acquisition of various movement abilities, and raised numerous questions concerning early practice and the acquistion of various movement abilities. The study of throwing behavior by Monica Wild (1938) marked the beginning of the study of developmental movement patterns in children. Unfortunately, however, after her study, which was outstanding in terms of depth and completeness, little interest was shown in the study of the various aspects of motor development for several decades. With the exceptions of the unpublished doctoral dissertation of Dorothy Deach (1951) and the continuing research of Espenschade, Rarick, and Glassow, little significant research was conducted until the early 1960s.

Since 1960 there has been a steadily growing knowledge base in the study of motor development. The work of Lolas Halverson and several of her graduate students at the University of Wisconsin on the acquisition of fundamental movement abilities did much to revive interest in children's research because of its emphasis on identifying the mechanisms behind the acquisition of skill instead of on the final skill itself. *Fundamental Motor Patterns* (1977) by Ralph Wickstrom and the excellent research conducted by Vern Seefeldt (1972) and his associates at Michigan State University on fundamental movement did much to set the stage for the research and study that are being conducted in the 1980s. Now, due in part to the youth sport phenomenon, and to the formation of the Motor Development Academy within the American Alliance for Health, Physical Education, Recreation, and Dance (AAHPERD), significant research is being conducted throughout North America and much of the rest of the world on the growth and motor development of children.

## Methods

There are two basic ways in which motor development is studied: the longitudinal study, and the cross-sectional study. Because motor development research involves the study of changes that occur in motor behavior over time, the longitudinal method of study is ideal in many ways. Longitudinal data collection attempts to explain behavior changes over time and involves charting various aspects of the individual's growth and/or motor performance for several years. The longitudinal approach allows one to observe changes over time on selected variables and although time consuming permits the study of motor development as a function of maturity rather than age. The Medford Boys Growth Study conducted by H. Harrison Clarke (1971) from 1956 to 1968 is one of the most complete longitudinal studies of growth ever carried out. The motor pattern development study begun in 1966 by Vern Seefeldt (1972) collected thousands of feet of film footage on children performing selected fundamental movement skills over several years and is a fine example of a longitudinal study of developmental movement.

It can easily be seen that the longitudinal method of data collection is very time consuming. The dropout rate because of children moving, illness, or disability is often great. Therefore, large numbers of children need to be tested in hopes of still having a representative sample at the end of the five- to ten-year study period. Problems in methodology and design are also likely to creep into the longitudinal study. The reliability and objectivity of changing testers over the course of the study period may cause problems in data interpretation. The potential learning effect over time from repeated performances on the measured items has also been shown to be a difficult variable to deal with (Beumen et al., 1980). Because of these difficulties many researchers have opted for the cross-sectional approach to studying motor development.

The cross-sectional method of study permits the researcher to collect data on different groups of people at varying age levels at the same point in time. Although this method yields only average changes in groups over time and not individual changes, the basic assumption is that random selection of subjects will provide a representative sample of the population for each age group tested. Cross-sectional studies can describe only typical behavior at the specific ages studied. The vast majority of research on motor development uses a cross-sectional approach. The reasons are obvious, but, most importantly, it is a simpler and more direct technique. It should be noted also that data collected from longitudinal studies, *in general*, do seem to substantiate the results of cross-sectional data collection studies even though the learning effects of repeated performances are still present (Wickstrom, 1977).

In recent years developmental psychologists and motor development researchers have begun to look more closely at the application of both cross-sectional and longitudinal research designs. This sequential method of studying development, or mixed-longitudinal method, as it is often termed, combines the best aspects of the cross-sectional and longitudinal methods in that it covers all of the possible data points necessary for both describing and explaining developmental change (Schaie and Baltes, 1975).

Both longitudinal and cross-sectional methods of study may be applied in a variety of research formats. Table 1.1 provides a brief overview of these formats for studying development. An investigation may take the form of an experimental study, the most powerful method because of the rigid controls required, or it may be cross-cultural, involve naturalistic observation, surveys, interviews, case history reports, or a combination of these techniques.

Over the years there has been a shift in the study of children's motor development from process to product and now back to process again. The early researchers emphasized the importance of studying the process of movement, that is, form and function. H.M. Halverson (Halverson et al., 1931; Halverson, 1937), Shirley (1931), and Wild (1938) all focused on the sequential acquisiton of movement patterns. Their suggestions for studying the process of motor skill development went largely unheeded until the 1960s when interest in such study was again revived; it has been a focus of motor skill development research in children ever since. The use of cinematography, electrogoniometry, and electromyographic techniques in conjunction with computer analysis has enhanced our knowledge of the process of movement.

Product-oriented research, or research on the performance capabilities of chil-

**Table 1.1   Primary Methods of Studying Child Behavior**

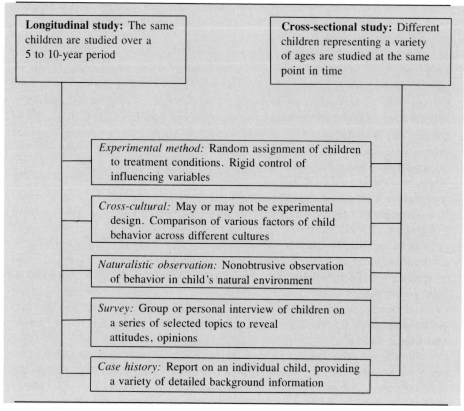

**Longitudinal study:** The same children are studied over a 5 to 10-year period

**Cross-sectional study:** Different children representing a variety of ages are studied at the same point in time

*Experimental method:* Random assignment of children to treatment conditions. Rigid control of influencing variables

*Cross-cultural:* May or may not be experimental design. Comparison of various factors of child behavior across different cultures

*Naturalistic observation:* Nonobtrusive observation of behavior in child's natural environment

*Survey:* Group or personal interview of children on a series of selected topics to reveal attitudes, opinions

*Case history:* Report on an individual child, providing a variety of detailed background information

dren, has been conducted for many years. This type of research is typically concerned with the outcome of the individual's performance. The distance a ball travels or the velocity with which it can be kicked are examples of performance scores. The strength, endurance, or flexibility of children as measured by a particular battery of tests can also be stated as performance scores.

The relationship between process and product, or form ratings and performance scores, is an interesting and largely unresearched area. Wickstrom (1977) has indicated, however, that "there is a positive but not direct causal relationship between form and performance. Mature form enhances performance, but good performance is not totally dependent upon mature form" (p. 5). The factors that influence performance, such as strength, speed of movement, agility, coordination, and reaction time have an impact on performance abilities but may not influence form to any significant degree.

## Problems

Data collection, whether it be product or process oriented, can be difficult and patience-trying when investigating infants and children. In fact, one of the chief causes of the lag in the motor development research information on infants and children is problems associated with data collection. Infants and preschoolers tend to be difficult subjects unless procedures are adopted that take into account their natural independent natures. The two primary problems associated with good data collection are inhibited or exaggerated performance, and inconsistency in performance. Special precautions must be taken to eliminate, as far as possible, the potential bias of the data caused by these factors. In an attempt to put the child at ease, time-consuming orientation periods, and modified data collection procedures that simulate a more naturalistic setting must be employed. This still will not ensure consistency in performance. For example, when asked to "throw the ball overhand as far as you can," the young child may throw first with the right hand and then just as casually begin throwing with the left. Some throws may be overhand, others sidearm or underhand, even after precise instructions as to the particular type of throw desired. Some throws may go several yards, others only a few feet. Some throws may closely approximate a mature pattern of action while others may look like a shot-put attempt or grenade-tossing exercise. As a result, the experimenter is required to exercise considerable patience and to work with the child until he or she has demonstrated what the experimenter judges to be a maximum or representative effort using the most characteristic pattern of movement. The potential problems that this may cause are serious. Learning and fatigue factors may contaminate the data, as may errors in experimenter judgment.

Another problem that plagues the developmental researcher is interrater consistency. It is crucial, for example, that observational assessment be systematically analyzed and that observers be carefully trained in how to observe and in what to look for. Still another problem, and potentially the most serious one facing the researcher involves the reliability and validity of the measuring instrument itself. A variety of motor development assessment devices are available. Some have been meticulously designed, while others represent a combination of measures for which there is only a vague notion as to their reliability with much less known about their validity.

The benefits to be gained from motor development research with infants and children far outweigh the problems and pitfalls. As information gradually accumulates and is replicated, we are gaining a more accurate picture of the processes involved in motor development in children. Research efforts that use longitudinal and cross-sectional approaches, that focus on form and performance, and that recognize the need for patient, unbiased data collection are making significant contributions to our understanding of motor development.

## TERMINOLOGY USED IN MOTOR DEVELOPMENT

A working knowledge of the terms commonly used in any area of study is an important first step in understanding that field. Whether it is medicine or law, special education or economics, there is jargon typical to each field of study, and motor development is no exception. Over the years a variety of terms have come into common usage. These terms are presented in this section. As with the jargon in most areas of study, agreement on the meaning of each term is not universal. We must strive for greater consistency of meaning. Words have meaning, and ideally their meanings should be universal. It is with this concept in mind that the following terms are presented.

### Growth and Development

The terms *growth* and *development* are often used interchangeably, but there is a difference in emphasis implied by each. In its purest sense, growth refers to an increase in the size of the body or its parts as the child progresses toward maturity. In other words, growth is an increase in the structure of the body brought about by the multiplication or enlargement of cells. The term growth, however, is often used to refer to the totality of physical change, and as a result it becomes more inclusive and takes on the same meaning as development.

Development, in its purest sense, refers to changes in the individual's level of functioning. It is the emerging and broadening of the child's ability to function on a higher level. The study of development is concerned with what occurs and how it occurs in the human organism in its journey from conception through maturity to death. It is a continuous process that encompasses all of the interrelated dimensions of our existence, and care must be taken not to consider each of these dimensions as autonomous.

The interwoven elements of maturation and experience play a key role in the developmental process. *Maturation* refers to qualitative changes that enable one to progress to higher levels of functioning. Maturation, when viewed from a biological perspective, is primarily innate; that is, it is genetically determined and resistant to external or environmental influences. Maturation is characterized by a fixed order of progression in which the pace may vary but the sequence of appearance of characteristics generally does not. For example, the progression and approximate ages at which an infant learns to sit, stand, and walk are highly influenced by maturation. The sequence of appearance of these abilities is fixed and resistant to change with only the rate of appearance being altered by the environmental influences of learning and experience.

*Experience* refers to factors within the environment that may alter or modify the appearance of various developmental characteristics through the process of learning. The experiences that children are exposed to may have an effect on the rate of onset of certain patterns of behavior.

The developmental aspects of both maturation and experience are interwoven. Determining the separate contribution of each of these processes is impossible. In fact, a heated debate in the literature over the relative importance of the two has raged for over a century. As a result, the term *adaptation* has come into vogue and is often used to refer to the complex interplay between forces within the individual and the environment. Figure 1.3 illustrates how the factors of growth, maturation, experience, and adaptation are all directly related to the developing child and to one another.

## Domains of Behavior

The classification of human behavior into domains or categories of behavior was first popularized by Bloom and his associates (1956) and Krathwohl, Bloom, and Masia (1964) in their pioneering attempt to establish a taxonomy of educational objectives. Their separation of behavior into cognitive (intellectual behavior), affective (social-emotional behavior), and psychomotor (motor behavior) has, unfortunately, caused many to deal with each domain as an independent entity of human development and learning. We must not lose sight of the interrelated nature of development and the three domains of human behavior even though we may tend to separate them for the sake of convenience in our discussion and study of children.

*Psychomotor development* involves the process of change and stabilization in physical structure and neuromuscular function. It is often referred to simply as motor development, and the two terms are used interchangeably throught the text. Psychomotor (motor) development is a lifelong process in the broadest sense of its definition. It encompasses all physical change and the acquisition, stabilization, or

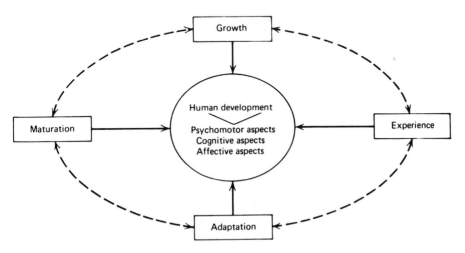

**Figure 1.3.** Interrelated components of human development.

diminution of motor skills. The motor development of children may be categorized into the development of physical abilities and the development of movement abilities. *Physical abilities,* or *motor abilities,* as they are sometimes called, is the term used to lump the various components of physical fitness (muscular strength, muscular endurance, cardiorespiratory endurance, and flexibility) and motor fitness (speed of movement, agility, coordination, balance, and power) together. Physical abilities are associated with the capacity to perform motor tasks. *Movement abilities,* on the other hand, is a comprehensive term used to group together the categories of movement (locomotor, manipulative, and stabilizing). Thus one may be interested in an aspect of motor development as it relates to understanding the physical abilities of children and as it applies to the performance of a variety of movement abilities across age, sex, or social class.

*Cognitive development* as applied to the study of movement behavior involves the functional relationship between mind and body. The reciprocal interaction of mind and body has been dealt with from as far back as the philosophical musings of Socrates and Plato to the developmental theorists of the twentieth century. Jean Piaget (1952), known for his theory of cognitive development, is an example of a modern theorist who recognized the important role of movement, particularly during the early years of life. Piaget's work has done much to spread the notions of perceptual-motor development and the development of academic concept readiness through the medium of movement. The term *perceptual-motor* has come into vogue in recent years to signify the important influence that sensory cues and the perceptual process have on motor activity. In its broadest sense a perceptual-motor act is any voluntary movement that relies on sensory data to process information used in the performance of that act. In other words, all voluntary movement may be viewed as perceptual-motor in nature. Movements that are subcortically controlled (reflexes) are the only forms of movement of the skeletal muscles that do not require some element of perception.

*Affective development* as related to the study of human movement involves feelings and emotions as applied to self and others through movement. Self-concept, peer relations, and play are areas of interest to students of motor development. *Self-concept* may be thought of as one's personal feelings of self-worth or worthlessness. It is influenced by a variety of factors, one of which is movement.

*Peer relations* refers to the level of social interaction evidenced by an individual. Play behavior has been shown to have a developmental base that manifests itself in changing peer relations and more sophisticated levels of functioning (Ellis, 1973).

These definitions of the psychomotor, cognitive, and affective domains as they influence, and are influenced by, developmental processes permit us to clarify a variety of terms that contain the word *motor* or *movement*. What follows is not a mere exercise in semantics. Words reflect concepts and are one of the few ways in which we can convey ideas. It is important that we impose similar meanings on them because subtle differences in words often make gigantic differences in the thought or concept being presented.

## Motor Development

The term *motor* when used by itself refers to the *underlying* biological and mechanical factors that influence movement. The term, however, is rarely used alone but serves as a suffix or prefix to such terms as : *psychomotor, perceptual-motor, sensorimotor, motor learning, motor control,* and, of course, *motor development*. The terms psychomotor, perceptual-motor, and sensorimotor have gained popularity in the jargon of psychologists and educators. Physical educators, on the other hand, have tended to limit use of the prefixes of these words to discussions that focus specifically on that aspect of the motor process. The term *motor* is used as a prefix to describe specific areas of study. The following is a brief description of several of these terms as they are commonly used.

*Learning* is defined as a relatively permanent change in behavior resulting from experience and training interacting with biological processes. *Motor learning* is that aspect of learning in which body movement plays a major part. *Motor behavior* is defined here as that aspect of motor learning that embodies learning and performance factors and maturational processes associated with movement performance. Motor behavior research is concerned with the study of changes in behavior and how these processes of change operate.

*Motor control* is that aspect of motor learning that deals with the study of isolated tasks under specific conditions. Study in this area is concerned with the underlying processes involved in the performance of a movement act that are consistent from trial to trial.

*Motor development* is that aspect of motor behavior and motor control that is primarily concerned with the study of changes in motor performance throughout the entire life span. Study of the underlying biological and environmental processes of motor development is typically viewed in stages (infancy, childhood, adolescence, adulthood, old age) that reflect the particular interest of the investigator.

The terms *motor pattern, fundamental motor pattern, motor skill,* and *perceptual-motor skill* all refer to the *underlying* sensory, integrative, and decision-making processes that precede the performance of an observable movement. Perception and cognition are important variables because they influence underlying motor processes. Underlying motor processes are involved in the performance of *all* voluntary movement.

## Movement Forms

The term *movement* refers to actual *observable* change in position of any part of the body. Movement is the culminating act of the underlying motor processes. The word movement is often linked with others to broaden or clarify its meaning, but in general it refers to the overt act of moving. The following is a brief description of some movement terms as they are commonly used.

A *movement pattern* as defined by Wickstrom (1977) is "a series of movements organized in a particular time-space sequence" (p. 3). A movement pattern is an organized series of related movements. More specifically, a movement pattern represents the performance of an isolated movement that in and of itself is too restricted to be classified as a fundamental movement pattern. For example, the sidearm, underarm, or overarm patterns of movement alone do not constitute the fundamental movements of throwing or striking but merely represent an organized series of movements. A *fundamental movement pattern*, therefore, refers to the observable performance of basic locomotor, manipulative, and stabilizing movements. Fundamental movement patterns involve the combination of movement patterns of two or more body segments. Running, jumping, striking, throwing, twisting, and turning are examples of fundamental movement patterns.

Although the terms movement pattern and movement skill are often used interchangeably, a *movement skill* is viewed here as a fundamental movement pattern performed with greater accuracy, percision, and control. In a movement skill, accuracy is stressed, and extraneous movement is therefore limited, whereas in a fundamental movement pattern, movement is stressed but accuracy is limited.

A *sport skill* is the combination of fundamental movement patterns or movement skills applied to the performance of sport related activities. Therefore, the fundamental movement patterns of twisting the body and striking may be developed to a high degree of precision and applied in their horizontal form to batting in the sport of baseball, or in their vertical form to playing golf or serving a tennis ball. The performance of a sport skill requires making increasingly precise alterations in the basic patterns of movement as higher levels of skill are achieved.

*Movement education* is a term that has been defined in a variety of ways all of which seem somewhat restrictive and shortsighted. It has been defined as a method, as a process, and as an aspect of the physical education program generally limited to children. Gilliom (1970) defines movement education as the "foundational structure and process portion of physical education" (p. 4). Logsdon et al. (1977) take a more global view of movement education as a "lifelong process of change" (p. 12). For the purpose of our discussion we will view movement education as the lifelong process of motor development as evidenced by changes in movement behavior. Input from a qualified physical education teacher, as well as use of the appropriate facilites and equipment, facilitates the process of movement education, but is not entirely restricted to these conditions nor to specific age ranges.

## Gross and Fine Movements

Movement, whether it takes the form of a movement pattern or a movement skill, may be classified in a variety of ways. There is not a clear delineation between the terms *gross* and *fine*, but movements are often classified as one or the other. A *gross motor movement* involves movement of the large muscles of the body. Most sport skills are classified as gross motor movements, with the exception perhaps of target shooting, archery, and a few others. *Fine motor movements* involve limited movements of parts of the body in the performance of precise movements. The manipulative movements of sewing, writing, and typing are generally thought of as fine motor movements.

## Discrete, Serial, and Continuous Movements

On the basis of its temporal aspects, movement may also be classified as discrete, serial, or continuous. A *discrete movement* has a very definite beginning and ending. Throwing, jumping, kicking, and striking a ball are examples of discrete movements. *Serial movements* involve the performance of a single, discrete movement several times in rapid succession. Rhythmical hopping, basketball dribbling, and a soccer or volleyball volley are typical serial tasks. *Continuous movements* are movements that are repeated for a specified period of time. Running, swimming, and cycling are common continuous movements.

## Open and Closed Movements

Fundamental movement patterns and movement skills are often referred to as open tasks or closed tasks. An *open task* is a movement task performed in an environment where the conditions are constantly changing. These changing conditions require the individual to make adjustments or modifications in the actual pattern of movement to suit the demands of the situation. Plasticity, or flexibility, in movement is required in the performance of an open skill. Most dual and group activities involve open skills that depend on external and internal feedback for their successful execution. For example, the child taking part in a typical game of tag, requiring running and dodging in varying directions, is never using the exact same patterns of movement during the game. The child is required to adapt to the demands of the activity through a variety of similar but different movements. Performance of an open movement task differs markedly from performance of a closed movement task.

*Closed movement tasks* may be thought of as movements that "require a constancy of movement pattern and are performed under an unchanging environment" (Sage, 1977, p. 338), A closed movement skill or fundamental movement pattern demands rigidity of performance. In other words, it depends on kinesthetic, rather than visual and auditory, feedback from the execution of the task. The child who is performing a headstand, throwing at a target, or doing a vertical jump is performing a closed movement task.

The reader is cautioned not to be arbitrary in the classification of movement as either gross or fine, discrete, serial, or continuous, and open or closed. The vast majority of movement involves some elements of each. Distinct separation and classification of movements is not always possible, nor is it always desirable. The child is a dynamic, moving being, constantly being acted upon and interacting with many subtle environmental factors. The arbitrary classification of movement should serve only to focus attention on the specific aspect of movement under consideration. Table 1.2 provides a schematic representation and brief description of terms commonly used in the study of learning and development. The reader will find it useful to carefully review these terms paying particular attention to their interrelatedness. The terms motor and movement, pattern and skill, which are commonly used interchangeably in the literature, have particularly subtle differences.

## Summary

A cursory look at most growth and development texts and many elementary physical education texts will reveal statements such as: "Children need plenty of daily vigorous physical activity in order to develop their movement abilities." Although a noble gesture for including physical activity as an important part of the child's day, and basically true, this statement needs to be qualified and broadened if it is to have *real* meaning. Children may, and generally can, have time during the course of the day to pursue vigorous activity. Often, however, they fail to take advantage of this time due to (1) lack of opportunities, (2) lack of motivation, and (3) lack of qualified instruction.

The daily routine of millions of children from the preschool years through the elementary grades has been programmed for them from the minute they wake up until the moment they go to sleep. Demands are constantly placed on their time in terms of eating, sleeping, school attendance, homework, and, of course, television. Little time is left for regular participation in vigorous physical activity, unless parents and teachers consciously help children program such activity into their daily schedule. Probably the easiest way to do so is to limit the amount of daily television watching and to instead use this time for play or active game participation. The best way to ensure that all have the opportunity to take part in regular vigorous physical activity is through the scheduling of a physical education period sometime during each school day.

Often, there is a lack of motivation on the part of both adults and children to be active. Although it is generally accepted that children are active, energetic, moving beings, the demands and constraints of our rapidly changing society, as well as the fascination with nonvigorous participatory devices such as computer games and television, often motivate the child away from active forms of participation and toward more sedentary activities. As adults, we need to be aware of the constant and often subtle societal and environmental pressures that lead to the inactivity of children. We need to temper these pressures and to develop techniques that encourage and motivate children to be active as a regular part of their daily life experience.

For too many years it has been assumed by parents and educators alike that

**Table 1.2   The Interrelated Nature of Terms Commonly Used in Motor Development**

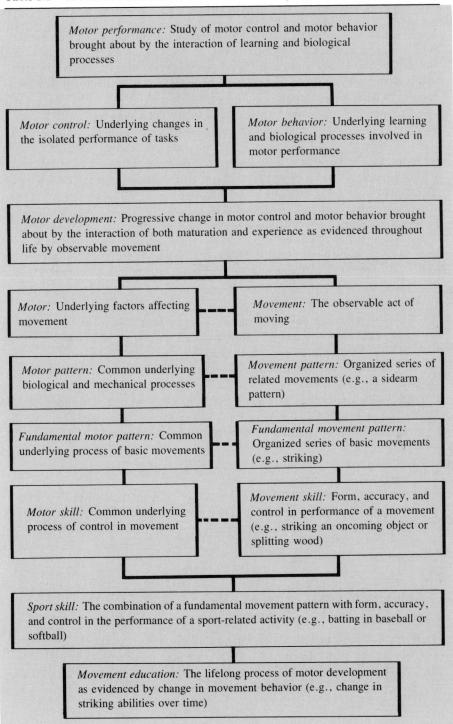

*Motor performance:* Study of motor control and motor behavior brought about by the interaction of learning and biological processes

*Motor control:* Underlying changes in the isolated performance of tasks

*Motor behavior:* Underlying learning and biological processes involved in motor performance

*Motor development:* Progressive change in motor control and motor behavior brought about by the interaction of both maturation and experience as evidenced throughout life by observable movement

*Motor:* Underlying factors affecting movement

*Movement:* The observable act of moving

*Motor pattern:* Common underlying biological and mechanical processes

*Movement pattern:* Organized series of related movements (e.g., a sidearm pattern)

*Fundamental motor pattern:* Common underlying process of basic movements

*Fundamental movement pattern:* Organized series of basic movements (e.g., striking)

*Motor skill:* Common underlying process of control in movement

*Movement skill:* Form, accuracy, and control in performance of a movement (e.g., striking an oncoming object or splitting wood)

*Sport skill:* The combination of a fundamental movement pattern with form, accuracy, and control in the performance of a sport-related activity (e.g., batting in baseball or softball)

*Movement education:* The lifelong process of motor development as evidenced by change in movement behavior (e.g., change in striking abilities over time)

through maturation children will *automatically* develop their movement abilities. Such a notion is absurd. There is little evidence to support the notion that fundamental movement abilities are developed automatically. Regular, systematic, quality instruction and supervised practice are crucial for most children if they are to develop their movement abilities to their mature form.

The physical education teacher or the classroom teacher with a sound background in the motor development and movement education of children can do much to provide children with the opportunities, motivation, and instruction necessary for the development of movement abilities. Therefore, the following modified statement seems more appropriate than the statement at the beginning of the section: *Children need plenty of opportunity, motivation, and instruction in a variety of daily vigorous physical activities in order to develop their unique movement abilities to an optimum level.*

## CHAPTER HIGHLIGHTS

1. Interest in the study of motor development begin in the 1930s but waned until the 1960s.
2. The study of motor development has, until recently, been overshadowed by study of the cognitive and affective processes of development.
3. There has been a rapidly expanding knowledge base in motor development over the past twenty five years, and it is now viewed as a cornerstone of the physical education profession.
4. Motor development research involves the use of a variety of techniques that depend on both longitudinal and cross-sectional data.
5. Data collection in controlled experiments is often very difficult with young children.
6. The terminology used in motor development must be understood in order to grasp the concepts being dealt with.
7. There is often overlap in the use of terms used to describe movement; yet there may be subtle differences involved.
8. Motor development is an important aspect of the individual's total development, which is viewed as a process of change beginning at conception and ending with death.

## CRITICAL READINGS

Lockhart, A.: "What's in a Name?" *Quest*, 2, 9–13, 1964.

Magill, R.A.: *Motor Learning: Concepts and Applications*, Dubuque, Iowa: W.C. Brown, 1980, Chapter 1.

Sage, G.H.: *Introduction to Motor Behavior: A Neuropsychological Approach*, Reading, Mass.: Addison-Wesley, 1977, Chapters 16–18.

Singer, R.N.: *Motor Learning and Human Performance*, New York: Macmillan, 1980, Chapters 1−2.
Wickstrom, R.L.: *Fundamental Motor Patterns*, Philadelphia: Lea and Febiger, 1977, Chapter 1.

# CHAPTER 2

# Models of Child Development

During the past half century several developmental theorists have closely studied the phenomena of human development. Sigmund Freud, Erik Erikson, Arnold Gesell, Robert Havighurst, and Jean Piaget have each made valuable contributions to our knowledge of child development. Each has constructed a theoretical model of development that depicts the many phases and stages that are passed through on the journey from childhood to maturity. Each of the models have several similarities but reflects its originator's philosophical leanings and particular interests in the study of development. This chapter will take a brief look at the models of growth and development proposed by these theorists. In order to provide a basis for a more detailed study of child development, we will also examine characteristic ways in which theorists view the phenomena of development and examine three of the most popular theories of development, namely those of Erik Erikson, Jean Piaget, and Robert Havighurst.

## THEORETICAL MODELS OF CHILD DEVELOPMENT

Sigmund Freud's (1962) psychoanalytic theory of human behavior may be viewed, in part, as a model of child development even though his work centered around personality and abnormal functioning in adults. His famous psychosexual stages of development reflected various zones of the body with which the child seeks gratification of the *id* (the unconscious source of motives, desires, passions, and pleasure seeking) at certain general age periods. The *ego* mediates between the pleasure-seeking behavior of the id and the *superego* (common sense, reason, and conscience). Freud's oral, anal, phallic, latency, and genital stages of personality development represent the terms applied to the pleasure-seeking zones of the body that come into play at different age periods. Each stage relies heavily on physical sensations and motor activity.

Psychoanalytic theory has received its share of criticism primarily due to the inability to scientifically objectify, quantify, and validate its concepts. It has, however, stimulated considerable research and study and served as the basis for the notable works of Erik Erikson.

Erikson (1963), a student of Freud's, focused on the influence of society, rather than of sex, on development. He described eight stages of the human life cycle and put them on a continuum, emphasizing factors in the environment, not heredity as facilitators of change. Erikson's view of human development acknowledges factors within the individual's experiential background as having a primary role in development. His view of the importance of motor development in childhood is more implicit than explicit, but he clearly points out the importance of success-oriented movement experiences as a means of reconciling the developmental crises that each child passes through.

Gesell's (1945) theory of growth and development also emphasizes the physical and motor components of human behavior. Gesell documented and described general age periods for the acquisition of a wide variety of rudimentary movement abilities and viewed these maturationally based tasks as important indicators of social and emotional growth. Gesell also described various ages when children are in "nodal" periods or when they are "out of focus" with their environment. A nodal stage is a maturational period during which the child exhibits a high degree of mastery over situations in the immediate environment, being balanced in behavior, and generally pleasant to be with. Being out of focus is just the opposite, namely, exhibiting a low degree of mastery over situations in the immediate environment, being unbalanced or troubled in behavior, and generally unpleasant to be with. Maturational theory is not widely accepted today, but it played a significant role in the evolution of child development as an area of study.

A fourth developmental model, that of Robert Havighurst (1952), views development as an interplay between biological, social, and cultural forces by means of which children are continually enhancing their abilities to function effectively in society. Havighurst viewed development as a series of tasks that must be achieved within a certain time frame to ensure the proper developmental progression of the individual. According to Havighurst's model, there are teachable moments when the body is ripe and when society requires successful completion of a task. As with the other models discussed, the tasks described by Havighurst rely heavily on movement, play, and physical activity for their development, particularly during infancy and childhood.

The last and currently most popular developmental theory among educators is that of Jean Piaget (1969). Piaget places primary emphasis on the acquisition of cognitive thought processes. He gained insight into the development of cognitive structures through careful observation of infants and children. The genius in Piaget's work lies in his uncanny ability to pick out subtle clues in children's behavior that give us indications of their cognitive functioning. Piaget views these subtle indicators as milestones in the hierarchy of cognitive development. Movement is emphasized as a primary agent in the acquisition of increased cognitive functioning, particularly during infancy and the preschool years. Piaget identified the developmental periods as sensorimotor (birth to 2 years), preoperational (2 to 7 years), concrete operations (7 to 11 years), and formal operations (12 years and over). Piaget did not directly concern himself with development beyond age 15 because he believed that highly sophisticated intellectual capabilities were developed by this time.

All theorists look at the phenomena of development from somewhat different points of view. However, close inspection reveals remarkable congruence on many aspects. Each theorist emphasizes movement, motor development, and play as important facilitators of enhanced functioning. Also, each tends to be more descriptive of human behavior than explanatory. They each differ, however, in the particular aspect of development emphasized. The multidimensional facets of development require a comprehensive model to explain behavior. In this regard, all of the theories have shortcomings, and care must therefore be taken not to subscribe to one to the exclusion of the others. We must be aware of the interrelatedness of children's behavior and dispel the notion that the psychomotor, cognitive, and affective domains of human behavior are independent of one another. Figure 2.1 illustrates the interrelatedness of each of the developmental models discussed and the particular area of interest of each theorist.

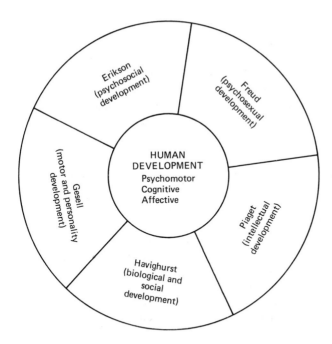

**Figure 2.1.** The interrelationship of theoretical models of child development.

## CONCEPTUAL VIEWPOINTS OF DEVELOPMENT

Close inspection of the five models of development just discussed as well as study of others reveals a distinct tendency for each to group around one of three similar but independent conceptual frameworks. These frameworks are classified here as (1) age-stage, (2) developmental task, or (3) developmental milestone, concepts of child development.

### Age-Stage Theory

The *age-stage concept* of development refers to periods that are characterized by certain types of behavior. These behaviors occur in phases or stages and last for arbitrary lengths of time. Each stage (i.e., typical behavior) generally covers a period of one year or more and may be accompanied by one or more other stages. Some theorists break particular phases into smaller stages. Others prefer to look at one phase typifying one particular stage. Most theorists who propose a phase/stage scheme have divided childhood, or even the entire life cycle, into ten periods or less. The age-stage concept is probably the most popular among parents and educators and is often reflected in our thinking and speech when we say, "she is just going through a stage'' or "I will be happy when he is out of that stage.'' Freud, Erikson, and Gesell each viewed child development as a stage-related process. Stages have been proposed for several fundamental movement tasks (Wild, 1938; Seefeldt et al., 1972, Wickstrom, 1977; McClenaghan and Gallahue, 1978a). However, Roberton (1977) questions the viability of a rigid stage theory of motor development and has suggested a more flexible stage model for motor development based on the components of a movement rather than on the total body form.

## Developmental Task Theory

A second conceptual viewpoint of child development is the *developmental task concept*. A developmental task is an important accomplishment that individuals must achieve by a certain time if they are to function effectively and meet the demands placed on them by society. Proponents of developmental task theory view the accomplishment of particular tasks within a certain time span as prerequisite to smooth progression to higher levels of functioning. This concept of development differs from the age-stage view in that it is predictive of later success or failure based on the individual's performance at an earlier stage and does not merely attempt to describe typical behavior at a particular age. Havighurst's view of child development uses the developmental task concept to describe and predict behavior during childhood.

## Developmental Milestone Theory

The *developmental milestone concept* is the third and final conceptual framework from which development is viewed. Developmental milestones are similar to developmental tasks except for their emphasis. Instead of referring to accomplishments that take place if the individual is to adapt to the environment, this concept refers to the strategic indicators of how far development has progressed. The accomplishment of a developmental milestone may or may not in itself be crucial to adjustment in the world as it is with a developmental task. Milestones are merely convenient guidelines by which the rate and extent of development can be gauged. As with age-stage concepts, they are more descriptive than predictive, but unlike age-stage concepts, they view development as a continual unfolding and intertwining of developmental processes, not as a neat transition from one stage to another.

Recognition of the fact that most models of child development tend to fall under one of these three concepts enables us to view the phenomena of growth and maturation more objectively. Each concept has merit and operates to a certain degree throughout the developmental process. The years of infancy and early childhood do, in fact, require the achievement of certain important tasks such as learning to walk, talk, and take solid foods by a certain age in order for normal functioning to be established. These years also encompass a variety of stages that all children pass through at more or less the same age in addition to a variety of milestones that are achieved as subtle indicators of how far development has progressed.

## THREE LEADING THEORIES OF CHILD DEVELOPMENT

In this section summaries of three theories, each representing a different conceptual point of view will be presented. The age-stage theory of Erik Erikson, the developmental milestone theory of Jean Piaget, and the developmental task theory of Robert Havighurst have been selected because of their thoroughness, popularity, and important implications for the motor development and movement education of children.

### Erik Erikson

The psychoanalytic theory of Erikson (1963) adheres to the age-stage concept of human development. It is an experience-based theory widely acclaimed by educators and psychologists. The following overview of Erikson's theory is presented in outline form for clarity and ease of understanding. Note the numerous implications for movement throughout the theory, particularly during the first four stages.

A. ACQUIRING A SENSE OF BASIC TRUST VERSUS MISTRUST (infancy).
   1. For the neonate, trust requires a feeling of physical comfort and a minimum of fear or uncertainty.
   2. A sense of basic trust helps the individual to accept new experiences willingly.
   3. Bodily experiences provide the basis for a psychological state of trust.
   4. The infant learns to trust "mother," oneself, and the environment through mother's perception of his or her needs and demands. Mutual trust and a willingness to face situations together are established between mother and child.
B. ACQUIRING A SENSE OF AUTONOMY VERSUS DOUBT AND SHAME (toddler).
   1. Continued dependency creates a sense of doubt about capacity.
   2. Children are bombarded by conflicting pulls of asserting themselves and denying themselves the right and capacity to make this assertion.
   3. Children need guidance and support lest they find themselves at a loss and become forced to turn against themselves with shame and doubt.
   4. Children explore and accomplish new feats.
   5. Proper development of the ego, which spells healthy growth, permits awareness of self as an autonomous unit.
   6. Children experience frustration as a reality of life (a natural part of life, not a total threat).
   7. Play allows children to develop autonomy within their own boundaries.
   8. Autonomy is developed in children through the realization that the environ-

ment and themselves can be controlled. Children develop concepts of forward, backward, upward, downward, and so on.

    **9.** Children violate mutual trust to establish autonomy in distinct areas.

**C.** ACQUIRING A SENSE OF INITIATIVE VERSUS GUILT (play age).

    **1.** Avid curiosity, feelings of guilt, and anxiety develop. The conscience is established.

    **2.** Specific tasks are mastered. Children assume responsibility for themselves and their world. They realize that life has a purpose.

    **3.** Children initiate behavior, the implications of which go beyond themselves. This includes feelings of discomfort and guilt through the frustration of the autonomy of others. Their guilt and desire to curtail all initiative conflict with the pull toward continuing their searching initiative.

    **4.** Children discover that in their greater mobility, they are not unlike the adults in their environment. Their use of language has improved, permitting them to expand their fields of activity and imagination.

    **5.** Children incorporate into their conscience what the parents really are as people and not merely what the parents try to teach them.

    **6.** Awareness of sex differences develops. Children find pleasurable accomplishment in manipulating meaningful toys.

    **7.** Most guilt and failure quickly become compensated for by a sense of accomplishment. The future absolves the past.

**D.** ACQUIRING A SENSE OF INDUSTRY VERSUS INFERIORITY (school age).

    **1.** This stage is marked by development of the skills necessary for life in general and preparation for marriage and family life.

    **2.** Children need to find a place among their peers instead of among adults.

    **3.** Children need to work on mastering social skills. They need to become competent and self-striving, and to obtain a sense of accomplishment for having done well. They ward off failure at any price.

    **4.** Activities tend to reflect competition.

    **5.** Boys and girls play separately. Play begins to lose importance at the end of this phase.

    **6.** Beginning with puberty, involvement in play merges into semiplayful and eventually real involvement in work.

    **7.** Children recognize that they must eventually break with accustomed family life.

    **8.** Dependence on parents as children's major influence shifts to dependence on social institutions.

**E.** ACQUIRING A SENSE OF IDENTITY VERSUS ROLE CONFUSION (puberty-adolescence).

    **1.** During this stage there is rapid body growth and sexual maturation. Masculine or feminine identity develops. Feelings of acceptance or rejection by peers are important. Conflict arises when peers say one thing and society says another.

2. Identity is essential for making adult decisions (vocation and marriage partner).
3. Youth will select as significant adults people who mean the most to them.
4. The individual slowly moves into society as an interdependent member.
5. A sense of identity assures the individual a definite place within his or her own corner of society.

F. ACQUIRING A SENSE OF INTIMACY VERSUS ISOLATION (young adult—late teens, early twenties).
   1. The individual accepts himself or herself and goes on to accept others by fusing his or her personality with others.
   2. Childhood and youth are at an end. The individual settles down to the task of full participation in the community, and begins to enjoy life with adult liberties and responsibilities.
   3. The individual shows readiness and ability to share mutual trust and to regulate cycles of work, procreation, and recreation.

G. ACQUIRING A SENSE OF GENERATIVITY VERSUS SELF-ABSORPTION (adulthood).
   1. The individual shows interest in the next generation rather than being caught up with his or her own problems (i.e., wants to advance the coming generation).
   2. Generativity refers to the course one establishes and pursues with one's mate in society in order to assure for the next generation the hope, virtues, and wisdom he or she has accumulated. It also includes parental responsibility for society's efforts and interests in child care, education, the arts and sciences, and traditions.

H. ACQUIRING A SENSE OF INTEGRITY VERSUS DESPAIR (mature adult, and old age).
   1. The individual accomplishes the fullest sense of trust as the assured reliance on another's integrity.
   2. A different love of one's parents is established. Integrity provides a successful solution to an opposing sense of despair.
   3. Fulfillment of this stage involves a sense of wisdom and a philosophy of life which often extends beyond the life cycle of the individual and which is directly related to the future of new developmental cycles.

## Jean Piaget

The developmental milestone theory of Jean Piaget (1952, 1954, 1957, 1969) is currently among the most popular of the theories postulated by experts in the field of child development because of it clarity, insight into, and understanding of the

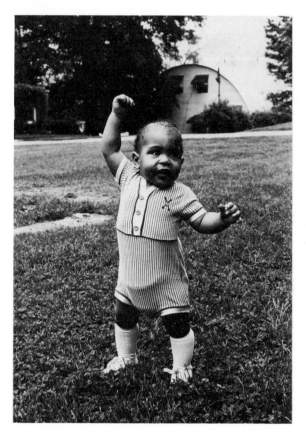

The sensorimotor phase is crucial to the motor as well as the cognitive development of the young child.

development of cognitive abilities. A summary of Piaget's theory presented in outline form follows. Note the numerous implications for movement throughout the phases of development, but particularly during the sensorimotor phase.

**A.** SENSORIMOTOR PHASE (birth to 2 years): The major developmental tasks are coordination of the infant's actions or motor activities and perceptions into a tenuous whole.

    **1.** *Use of reflexes* (birth to 1 month): There is a continuation of prenatal reflexes. They are spontaneous repetitions caused by internal and external stimulation. Rhythm is established through practice, and habits are formed that later emerge as voluntary movements.

    **2.** *Primary circular reactions* (1 to 3 months).

        **a.** Reflexive movement is gradually replaced by voluntary movements.

  **b.** Neurological maturity must be reached before sensations can be understood.

  **c.** What previously had been automatic behavior is repeated voluntarily.

  **d.** More than one sensory modality can be used at a time.

  **e.** Accidentally acquired responses become new sensorimotor habits.

  **f.** Primary circular reactions refer to the assimilation (i.e., the taking in of new information) of a previous experience and the recognition of the stimulus that triggers the reaction.

  **g.** New or past experiences have no meaning unless they become part of the primary circular reaction pattern.

**3.** *Secondary circular reactions* (3 to 9 months).

  **a.** The infant tries to make events last and tries to make events occur.

  **b.** The focus of the infant is on retention, not repetition.

  **c.** The infant tries to create a state of permanency.

  **d.** Primary circular reactions are repeated and prolonged by secondary reactions.

  **e.** Two or more sensorimotor experiences as related to one experiential sequence or schema. (*Schema* is Piaget's term for a pattern of physical or motor action.)

  **f.** Vision is the prime coordinator, but other sensory modalities are also used.

  **g.** Imitation, play, and emotion begin to appear at this stage.

**4.** *Application of the secondary schemata to new situations* (8 to 12 months).

  **a.** This is characterized by the child's ability to distinguish means from ends (i.e., producing the same result more than one way).

  **b.** Children use previous behavioral achievements primarily as the basis for adding new achievements to their expanding repertoire.

  **c.** There is increased experimentation; ends and means are differentiated by experimenting.

  **d.** Accommodation (i.e., adaptation that the child must make to the environment when new and incongruent information is added to the repertoire) is a result of experimentation.

  **e.** The infant can experience action by observation.

**5.** *Tertiary circular reactions* (12 to 18 months).

  **a.** Discovery of new means through active experimentation.

  **b.** Curiosity and novelty-seeking behavior are developing.

  **c.** Reasoning comes into play and is developed.

  **d.** Failure to remember is failure to understand.

  **e.** The infant develops spatial relationships upon discovering objects as objects.

  **f.** Imitation develops.

  **g.** Play is very important because it repeats the action phase.

**6.** *Invention of new means through mental combinations* (12 to 24 months).

   **a.** There is a shift from sensorimotor experiences to an increased reflection about these experiences. This is the steppingstone to the next phase, which is an advanced level of intellectual behavior.

   **b.** Children discern themselves as one object among many. They perceive and use objects for their own intrinsic qualities.

   **c.** Children begin to relate the objects to new actions without actually perceiving all of the actions.

   **d.** Sensorimotor patterns are slowly replaced by semi-mental functionings.

   **e.** Imitation copies the action itself or the symbol of the action.

   **f.** Parallel play appears.

   **g.** Identification, as a mental process, becomes evident at the end of this phase. It depends on the level of intellectual development of the child.

   **h.** This period is characterized by the creation of means and not merely the discovery of means (insight begins).

**B.** PREOPERATIONAL PHASE (2 to 7 years).

   **1.** This is a period of transition from self-satisfying behavior to rudimentary socialized behavior.

   **2.** Continuous investigation of one's world develops.

   **3.** The child knows the world only as he or she sees it.

   **4.** The child is egocentric rather than autistic, as in the sensorimotor phase.

   **5.** Assimilation is the paramount task of the child.

   **6.** Play occupies most of the waking hours. Emphasis on ''how'' and ''why'' becomes a primary tool for adaptation.

   **7.** Imaginary play is important.

   **8.** Language begins to repeat and replace sensorimotor activity.

   **9.** Events are judged by outward appearance regardless of their objective logic.

   **10.** Either the qualitative or quantitative aspects of an event are experienced, but not both simultaneously. The child cannot merge concepts of objects, space, and causality into interrelationships with a concept of time.

   **11.** There is widening social interest in the world about the child.

   **12.** Egocentricity is reduced and social participation increases.

   **13.** The first real beginning of cognition occurs.

   **14.** Speech replaces movement to express thinking.

   **15.** The child can think of only one idea at a time.

   **16.** The child tries to adjust new experiences to previous patterns of thinking.

   **17.** The child becomes aware of relationships.

   **18.** Conservation of quantity (i.e., object permanence), such as permanence and continuity, must be mastered before a concept of numbers can be developed.

   **19.** Play enacts the rules and values of elders.

   **20.** Parallel play continues.

**C.** CONCRETE OPERATIONS PHASE (7 to 11 years).
  **1.** The child becomes aware of alternative solutions.
  **2.** The child acquires reversibility—the capacity to relate an event or thought to a total system of interrelated parts in order to consider the event or thought from beginning to end or from end to beginning.
  **3.** Operational thought develops mental capacity. It is the capacity to order and relate experience to an organized whole.
  **4.** The concrete operational thought level presupposes that mental experimentation still depends on perception.
  **5.** The child examines parts to gain knowledge of the whole.
  **6.** The child establishes systems of classifications of organizing parts into a hierarchical system.
  **7.** Perceptions are more accurate.
  **8.** The child applies interpretation of perceptions of the environment knowingly.
  **9.** Play is used for understanding the physical and social world.
  **10.** Play loses its assimilative characteristics and becomes a balanced subordinate process of cognitive thought.
  **11.** Curiosity finds expression in intellectual experimentation instead of in active play.
  **12.** The child becomes interested in rules and regulations.
**D.** FORMAL OPERATIONS PHASE (12 to 15 years).
  **1.** Childhood ends and youth begins.
  **2.** The individual enters the world of ideas.
  **3.** There is a systematic approach to problems.
  **4.** There is logical deduction by implication.
  **5.** The individual thinks beyond the present (vertically).
  **6.** The individual can dream and does not need reality.
  **7.** Deduction by hypothesis and judgment by implication enable reasoning beyond cause and effect.

### Robert Havighurst

The theory of Robert Havighurst (1952, 1953, 1972; Havighurst and Levine, 1979) is based on the concept that successful achievement of developmental tasks leads to happiness and success with later tasks, whereas failure leads to unhappiness, social disapproval, and difficulty with later tasks. It is interesting to note his disagreement with any theory that proposes an innate basis of growth and development. He believes that living is learning and growing is learning (1972). Development, then, according to Havighurst, is the process of *learning* one's way through life.

Havighurst conceives of successful dvelopment as requiring mastery of a series of tasks. At each level of development the child encounters new social demands. These demands, or tasks, arise out of three sources. First, tasks arise from physical maturation. Such things as learning to walk and talk and to get along with one's age-mates are maturation-based tasks. Second, tasks arise out of the cultural pressures of society, such as learning how to read and learning to be a responsible citizen. The third source is oneself. Tasks arise out of the maturing personality and the individual's values and unique aspirations.

Havighurst's theory has implications for all age levels. His theory is of particular importance to educators because it emphasizes that when the body is "ripe," when society requires, and when the self is ready to achieve a certain task, the teachable moment (readiness period) has arrived. Therefore, we can better time our efforts at teaching by identifying the tasks that are suitable for a particular level of development, being fully aware that one's level of readiness is influenced by biological, cultural, and self factors all interacting with one another.

Havighurst has suggested six major periods of development: infancy and early childhood (birth through 5 years), middle childhood (6 through 12 years), adolescence (13 through 18 years), early adulthood (19 through 29 years), middle adulthood (30 through 60 years), and later maturity (61 years and up). A summary of Havighurst's developmental tasks in outline form follows. The reader is cautioned to be flexible in the interpretation of these tasks with respect to age. Ages are only convenient approximations and should not be viewed as rigid time frames. Significant deviation beyond these age boundaries would, however, according to Havighurst, represent failure in a developmental task, with resulting unhappiness and difficulty with succeeding tasks.

A. INFANCY AND EARLY CHILDHOOD (birth to 5 years).
   1. Learning to walk.
   2. Learning to take solid foods.
   3. Learning to talk.
   4. Learning to control the elimination of bodily wastes.
   5. Learning sex differences and sexual modesty.
   6. Acquiring concepts and language to describe social and physical reality.
   7. Readiness for reading.
   8. Learning to distinguish right from wrong and developing a conscience.
B. MIDDLE CHILDHOOD (6 to 12 years).
   1. Learning physical skills necessary for ordinary games.
   2. Building a wholesome attitude toward oneself.
   3. Learning to get along with age-mates.
   4. Learning an appropriate sex role.
   5. Developing fundamental skills in reading, writing, and calculating.
   6. Developing concepts necessary for everyday living.

    **7.** Developing a conscience, morality, and a scale of values.

    **8.** Achieving personal independence.

    **9.** Developing acceptable attitudes toward society.

**C.** ADOLESCENCE (13 to 18 years).

    **1.** Achieving mature relations with both sexes.

    **2.** Achieving a masculine or feminine social role.

    **3.** Accepting one's physique.

    **4.** Achieving emotional independence of adults.

    **5.** Preparing for marriage and family life.

    **6.** Preparing for an economic career.

    **7.** Acquiring values and an ethical system to guide behavior.

    **8.** Desiring and achieving socially responsible behavior.

**D.** EARLY ADULTHOOD (19 to 29 years).

    **1.** Selecting a mate.

    **2.** Learning to live with a partner.

    **3.** Starting a family.

    **4.** Rearing children.

    **5.** Managing a home.

    **6.** Starting an occupation.

    **7.** Assuming civic responsibility.

**E.** MIDDLE ADULTHOOD (30 to 60 years).

    **1.** Helping teenage children to become happy and responsible adults.

    **2.** Achieving adult social and civic responsibility.

    **3.** Satisfactory career achievement.

    **4.** Developing adult leisure-time activities.

    **5.** Relating to one's spouse as a person.

    **6.** Accepting the physiological changes of middle age.

    **7.** Adjusting to aging parents.

**F.** LATER MATURITY (61 years and up).

    **1.** Adjusting to decreasing strength and health.

    **2.** Adjusting to retirement and reduced income.

    **3.** Adjusting to death of spouse.

    **4.** Establishing relations with one's own age group.

    **5.** Meeting social and civic obligations.

    **6.** Establishing satisfactory living quarters.

**Summary**

The process of development is commonly viewed as hierarchical. That is, the individual proceeds from *general* to *specific*, and from *simple* to *complex*, in gaining mastery and control over his or her environment. Erik Erikson's age-stage theory, Jean Piaget's developmental milestone theory, and Robert Havighurst's developmental task theory make it obvious that the human organism throughout all aspects of its development is moving from comparatively simple forms of existence to more complex and sophisticated levels of development. These levels of development have been expressed primarily in terms of the cognitive and affective behaviors of the individual, with only indirect attention given to motor development.

Although the theoretical formulations of Erikson, Piaget, and Havighurst are of value, none adequately addresses motor development. It is, therefore, appropriate that a theoretical model of motor development be put forth in order that we may describe and explain this important aspect of development. The following chapter is dedicated to this end.

## CHAPTER HIGHLIGHTS

1. There are numerous theories of development, each of which reflects the originator's interests and biases.
2. Theories of development are molar in nature. That is, they attempt to explain *all* aspects of behavior, and, by necessity, break down at some point.
3. No one theory of development is complete or totally accurate. Each offers us a better but still incomplete understanding of the child and should generate testable hypotheses.
4. Most theories of development do not deal with movement as an integral part of the model but view it instead in terms of how it impacts on cognition and affective development.
5. Developmental theory may be subdivided into three distinct conceptual viewpoints (age-stage, developmental task, developmental milestone theories).
6. Erik Erikson is a leading proponent of the age-stage view. Jean Piaget is a leader of developmental milestone theory. Robert Havighurst is an advocate of the developmental task model.
7. Erikson's theory focuses on the affective development of the individual throughout life and has numerous implications for movement.
8. Piaget's theory focuses on the cognitive development of the individual from birth to about age 15. The sensorimotor phase has particular implications for the child's motor development.
9. Robert Havighurst focuses on crucial tasks throughout life that impact on later development, in the cognitive, affective, and psychomotor domains.
10. Close examination of developmental theories provies us with a clearer understanding of the intricate physical and mental processes involved in development and help us construct theoretical models for the process of motor development.

## CRITICAL READINGS

Erikson, E.: *Childhood and Society,* New York: Norton, 1963.

Havighurst, R.: *Developmental Tasks and Education,* New York: David McKay, 1972.

Lerner, R.M.: *Concepts and Theories of Human Development,* Reading, Mass.: Addison-Wesley, 1976, Chapters 6−8.

Maier, H.W.: *Three Theories of Child Development,* New York: Harper & Row, 1978, Chapters 2−3.

## CHAPTER 3

# Motor Development: A Theoretical Model

Summary
Chapter Highlights
Critical Readings

A major function of theory is to integrate existing facts, to organize them in such a way as to give them meaning. Theories of development take existing facts about the human organism and provide a developmental model congruent with these facts. Therefore, theory formulation serves as a basis for fact testing, and vice versa. Facts are important, but they alone do not constitute a science. The development of a science depends on the advancement of theory as well as on the accumulation of facts. In the study of human behavior, especially in the areas of cognitive and affective development, theory formulation has gained increased importance over the past several years. Theory has played a critical dual role in both of these areas; namely, it has served and continues to serve as an integrator of existing facts *and* as a basis for the derivation of new facts. Unfortunately, the recent surge of interest in motor development has been concerned primarily with describing and cataloguing data, with little interest in developmental models leading to a theoretical explanation of behavior. This research has been necessary and very important to our knowedge base, but at present only a limited number of comprehensive developmental models exist and there is no comprehensive theory of motor development. Researchers and scholars have focused on the performance of specific movement tasks at specific developmental levels. This research has produced both *process*-oriented information (i.e., biomechanical and observational assessment along various levels) and *product*-oriented information (i.e., normative data on the physcial and movement abilities of specific age groups). At this point in our knowledge of human motor development, it is appropriate that a comprehensive model leading to a theory of motor development be put forth in an effort to explain motor development and to generate new facts about this aspect of behavior.

The first function of a theory of motor development should be to integrate the existing facts encompassed by the area of study. The second function should be to generate new facts. One might argue that the facts could be interpreted in more than one way, that is, from different theoretical perspectives. This is entirely possible and, in fact, desirable. Different view points generate theoretical arguments and debates—the very spark for the initiation of research to shed new light on differing theoretical interpretations. Even if theoretical differences do not exist, research should be undertaken to determine whether the hypotheses derived from the theory can be experimentally supported.

Theory should undergird all research and science, and the study of motor development is no exception. Without a theoretical base of operation, research in motor development often tends to yield little more than isolated facts. Without an existing body of knowledge (facts), we cannot formulate theory, but without the formulation and constant testing of theory we cannot hope for a higher level of understanding and awareness of the phenomenon that we call motor development.

A theory is a group of statements, concepts, or principles that integrate existing facts and lead to the generation of new facts. The model of The Phases Of Motor Development presented in this chapter is not based solely on the accumulation of facts. Such a model would result from using an inductive method of theory formulation. That is, in the inductive method the researcher first starts with a set of facts and then tries to find a conceptual framework to organize and explain them. The deductive model of theory formulation, as used here, is based on inference and has three qualifications: (1) The theory should integrate existing facts and account for existing empirical evidence that bears on the content of the theory. (2) The theory should lend itself to the formulation of testable hypotheses in the form: If _____, then _____. (3) The theory should meet the empirical test; that is, hypotheses that are experimentally tested should yield results that lend further support to the theory (Lerner, 1976).

The use of a deductive, rather than an inductive, model enables us to see how well these accumulated facts fit together into a cohesive, understandable whole. It also enables us to identify the information that is needed to fill in gaps in the theory or to clarify or refine it. The Phases Of Motor Development outlined here are deductively based and serve as a model for theory formulation. In Section IV each phase will be dealt with in greater detail.

## THE PHASES OF MOTOR DEVELOPMENT

The process of motor development reveals itself primarily through changes in movement behavior. Children of preschool and elementary school age are primarily involved in learning how to move efficiently. We are able to see developmental differences in their movement behavior, brought about by biological and environmental factors, through observation of changes in process (form) and product (performance). Therefore, a primary means by which the process of motor development may be viewed is through the progressive development of movement abilities. In other words, the "window" to the *process* of motor development is provided through the the child's actual observable movement behavior (Figure 3.1). These observable behaviors give us a clue to underlying motor processes. A variety of cognitive, affective, and psychomotor factors will influence and are influenced by the development of movement abilities and are worthy of study. As teachers, our primary focus is, however, on the process of movement itself.

Observable movement takes many forms. Movement may be categorized as nonlocomotor (or stabilizing), locomotor, or manipulative, or any combination of the three. In the broadest sense, a stability movement is any movement in which

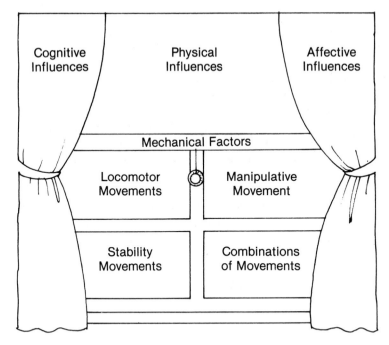

**Figure 3.1.** "The window dressing" of influences on the "window" of movement abilities (i.e. factors influencing the development of movement abilities.)

some degree of balance is required (i.e., virtually all gross motor activity). In a narrower sense, a stability movement is a movement that is both nonlocomotor and nonmanipulative. In other words, it often serves as a convenient category for movements such as twisting, turning, pushing, and pulling that cannot be classified as locomotor or manipulative. In this book stability as a category of movement is viewed as more than a convenient catchall term, but as less than a global term applicable to all movement. Stability, then, refers to any movement that places a *premium* on gaining and maintaining one's equilibrium in relation to the force of gravity. Thus axial movements (another term sometimes used for nonlocomotor movements) as well as inverted and body rolling postures are considered here as stability movements.

The locomotor category of movement refers to movements that involve a change in location of the body relative to a fixed point on the surface. To walk, run, jump, hop, skip, or leap is to perform a locomotor task. In our use of the term such activities as the forward roll and backward roll may be considered to be both locomotor and stability movements—locomotor because the body is moving from point to point, stability because of the premium placed on maintaining equilibrium in an unusual balancing situation.

The manipulative category of movement refers to gross motor manipulation. The tasks of throwing, catching, kicking, and striking an object are all considered to be gross motor manipulative movements. Sewing, cutting with scissors, and typing are fine motor manipulative movements. A large number of our movements involve a combination of stability, locomotor, and/or manipulative movements. For example, jumping rope involves locomotion (jumping), manipulation (turning the rope), and stability (maintaining balance). Likewise, playing soccer involves locomotor skills (running and jumping), manipulative skills (dribbling, passing, kicking, and heading), and stability skills (dodging, reaching, sliding, turning, and twisting).

In summary, if movement serves as a window to the process of motor development, then one way of studying this process is through the study of the sequential progression of movement abilities throughout the entire life span. The following Phases Of Motor Development and the developmental stages within each phase are designed to serve as a model for this study. (See Figure 3.2 for a visual representation of the four phases and their corresponding stages.)

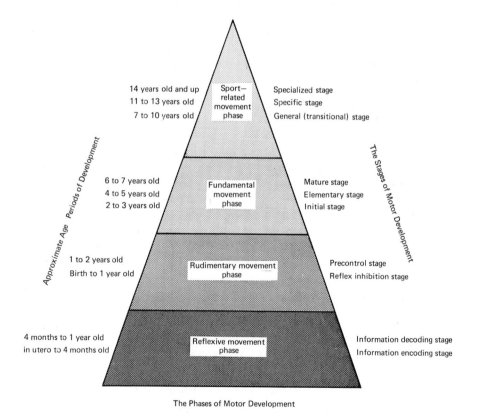

Figure 3.2 The phases of motor development.

## Reflexive Movement Phase

The very first movements the fetus makes are reflexive. These involuntary, subcortically controlled movements form the basis for the phases of motor development. Through reflex activity the infant gains information about the immediate environment. The infant's reactions to touch, light, sounds, and changes in pressure trigger involuntary movement activity. These involuntary movements, coupled with the increasing cortical sophistication in the early months of life, play an important role in helping the child learn more about his or her body and the outside world. Reflexes may be classified as information gathering, nourishment seeking, and protective. They are information gathering in that they help stimulate cortical activity and development. They are nourishment seeking and protective because there is some evidence that they are phylogenetic in nature. Primitive reflexes such as the rooting and sucking reflexes are thought by some to be primitive survival mechanisms. Without them, the newborn would be unable to obtain nourishment.

Postural reflexes are the second form of involuntary movement. They are remarkably similar in appearance to later voluntary behaviors but are entirely involuntary. According to Wyke (1975), these reflexes seem to serve as a "neuromotor testing time" for locomotor, manipulative, and stability mechanisms that will be used later with conscious control. The primary stepping reflex and the crawling reflex, for example, closely resemble later voluntary walking and crawling behaviors. The palmar grasping reflex is closely related to later voluntary grasping and releasing behaviors. The labyrinthine righting reflex and the propping reflexes are related to later balancing abilities. The reflexive phase of motor development may be divided into two overlapping stages.

**Information Encoding Stage.** The information encoding (gathering) stage of the reflexive movement phase is characterized by observable involuntary movement activity during the fetal period until about the fourth month of infancy. During this stage lower brain centers are more highly developed than the motor cortex and are essentially in command of fetal and neonatal movement. These brain centers are capable of causing involuntary reactions to a variety of stimuli of varying intensity and duration. During this stage reflexes serve as the primary means by which the infant is able to gather information, to seek nourishment, and to seek protection through movement.

**Information Decoding Stage.** The information decoding (processing) stage of the reflex phase begins around the fourth month. During this time there is a gradual inhibition of many reflexes as higher brain centers continue to develop. Lower brain centers gradually relinquish control over skeletal movements and are replaced by voluntary movement activity mediated by the motor area of the cerebral cortex. The decoding stage replaces sensorimotor activity with perceptual-motor behavior. That is, the infant's development of voluntary control of skeletal movements involves processing sensory stimuli with stored information, not merely reacting to stimuli.

Chapter 9 focuses on primitive and postural reflexes as they are related to the information encoding and decoding stages. Special attention is given to the relationship between the reflex phase of development and voluntary movement.

## Rudimentary Movement Phase

The first forms of voluntary movement are rudimentary movements. They are seen in the infant beginning at birth up to about age 2. Rudimentary movements are maturationally determined and are characterized by a highly predictable sequence in their appearance. This sequence is resistant to change under normal conditions. The rate at which these abilities appear will, however, vary from child to child and is dependent on both biological and environmental factors. The rudimentary movement abilities of the infant represent the basic forms of voluntary movement that are required for survival. They involve stability movements such as gaining control of the head, neck, and trunk muscles; the manipulative tasks of reach, grasp, and release; and the locomotor movements of creeping, crawling, and walking. The rudimentary movement phase of development may be subdivided into two stages that represent progressively higher orders of movement control.

**Reflex Inhibition Stage.** The reflex inhibition stage of the rudimentary movement ability phase may be thought of as beginning at birth. At birth, reflexes dominate the infant's movement repertoire. From then on, however, the infant's movements are increasingly influenced by the developing cortex. Development of the cortex causes several reflexes to be inhibited and gradually to disappear. The primitive and postural reflexes are replaced by voluntary movement behavior. At the reflex inhibition level, voluntary movement is poorly differentiated and integrated. That is, the neuromotor apparatus of the infant is still at a rudimentary stage of development. Movements, though purposeful, appear uncontrolled and unrefined. If the infant wishes to make contact with an object, there will be global activity of the entire hand, wrist, arm, shoulder, and even trunk. In other words, the process of moving the hand into contact with the object, although voluntary, lacks control.

**Precontrol Stage.** Around 1 year of age, children begin to bring greater precision and control to their movements. The process of differentiating between sensory and motor systems and integrating perceptual and motor information into a more meaningful and congruent whole takes place. The rapid development of higher cognitive processes as well as motor processes makes for rapid gains in rudimentary movement abilities during this stage. During the movement control stage children learn to gain and maintain their equilibrium, to manipulate objects, and to locomote throughout the environment with an amazing degree of proficiency and control considering the short time they have had to develop these abilities. The maturational process may explain the rapidity and extent of development of movement control during this phase, but the growth of motor proficiency is no less amazing.

Chapter 10 provides a detailed explanation of the development of rudimentary movement abilities. Particular attention is paid to the interrelationship between the stages within this phase and the stages within the reflexive phase of development. Attention is also focused on the critical function that the rudimentary movement phase serves in preparing the child for the development of fundamental movement abilities.

## Fundamental Movement Phase

The fundamental movement abilities of early childhood are an outgrowth of the rudimentary movement phase of infancy. This phase of motor development represents a time in which young children are actively involved in exploring and experimenting with the movement capabilities of their bodies. It is a time for discovering how to perform a variety of locomotor, stability, and manipulative movements, first in isolation and then in combination with one another. Children who are developing fundamental patterns of movement are learning how to respond with adaptability and versatility to a variety of stimuli. They are gaining increased control in the performance of discrete, serial, and continuous movements as evidenced by increased fluidity and control in movement. Fundamental movement patterns are basic observable patterns of behavior. Locomotor activities such as running and jumping, manipulative activities such as throwing and catching, and stability activities such as the beam walk and stick balance are examples of fundamental movement abilities that should be developed during the early childhood years.

A major misconception about the developmental concept of the fundamental movement ability phase is the notion that these abilities are maturationally determined and are little influenced by environmental factors. Some child development experts (not in the motor development area) have written repeatedly about the "natural" unfolding of the child's movement or play skills and the idea that merely by growing older (maturation), these abilities will develop. Maturation does, in fact, play a role in the development of fundamental movement abilities. It should not, however, be viewed as the only influencing factor. The factors of opportunity, motivation, and instruction all play important roles in the degree to which fundamental movement abilities develop. (Refer to the section Critical Learning Periods in Chapter 5 for a discussion of *when* these factors are of primary importance.)

Several investigators and assessment instrument developers have attempted to subdivide fundamental movements into a series of identifiable sequential stages. For the purposes of our model we will view the entire fundamental movement phase as having three separate but often overlapping stages, namely the initial, elementary and mature stages.* These stages are dealt with briefly here and in greater detail in Chapter 11.

*Bruce McClenaghan (1976) is credited with the popularization of these terms.

**Initial Stage.** The initial stage of a fundamental movement ability phase represents the child's first goal-oriented attempts at performing a fundamental skill. Movement itself is characterized by missing or improperly sequenced parts, markedly restricted or exaggerated use of the body, and poor rhythmical flow and coordination. In other words, spatial and temporal integration of movement are poor during this stage. Typically, the locomotor, manipulative, and stability movements of the 2-year-old are at the initial level. Some children may be beyond this level in the performance of some patterns of movement, but most are at the initial stage.

**Elementary Stage.** The elementary stage involves greater control and better rhythmical coordination of fundamental movements. The temporal and spatial elements of movement are better coordinated, but patterns of movement at this stage are still generally restricted or exaggerated, although better coordinated. Children of normal intelligence and physical functioning tend to advance to the elementary stage primarily through the process of maturation. (McClenaghan and Gallahue, 1978a). Observation of the typical 3- or 4-year-old child reveals a variety of abilities at the elementary stage. Many individuals fail to develop beyond the elementary stage in many patterns of movement and remain at this stage throughout life due to a lack of opportunities for practice, motivation, and qualified instruction.

**Mature Stage.** The mature stage within the fundamental movement phase is characterized by mechanically efficient, coordinated, and controlled performances. The majority of available data on the acquisition of fundamental movement skills suggest that children can and *should* be at the mature stage by age 5 or 6. Even a casual glance at the movements of children and adults reveals that a great many have not developed their fundamental movement abilities to the mature level. Although some children may reach this stage primarily through maturation and a minimum of environmental influences, the vast majority require opportunity for practice, motivation to learn, and instruction. Failure to include these factors in the lives of individuals makes it virtually impossible for them to achieve the mature stage within this phase and will inhibit complete development in the next phase.

### Sport-Related Movement Phase

The sport-related† phase of motor development is an outgrowth of the fundamental movement phase. During this phase, movement, instead of continuing to be closely identified with learning to move for the sake of movement, now becomes a tool that may be applied to a variety of competitive and cooperative games, sports, dances, and related recreational activities. It is a period when basic locomotor, manipula-

---

†The term *sport* is used in its broadest sense. It should not be construed to apply solely to competitive sports but also encompasses rhythmical and recreational activities and games of a gross motor nature.

tion, and stability skills are progressively refined, combined, and elaborated upon in order that they may be used in increasingly demanding activities. The fundamental movements of hopping and jumping, for example, are now applied to rope-jumping activities, to performing the folk dance known as seven jumps, and to performing the triple jump (hop-step-jump) in track.

The onset and extent of skill development within the sport-related phase depends on a variety of cognitive, affective, and psychomotor factors. Reaction time and movement speed, coordination, body type, height and weight, customs, peer pressure, and emotional makeup are but a few of the factors. There appear to be three stages within the sport-related phase.

**General or Transitional Stage.** Somewhere around the seventh or eighth year of life, children commonly enter a transitional,‡ or general movement, skill stage. During the general movement stage the individual begins to combine and apply fundamental movement skills to the performance of sport-related skills. Walking on a rope bridge, jumping rope, and playing kickball are examples of common transitional skills. General movement skills contain the same elements as fundamental movements but greater form, accuracy, and control of movement are now evident. The fundamental movement abilities that were developed and refined for their own sake during the previous stage are now applied in play and game situations. General sport skills are simply an application of fundamental movements in somewhat more complex and specific forms.

The general stage is an exciting time for the parent and the teacher as well as for the child. During this stage children are actively involved in discovering and combining numerous movement patterns and skills and are often elated by their rapidly expanding abilities. The goal of the concerned parent and teacher during this stage should be to help the child develop and expand his or her abilities in a *wide variety* of sport-related activities. Care must be taken not to cause the child to specialize or restrict his or her activity involvement. A narrow focus on skills during this stage is likely to have undesirable effects on the last two stages of the sport related phase. In fact, Schmidt (1977) has stated that "a variety of movement experiences produces an increased capacity to move" (p. 37).

**Specific Movement Skill Stage.** From about age 11 to age 13 (the middle school years) interesting changes take place in the skill development of the individual. During the previous stage the limited cognitive abilities, affective abilities, and experiences of the child, coupled with a natural eagerness to be active, caused the normal focus (without adult interference) on movement to be broad and generalized to "all" activity. During the specific movement skill stage, increased cognitive sophistication and a broadened experience base enable the individual to make

---

‡Vern Seefeldt (1980a) is credited with the popularization of this term.

numerous learning and participation decisions based on a variety of factors. For example, the 5 ft. 10 in. tall 12-year-old who likes team activities and applying strategy to games, who has reasonably good coordination and agility, and who lives in Indiana may, based on specific physical, cognitive, and cultural factors, choose to specialize in the development of basketball playing abilities. A similar child who does not really enjoy team efforts may choose to specialize in improving his or her abilities in a variety of track and field activities. In other words, the individual begins to make conscious decisions based on a variety of likes and dislikes, strengths and weaknesses, opportunities and restrictions, to narrow his or her activity base. The child begins to seek out or avoid participation in specific activities. Increased emphasis should now be placed on form, skill, and accuracy of performance. This is a time for more complex skills to be refined and used in the performance of advanced lead-up activities and in the chosen sport itself.

**Specialized Movement Skill Stage.** The specialized stage of the sport-related phase of motor development begins around the fourteenth year of life and continues through adulthood. The specialized stage represents the pinnacle of the development process and is characterized by the individual's desire to participate in a limited number of movement activities over a period of years. The interests, abilities, and choices made during the previous stage are carried over to this stage and further refined. Factors such as available time and money, equipment, and facilities for participation affect this stage. The *level* of activity participation will depend on the individual's talents, opportunities, physical condition, and motivation. One's lifetime performance level may range anywhere from the professional levels and the Olympics, to intercollegiate and interscholastic competition, to participation in organized or unorganized, competitive or cooperative, recreational sports.

In essence, the specialized stage represents a culmination of all preceding stages and phases. It should, however, be viewed as a continuation of a lifetime process. One of the primary goals of education is to develop individuals to a point that they become happy, healthy, contributing members of society. We must not lose sight of this lofty but worthy goal. We must view the hierarchical development of movement abilities as stepping-stones to the specialized movement skill level. We must cease to view young children as miniature adults who can be programmed to perform at this stage in such potentially high-pressure, physiologically and psychologically questionable activities as Little League Baseball and Pee Wee Football. We must view children as developmentally immature individuals, and structure meaningful movement experiences appropriate for their particular developmental level. Only when we recognize that the progressive development of movement abilities in a developmentally appropriate sequence is imperative to the balanced motor development of children will we begin making significant contributions to the total development of the individual. Specialized skill development can and should play a role in our lives, but it is unfair to require of children that they specialize in one or two skill areas at the expense of developing their abilities in and appreciation for many other areas. Chapter 12 focuses on the specialized movement skill stage.

The age ranges for each phase of motor development should be viewed as general boundaries only. Children will often be functioning at different phases depending on their experiential background and genetic makeup. For example, it is entirely possible for a 10-year-old to function in the sport-related phase at the specialized movement skill stage in stability activities involving gymnastic movements but only at the elementary stage of the fundamental movement phase in manipulative or locomotor activities such as throwing, catching, or running. Although we should continue to encourage this precocious behavior in gymnastics, we should also be concerned that the child catches up to his or her age-mates in the other areas and develops an acceptable level of proficiency in this stage as well. Rigid adherence to age classifications is unwise and in direct conflict with the principle of individual differences. Development is a lifelong process and so too should be the development of movement skills that have utility throughout life.

## PHYSICAL FACTORS AFFECTING MOTOR DEVELOPMENT

It has been stated repeatedly that the development of one's movement abilities does not occur in a vacuum. A wide variety of factors from all three domains of human behavior influence development. Factors within the psychomotor domain are termed *physical abilities*. Physical abilities are distinguished from movement abilities in that *physical fitness* and *motor fitness* abilities—which make up physical abilities—affect the performance level of one's locomotor, manipulative, and stability movements. Figure 3.3 illustrates this concept.

### Physical Fitness Factors

The physical development aspects of the motor domain may be divided into health-related physical fitness factors and performance-related physical fitness (namely, motor fitness) factors that influence performance in each of the four phases of motor development (Falls, 1980). These terms, however, are difficult to define to the mutual satisfaction of experts in the field. Physical fitness is generally defined in broad terms because the level of fitness required of one individual may not be the same as that required of another. Hence physical fitness is generally considered to be the health-related aspects of one's existence that influence the ability to perform one's daily tasks at an acceptable level without undue stress. It also is a state in which ample reserves of energy are available for recreational pursuits and emergency needs. *Muscular strength, muscular endurance, circulatory-respiratory endurance,* and *muscular flexibility* are usually considered to be the components of health-related physical fitness. The extent to which each of these factors is

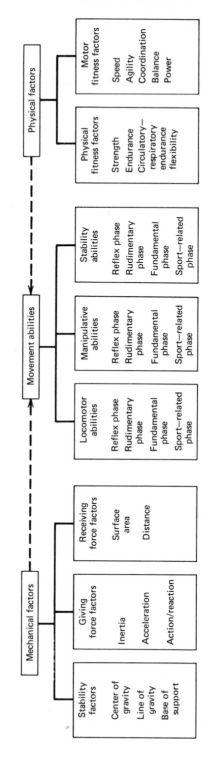

**Figure 3.3.** Physical and mechanical factors affect the development of movement abilities at all phases of motor development.

possessed will influence the individual's performance capabilities in movement. For example, how far or how fast one can run or ride a bicycle is related to the individual's level of muscular strength and endurance as well as to the general cardiovascular endurance.

## Motor Fitness Factors

Motor ability, or motor fitness, as it is often termed, is the performance-related aspect of physical fitness. It is also an elusive concept that has been studied extensively over the past several years and is classified as being a part of the global concept of fitness. Hockey's (1973) statement probably best summarizes the debate:

> Many factors associated with the development of skill have erroneously been referred to as physical fitness components. It should be kept in mind that only factors that relate to the development of health and increase the functional capacity of the body should be classified as physical fitness components. Those that are necessary for skillful performance of an activity should be classified as motor ability components. (p. 6)

Motor fitness (motor ability) is generally thought of as one's performance abilities as influenced by factors such as movement, speed, agility, balance, coordination, and power. (Hockey, 1981).

The generality and specificity of motor abilities have been debated and researched for years, with the bulk of research evidence in favor of its specificity (Henry, 1960; Henry and Rogers, 1960). For years many physical educators believed that motor abilities were general in nature; as a result, the term *general motor ability* came into vogue. It was assumed that because an individual excelled in a certain sport, corresponding ability would be automatically carried over to other activities. Although this often does occur, it is probably due to the individual's personal motivation, numerous activity experiences, and several specific sport aptitudes, not to transfer or carryover of skills from one activity to another. In an effort to avoid confusion between the terms motor ability and general motor ability, we will instead refer to factors of movement as elements of *motor fitness*. One's motor fitness abilities will have a definite effect on the performance of any movement activity that requires quick reactions, speed of movement, agility and coordination of movement, explosive power and balance. Chapter 13 focuses on the performance abilities of children in relation to their levels of physical and motor fitness.

## MECHANICAL FACTORS AFFECTING MOVEMENT

Before embarking on a detailed discussion of motor development, it will be useful to review some mechanical principles of movement as they relate to stability, locomotion, and manipulation. There are numerous ways in which the human body is capable of moving. At first glance it may appear to be an impossible task to learn all of the skills that are involved in the performance of the numerous game, sport, and dance activities engaged in by children. Closer inspection of the total spectrum of movement will reveal, however, that there are fundamental mechanical laws affecting all human movement. Selected mechanical principles are considered here to serve as basic preparation for the chapters that follow.

## Balance

All masses that are within the gravitational pull of the earth are subjected to the force of gravity. The three primary factors of concern in the study of balance principles are (1) center of gravity, (2) line of gravity, and (3) base of support.

A *center of gravity* exists within all objects. In geometric shapes it is located in the exact center of the object. In asymmetrical objects (e.g., our bodies) it is constantly changing during movement. The center of gravity of our bodies always shifts in the direction of the movement or the additional weight. The center of gravity of a child standing in an erect positon is approximately at the top of the hips between the front and the back of the trunk. In activities in which the center of gravity remains in a stable positon, as with standing on one foot or performing a headstand, we refer to them as static balance activities. If the center of gravity is constantly shifting, as with jumping rope, walking, or doing a forward roll, we refer to the activities as dynamic balance movements (Figure 3.4).

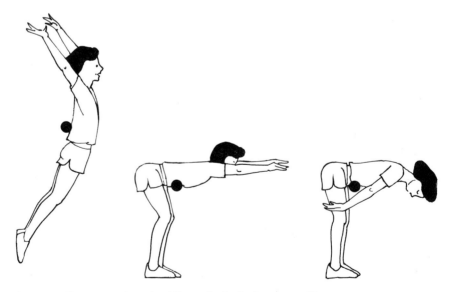

**Figure 3.4.** The center of gravity shifts as the body changes position.

The *line of gravity* is an imaginary line that extends vertically through the center of gravity to the center of the earth. The interrelationship of the center of gravity and the line of gravity to the base of support determines the degree of stability or instability of the body (Figure 3.5).

The *base of support* is the part of the body that comes into contact with the supporting surface. If the line of gravity falls within the base of support, the body will be in balance. If it falls outside the base, it is out of balance. The wider the base of support, the greater the stability, as can be seen when balancing on two feet as opposed to balancing on one foot. The nearer the base of support to the center of gravity, the greater the stability. This may be readily observed by attempting to push someone off balance from an erect standing position and then repeating the act from the referee's position in wrestling or lineman's stance in football. The nearer the center of gravity to the center of the base of support the greater the stability. A foot position that allows for a larger base of support in the direction of the movement gives additonal stability. This principle is illustrated by the foot position of a runner who is attempting to stop or of a catcher who is trying to receive and control a heavy object.

## Giving Force

*Force* is one of the basic concepts of movement and body mechanics. Force is the instigator of all movement and may be defined as the effort that one mass exerts on another. The result may be (1) movement, (2) cessation of movement, or (3) merely

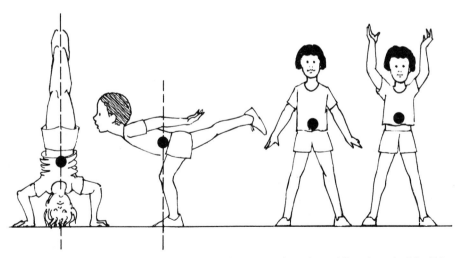

**Figure 3.5.** The body remains balanced when the center of gravity and line of gravity fall within the base of support.

resistance of one body against another. There may be force without motion, as is seen in isometric activities, but motion is impossible without some form of force being applied. Three forces relative to the human body are of concern to us: (1) force produced by muscles, (2) force produced by the gravitational pull of the earth, and (3) momentum. The entire science of force is based on Newton's three laws of motion, namely, the law of inertia, the law of acceleration, and the law of action and reaction.

The *law of inertia* states that a body at rest will remain at rest and a body in motion will remain in motion at the same speed in a straight line unless acted upon by an outside force. In other words, in order for movement to occur a force must act upon a body sufficiently to overcome that object's inertia. If the applied force is less than the resistance offered by the object, motion will not occur. Large muscles can produce more force than small muscles, as is seen with the amount of force generated by the legs as opposed to the arms. Once an object is in motion, it will take less force to maintain its speed and direction (i.e., momentum). This may be readily observed in snow skiing, the glide in swimming, or rolling a ball. The heavier the object and the faster it is moving, the more force that is required to overcome its moving inertia or to absorb its momentum, as is seen in catching a heavy object as opposed to catching a light object.

The *law of acceleration* states that the change in the velocity of an object is directly proportional to the force producing the velocity and inversely proportional to the object's mass. the heavier an object, the more force that is needed to accelerate or deccelerate it. This may be observed when throwing a heavy object (shot put) and a light object (softball) a given distance. an inccease in speed is proportional to the amount of force that is applied. The greater the amount of force imparted to an object, the greater the speed at which the object will travel. If the same amount of force is exerted on two bodies with a different mass, greater acceleration will be produced on the lighter or less massive object. The heavier object will, however, have greater momentum once inertia is overcome and will exert a greater force than the lighter object on something that it contacts (Figure 3.6).

The *law of action and reaction* states that for every action there is an equal and opposite reaction. This principle of cmunterforce is the basis for all locomotion and may be observed by the depressions left behind while walking in sand. This principle applies to both linear and angular motion. Its application requires that adjustments be made by the individual to sustain the value of the primary forces in any movement. For example, the use of opposition in the running pattern counters the action of one part of the body with that of another (Figure 3.7).

## Receiving Force

In order to stop a moving object or our bodies, we absorb the force over the greatest distance possible and with the largest surface area possible. The greater the distance

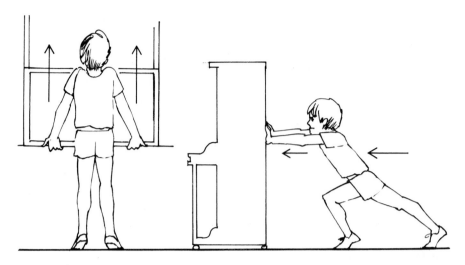

**Figure 3.6.** Exert the applied force in the direction of the intended movement.

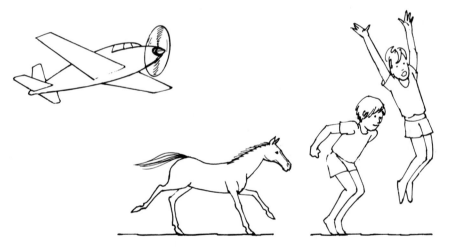

**Figure 3.7.** The law of action and reaction permits movement through space.

over which the force is absorbed, the less will be the impact on the part of the body that receives the force. This may be demonstrated by attempting to catch a ball by keeping the arms straight out in front of the body and then repeating the task by bending the arms as the ball is being caught. The same thing may be observed in landing with the legs bent from a jump as opposed to landing with the legs straight. Forces should be absorbed over as large a surface area as possible. In this way the impact is reduced in proportion to the size of the surface area and the likelihood of injury is reduced. For example, keeping the arms extended and trying to absorb the shock of a fall with the hands will probably result in injury because the small surface area of the hand must receive the entire impact. It is far better to let as much of the body as possible absorb the impact.

The final direction of a moving object or our bodies depends on the magnitude and the direction of all of the forces that have been applied. Therefore, whenever we kick, strike, or throw an object, its accuracy and the distance traveled are dependent on the forces acting on it. If we are performing a vertical jump, we must work for a summation of forces in a vertical direction, whereas a good performance in the long jump requires a summation of horizontal and vertical forces so that the takeoff is at the appropriate angle.

Separate discussion of the principles of balance, giving force, and receiving forces should not be taken to mean that one is used in the absence of the others. Most of our movements combine all three. An element of balance is involved in almost all of our movements, and we both give force to the body and receive force from the body whenever we perform any locomotor or manipulative movement. A gymnast, for example, must maintain his or her equilibrium when performing a tumbling trick such as a front flip, and also must absorb force from the body (on the landing). A handball player must move to a position of readiness (giving to and receiving force from the body), contact the ball (giving force to an object), and maintain balance throughout the act. Although each of the movement patterns and skills discussed in the following chapters involve a specific sequence of movements, all incorporate the basic mechanics of movement discussed here because these mechanical principles are common to all movement situations.

## Summary

The development of movement abilities is an extensive process beginning with the early reflexive movements of the newborn and culminating with the refined sport skill abilities of the adolescent and adult. The process by which an individual progresses from the reflexive movement phase, through the rudimentary and fundamental movement phases, and finally to the sport skill phase of development is influenced by both hereditary and environmental factors.

Reflexes and rudimentary movement abilities are largely maturationally based. They appear and disappear in a fairly rigid sequence deviating only in the rate of their appearance. They do, however, form an important base upon which fundamental movement abilities are developed.

Fundamental movement abilities are basic movement patterns that begin developing around the same time that the child is able to walk independently and move freely through his or her environment. These basic locomotor, manipulative, and stability abilities go through a definite, observable, process from immaturity to maturity. A variety of stages within this phase have been identified for a number of fundamental movements; these are initial, elementary, and mature stages. Attainment of the mature level is influenced greatly by opportunities for practice, encouragement, and motivation. All indications are that given the proper environment, children are capable of performing at the mature stage in the vast majority of fundamental movement abilities by age 6. Therefore, the elementary school years may be more properly viewed as a time for skill refinement rather than for new skill acquisition. The fundamental movement abilities of children entering school are too often incompletely developed. Therefore, the primary grades offer an excellent opportunity to develop fundamental movement abilities to their mature level. It is these same fundamental skills that will be elaborated on and refined to form the sport skill abilities so highly valued by our society.

The sport-related movement phase of development is in essence an elaboration of the fundamental phase. Sport skills are more precise than fundamental skills. They often involve a combination of fundamental movement abilities and require a greater degree of exactness in performance. Sport skills have three related stages. The general sport skill stage is typically the level of the girl or boy in grades three through five. At this level, children are involved in their first real application of fundamental movements to sport. If the fundamental abilities used in the particular sport activity are not at the mature level, the child will have to resort to the use of less mature or elementary patterns of movement. It should be obvious that involving the children in sport skill refinement prior to achieving a mature level of ability in prerequisite fundamentals is unwise. When this happens, any of the immature movements found in the basic patterns are carried over to those related sport skills. The child will in fact regress to his or her characteristic pattern. It is important that sensitive teaching and coaching be incorporated at this point. Today, children are often not completely ready motorically when they are thrust into youth sport activities. If these activities are to be of any real benefit to children the teacher/coach must ensure that the mature fundamental movement pattern is completely developed and that the transition to the general sport skill is based on sound teaching and coaching. In defense of this point of view Wickstrom (1977) has stated:

> The major consequences of accelerated progression into sport skills should be considered carefully. If immature movements become a permanent part of a sport skill pattern, premature encounter with the sport is undesirable. However, if immature movements become modified positively by encouragement and the challenge of the more difficult task, the eventual result is beneficial to motor skill development. The question of when to move on to more difficult tasks is an important one with the fate of optimal motor development possibly being in the balance. Unfortunately, a patent answer to the question does not exist. (p. 13)

The fundamental and sport skill abilities of children and youth are influenced by a wide variety of physical and mechanical factors. The physical factors of strength, coordination, speed of movement, and others all have a profound effect on the ultimate performance potential of the individual. The mechanical factors of movement play the determining role in the form with which a movement may be executed. Except for stylistic variations in an individual's movement and performance, there is little difference between fundamental movement abilities and sport skill abilities. The motor development specialist interested in the physical education of children will pay close attention to the development and refinement of fundamental movement abilities, being concerned first with process (form) and concentrating on the product (performance) only after mature levels have been achieved.

## CHAPTER HIGHLIGHTS

1. No comprehensive theory of motor development exists.
2. A theoretical model of motor development should integrate existing facts and stimulate the generation of new facts.
3. Development of theoretical models can use inductive or deductive approaches to theory formulation.
4. The Phases Of Motor Development presented here utilize a deductive means of theory formulation.
5. The human organism progresses from the simple to the complex and moves from the general to the specific in the development of movement abilities.
6. Four phases of motor development, each containing two or three stages, make up the hierarchical sequence of motor development.
7. Each successfully completed phase and stage of development leads to higher levels of functioning.
8. Difficulty in the performance of a specific skill at one stage of development will lead to difficulty or inability in progressing to subsequent stages.
9. Individuals are often at different stages of development within tasks and between tasks.
10. A variety of physical fitness and motor fitness factors influence the ultimate performance level of a movement task by an individual.
11. Numerous mechanical principles influence the actual performance of all movement tasks.
12. The interaction of factors in the phases and stages of motor development make each individual's developmental schedule unique.
13. Numerous cognitive, affective, and physical factors influence the stages of motor development of each individual.
14. Opportunity for practice, encouragement, and instruction play a key role in the individual's progress through the phases of motor development.

## CRITICAL READINGS

Holle, B.: Motor Development In Children: Normal and Retarded, Copenhagen: Munksgaard, 1976.

Lerner, R.M.: *Concepts and Theories of Human Development*, Reading, Mass.: Addison-Wesley, 1976, Chapter 1.

Seefeldt, V.: "Physical Fitness Guidelines for Preschool Children" in *Proceedings of the National Conference on Physical Fitness and Sports For All*, Washington, D.C., The President's Council on Physical Fitness and Sports, 1980, pp. 5–19.

# SECTION TWO

# FACTORS AFFECTING MOTOR DEVELOPMENT

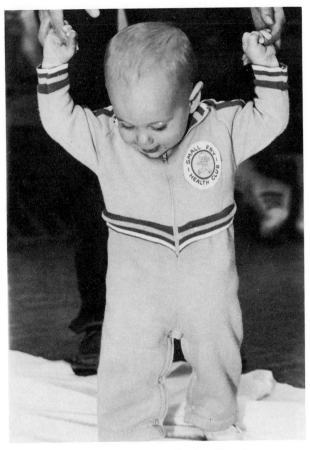

**Chapter 4** Prenatal Factors Affecting Development
**Chapter 5** Infant and Childhood Factors Affecting Development

# Prenatal Factors Affecting Development

Among the most positive contributions of medical technology are the advances that have been made in reducing infant mortality. As little as two generations ago prenatal and neonatal illness, disease, and death were common in North America. One need, however, only look at less advanced cultures throughout the world, and among the poor, deprived, and neglected in our society, to see that the threat of severely handicapping conditions resulting from a variety of prenatal factors still exists. Hagberg (1975) reported that the current leading cause of severe impairment, among rich and poor, stems from prenatal factors. Although only about 1 percent of the population shows moderate to severe problems in the years before school (Mercer, 1973), Hagberg estimates that 85 to 90 percent of these intellectual and neurological problems stem from prenatal causes. In a country whose population will exceed 230 million by 1985, and 260 million by the year 2000 it seems important, therefore, that as many prenatal factors that adversely affect later growth and development be identified and eliminated as possible (U.S. Bureau of the Census, 1980). It is staggering to contemplate that over 2 million Americans have *severe* afflictions because of conditions over which they have absolutely no control. It is doubly staggering when we speculate on the number of individuals that have been only moderately or slightly affected by these conditions.

Growth and motor development are processes that begin at conception and are influenced by numerous factors. In this chapter we will examine several of the prenatal factors that may inhibit normal growth and development. Attention will also be given to the influences of medication administered during the birth process and to various methods of childbearing.

## NUTRITIONAL AND CHEMICAL FACTORS

What the expectant mother ingests will affect the unborn child in some way. Whether these effects are harmful and will have lasting consequences depends on a variety of circumstances. The condition of the fetus, degree of nutritional or chemical abuse, amount or dosage, period of pregnancy, and the presence of other influencing factors are but a few of the circumstances that influence the probability of birth defects. The fetus is potentially at risk, however, when any one or more of the following nutritional or chemical factors are present.

### Maternal Nutrition

The fetus depends on the mother's blood supply and the osmotic action of the placenta and umbilical cord for its nutrients. Because of this, deficiencies in the mother's diet both prior to and during pregnancy can have a harmful effect on the child. A sound, nutritious diet is absolutely essential for the mother's health and that of her unborn child.

Although most of us, at least for now, in our Western culture enjoy an abundance of food, *malnourishment,* and not undernourishment, is an area of concern among nutritionists and specialists in child development. The fact is that literally millions of women of childbearing age are malnourished worldwide. In other words, they are not receiving the proper nutrients through their normal daily intake of food. The mother-to-be who is malnourished may be so for reasons ranging from the potentially easy to alter esthetic reasons and the lifelong "junk" food, "fast" food habits of millions, to the more difficult to deal with reasons of poverty, low socioeconomic class, anxiety, stress, and trauma.

The sharpest contrasts in maternal malnutrition and normal nutrition are seen between poor and nonpoor mothers. Naeye et al. (1969) studied 252 infants who were stillborn or died within two days of birth. His survey indicated that infants who were "below the poverty level" were 15 percent smaller than nonpoverty infants. Also, a higher percentage of stillborn children were born to impoverished mothers. Maternal malnutrition may account for the fact that low socioeconomic families have a higher percentage of children with birth defects than do families with higher and generally more adequate nutrition (Hepner, 1958; McGarrity et al., 1958).

Inadequate nutrition has been shown to be a major factor in low-birthweight infants. Low-birthweight babies are much more susceptible to a variety of developmental abnormalities and have a higher mortality rate than normal birthweight infants. Figure 4.1 shows that the mortality rate for low-birthweight babies is significantly higher than for those of normal weight.

Lack of vitamins C, B-complex, D, K, and E as well as protein deficiencies may result in serious physical and mental damage or even death to the unborn child

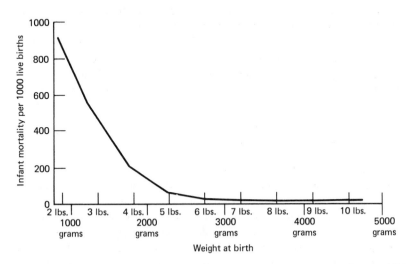

**Figure 4.1.** *Relationship between infant mortality and birth weight. (Source:* White House Conference on Children, 1970.)

(Litch, 1978). Information, through experimentation, is difficult to gather as to the effect of specific vitamin and mineral deficiencies in the diet of the expectant mother and mother-to-be. It is unethical to study the effects of malnutrition by purposely depriving expectant mothers. It is also difficult to compare mothers with inadequate diets against those who have adequate nutrition because of confounding variables such as extreme anxiety, stress, poverty, and poor nutritional habits.

## Common Maternal Drugs

The wall of the placenta is porous, and chemicals may penetrate it with tragic results to the unborn child. The drugs found in the average person's medicine cabinet are potentially destructive to the fetus. Every drug has side effects. Whether it is a prescription or nonprescription drug and whether the drug has been given during pregnancy without serious side effects in others do not imply that it is safe for all unborn children. The following factors need to be considered whenever the influence of a drug on an unborn child is determined.

1. The time of pregnancy during which the drug is taken.
2. The dosage of the drug.
3. The length of time the drug is taken.
4. The genetic predisposition of the fetus.
5. How these four factors interact.

There are various ways in which a drug may affect the unborn child. Drugs may interfere with organ growth or cell differentiation and result in deviations from normal development. The penetrability of the placenta may be altered and reduce the flow of oxygen and nutrients or magnify the drug concentration flowing to the fetus. Drugs may impair development and functioning of the liver, which balances blood waste products called bilirubin. The inability of the biliary ducts to excrete bilirubin efficiently results in jaundice. Excessive jaundice is called kernicterus. Kernicterus can cause permanent and devastating brain damage. Table 4.1 provides a few examples of common drugs taken during pregnancy and the associated risk factors.

## "Necessary" Maternal Drugs

During pregnancy the expectant mother may be under the care of a physician because of an illness or disease. Good, consistant medical care is doubly important because the developing fetus inside a mother with a special medical condition may have special needs. The medication prescribed for the mother may have to be modified to protect the unborn child. A mother being treated for epilepsy for example, should avoid the use of Dilantin and phenobarbital and other drugs used for seizure control. Although she may not be able to completely discontinue the use

**Table 4.1   The Effect of Common Drugs on the Unborn Child**

| Drug | Use | Possible Effects |
| --- | --- | --- |
| Coumadin | An anticoagulant used for blood clots | May cause bleeding before or during birth, resulting in brain damage |
| Diuretics | To treat toxemia, particularly water retention | Water and salt imbalance. An electrolyte imbalance may result in brain damage |
| Streptomycin | To treat infection in the mother | Impairment of kidneys, hearing, and balance |
| Aspirin | For aches, pain, fever. Almost 80% of over-the-counter drugs contain aspirin | Death; congenital deformities; bleeding under the skull, causing brain damage; hemorrhaging during birth |
| Tetracyclines | For acne | Stunts bone and teeth growth |

of medication, the drug should not continue to be taken automatically and the dosage may need modification under medical supervision.

The expectant mother with cancer is at risk when chemotherapy is being used to decrease the rate of malignant cell growth, particularly during the first three months of pregnancy. Also, the use of progesterone to correct menstrual cycle abnormalities and to prevent miscarriage should be avoided in all expectant mothers because of the potentially harmful effects on the newborn.

The unborn child of a diabetic mother-to-be is particularly vulnerable. "One out of every four babies dies in the womb [of diabetic mothers] if the mother is not under excellent medical care" (Litch, 1978, p. 172). Table 4.2 provides a brief overview of some common medical conditions of the expectant mother that may affect later development.

## Mind-Altering Drugs

During the past decade there has been an increase in the habitual use of mind-altering drugs by women of childbearing age. The use of opiates (opium, heroin), cocaine, amphetamines ("speed"), lysergic acid diethylamide (LSD), and cannabis (hashish, marijuana) has been of great concern to those interested in the well-being of the unborn child. Because of legal, moral, and ethical reasons, it is impossible to conduct controlled experiments on the effects of these mind-altering drugs on fetal development. Our knowledge is limited to laboratory settings with animals. The results of two carefully controlled studies with mice indicated that LSD produced a much higher incidence of birth defects (Alexander et al., 1967) and that cannabis produced a high number of stillbirths (Harbison, and Mantilla-

**Table 4.2   Common Drugs for Medical Conditions During Pregnancy and the Possible Effects on the Unborn Child**

| Maternal Condition | Drug | Possible Effects on the Unborn Child |
|---|---|---|
| Hypertension | Resperine | Choking, gasping, nasal congestion at birth |
| Thyroid | Thiouracile Iodides Radioactive iodine | Thyroid abnormalities in child: cretinism (hypothyrodism) |
| Diabetes | Insulin | Excessive birthweight, prematurity, heart defects, jaundice, low blood sugar, convulsions, mental and physical retardation |
| Menstrual abnormality | Progesterone | Gross deformities, masculinization of female organs |
| Allergy or cold | Antihistamines | Deformities (in animal studies) |
| Epilepsy | Seizure control drugs | Cleft palate and other malformations |

Plata, 1972). Houston's (1969) research suggests that hallucinogens produce birth defects when taken early in pregnancy. Persons taking LSD are much more likely to have chromosome abnormalities than are nonusers. Although available research is limited to animals and only correlational in nature, it seems reasonable to assume that mind-altering drugs are likely to adversely affect the unborn child. Table 4.3 provides an overview of the possible effects of some mind-altering drugs on the newborn child.

## Alcohol and Tobacco

Although alcohol and tobacco are considered by some to be mind- or mood-altering drugs, they have been separated here because of the frequency of their usage and in order to amplify their potential hazards. It has been variously reported that there are over 1 million alcoholics of childbearing age. The fetus is affected twice as fast as the mother by her alcohol consumption and at the same level of concentration. Until recently, the widespread myth that the fetus will take what it needs from its mother and be uninfluenced by her consumption of foods and beverages caused expectant mothers to be unconcerned about their alcohol consumption. The potential dangers of alcohol to the unborn child were recognized, however, as far back as the Greek era, when newly married couples were forbidden to consume alcohol in order to prevent conception while intoxicated.

**Table 4.3    Possible Effects of Mind-Altering Drugs on the Development of the Unborn Child**

| Drug | Possible Effects on the Unborn Child |
|------|--------------------------------------|
| Heroin and morphine | Irritable. Sleeps poorly. High-pitched cry. Vomiting and diarrhea. Marked physiological withdrawal symptoms. Decreased oxygen in the blood tissues. Hepatitis from unclean needle. Susceptible to infection. Complications in 40 percent of addicted: 1. Toxemia. 2. Breach birth. 3. Prematurity. 4. Small for date of birth. 5. Premature separation of the placenta. Complications if not treated: 1. Dehydration. 2. Respiratory distress. 3. Shock. 4. Coma. 5. Mineral imbalance. |
| Amphetamines and barbiturates | Miscarriage. Birth defects. |
| Tranquilizers | Such drugs as Sominex, Nytol, Sleep-Eze and Compoz contain two antihistamines that have produced congenital deformities in animals. |
| LSD (lysergic acid diethylamide) | *May* cause chromosome damage. *Sometimes* contaminated with quinine or other materials that may harm the unborn child. A few surveys have found a higher incidence of congenital defects in children of LSD users. |

In the 1890's William Sullivan, a physician at a Liverpool, England, prison for women was the first to carefully document the effects of chronic alcoholism on the offspring of 120 alcoholic inmates. This early study revealed a significantly higher mortality rate among the 600 offspring and a much greater number of developmental difficulties of the infants (cited in Rosett and Sander, 1979). Further research into the effects of maternal alcoholism lagged in the United States and Great Britain after 1920, following the enactment of Prohibition, although some research continued in France and Germany. It was not until 1970 that the actual "discovery" and labeling of fetal alcohol syndrome took place (Witti, 1978).

Alcohol is now recognized as the third leading cause of birth defects (Litch, 1978). The other two are Down's syndrome and spina bifida. Fetal alcohol syndrome is the only cause that offers a possibility of prevention. Forty to 50 percent of infants born to mothers who are chronic alcoholics (with a consumption level of three or more average-size drinks per day) or who go on drinking binges are born mentally retarded or with marked physical defects. Table 4.4 summarizes some of the potential dangers of fetal alcohol syndrome.

Alcohol in the mother's blood is passed directly through the placenta to the fetus. Current evidence shows that the fetus does not have any ethanol-oxidizing or alcohol dehydrogenasic abilities, and therefore the alcohol is fed directly into its system (Brown et al., 1979). Evidence on the exact amounts of alcohol that are harmful to the fetus and on the critical periods during which it should be avoided is unclear. Also, social drinking during pregnancy has not been clearly associated with an increase in risk. Witti (1978), however, states that "until the answers are in on the key questions of exactly how much or when alcohol is safe to drink during pregnancy, medical authorities agree that it is wise to be cautious" (p. 23).

**Table 4.4   Characteristics of Fetal Alcohol Syndrome**

| | |
|---|---|
| Growth | Growth failure before birth. |
| | Growth failure after birth. |
| | Skull that is too small for the brain. |
| | Small in length compared to weight. |
| Eyes | Lesions in the eyelids. |
| | Fold of the skin in the corner of the eye. |
| | Perceptual problems. |
| | Narrow eyes. |
| Face | Low nasal bridge. |
| | Short, upturned nose. |
| | Outer ear deformity. |
| | Underdevelopment of the jaw. |
| Other | Heart defects. |
| | Hip dislocation. |
| | Skeletal defects. |
| | Decrease in joint mobility. |
| | Motor development delay. |
| | Abnormal creases in the palm of the hand. |
| | Female genital defects. |
| Behavior | Jittery. |
| | Hyperactive. |
| | Weak grasp, poor coordination. |
| | Poor sucking. |
| | Irregular sleeping. |
| | Self-stimulator. |
| Intellectual | Mentally retarded: borderline to moderate. |

Smoking has been implicated in numerous studies as a cause of low birthweight in infants (Meredith, 1975; Pasamanuck and Knoblach, 1966). The National Foundation/March of Dimes (1977) has indicated that women who smoke a pack of cigarettes or more a day tend to have low birthweight babies and a greater tendency toward stillbirths and early infant mortality. Maternal smoking speeds up the fetal heart rate and has an adverse effect on central nervous system integration of the newborn. A survey of children born to nicotine-addicted mothers showed that they tend to rate lower on behavior assessment scales than other newborns. They tend to be more fretful, less coordinated, less alert, less responsive to cuddling (Strauss et al., 1975). Butler et al. (1972), however, found that women who stop smoking before the fourth month of pregnancy are no more likely than nonsmoking mothers to have a low birthweight baby. Therefore, there may be cause for cautious optimism, in that the effects of smoking may not be cumulative, and their impact on the unborn child may be negligible if smoking ceases early in pregnancy. Verification of this awaits further research.

## HEREDITARY FACTORS

Until relatively recently the study of heredity through the science of genetics was only a matter of theory and speculation. Today, however, we have more precise and experimentally verifiable knowledge of heredity. Since it is impossible to discuss it in detail within the confines of this chapter, we will, concern ourselves with the potential impact of various hereditary factors on later development.

The union of a sperm with an egg begins the process of development. The sperm carries twenty-three chromosomes, which contain all of the hereditary material that the father contributes. The egg also contains twenty-three chromosomes, the mother's contribution to the child's heredity. The new fetus, therefore, contains a total of forty-six chromosomes (twenty-three pairs). Each chromosome, by the process of cell division (mitosis), has a replica in every cell of the body. Genes are found on each chromosome. It has been estimated that each chromosome may contain up to 20,000 genes (Whithurst and Varta, 1977). The genes determine the vast variety of individual characteristics such as sex, hair and eye color, body size and structure.

Under most conditions the chromosomes and genes remain unaltered throughout the prenatal period. (There is growing speculation that certain chemical substances may cause chromosomal damage after conception.) A variety of genetic factors prior to conception, however, have been shown to alter the normal process of development.

### Chromosome-Based Disorders

It has been estimated that between 3 and 6 percent of all conceptions show evidence of chromosome damage, and of these about 90 percent will be spontaneously aborted (Ford, 1973). Most chromosome variations are so potent that they are rarely seen in surviving newborns, but fully 1 percent of live infants show evidence of chromosomal damage, according to Ford (1973).

Probably the most common chromosomal alteration is that of Down's syndrome. Down's syndrome is the result of an error in which forty-seven chromosomes are present rather than the standard forty-six. Down's syndrome occurs in approximately 1 out of every 500 to 700 live births (Thompson and Thompson, 1973). The rate of incidence seems, however, to be age related and shows dramatic increases in births occurring in women over forty-five years of age. In fact, the frequency of women under 30 is about 1 in 1500, while women over 45 years of age have a 1-in-65 chance of giving birth to a child with Down's syndrome (Smart and Smart, 1973a).

Down's syndrome children are often born prematurely. Their rate of growth is slower than normal, often resulting in shorter stature. The nose, chin, and ears tend to be small, along with poor development of the teeth and poor eyesight. Poor balance, hypotonus, short arms and legs, and nonelastic skin are other characteristics of the Down's child. Cardiovascular defects resulting in frequent respiratory ailments are common, along with limited intellectual functioning. Language and conceptualization skills are generally poor. Motor development proceeds in the same manner as for the normal infant but at a slower rate.

Chromosome-linked disorders other than Down's syndrome sometimes occur. Fortunately conditions such as Patau's syndrome and Edward's syndrome are rare. Little is known about them other than that they are also associated with an extra chromosome and that they result in severe deformities, retardation, and early mortality (Kopp and Parmelee, 1979).

## Gene-Based Disorders

Genetic defects vary widely in their consequences. The severity of the defect is dependent on whether the mutant gene is on an autosomal or on a sex-linked chromosome and whether it is on a single gene (heterozygous) or also on its mate (homozygous). Kopp and Parmelee (1979) have reported:

> Infants with a recognized autosomal dominant syndrome have inherited mutant genes from only *one* affected parent; as such the dosage they receive is single (heterozygous). In general, these infants will be less severely affected than those diagnosed with autosomal recessive conditions, in the latter conditions mutant genes are inherited from *both* parents and thus the dosage is double (homozygous). (p. 35)

Delay and retardation in motor and cognitive functioning are not usually present in autosomal dominant mutations. Autosomal recessive mutations, however, are often associated with mental retardation and problems in motor development. Nora and Fraser (1974) list sixty-one autosomal syndromes, one third of which are associated with mental retardation and other developmental abnormalities that interfere with the normal process of motor development. Among the more common autosomal recessive mutations are Hurler's syndrome, genetic thyroid defects, maple syrup urine disease, and phenyloketonuria (PKU). Many of these diseases can be treated effectively through dietary and chemical means if diagnosed early in life.

The environment's influence on heredity is no more clearly indicated than when we consider the effects of ionizing radiation on gene mutation. The cumulative effects of radiation exposure, even through routine dental and physical x-rays, have been shown to be related to later developmental abnormalities, including malformations and microcephaly (Plummer, 1952).

## MEDICAL PROBLEMS

The causes and effects of developmental difficulties in the offspring of mothers with various maternal infections, hormonal and chemical imbalances, Rh incompatibility, and severe maternal stress are being researched. These conditions play a significant role in placing the unborn child at risk.

### Maternal Infections

Perhaps the most significant diseases contracted by the mother that adversely affect the fetus are cytomegalovirus (CMV), rubella (German measles) contracted during the first trimester of pregnancy, diabetes, and syphilis. All of these diseases pass through the placenta to the fetus and can have serious debilitating effects. CMV is a common infectious cause of birth defects including blindness, deafness, and mental retardation. Very little is known about this virus and its effects. It is still unclear whether the virus is introduced into the fetus by a primary infection to the mother during pregnancy or whether it may already be present genetically but in latent form (Marx, 1975). On the other hand, much is known about the causes and results of rubella. The child born after its mother has had rubella is likely to be deaf, blind, or mentally retarded due to interference with sensory and/or cognitive development during the embryonic, or early fetal period. The newborn with congenital syphilis is likely to be born displaying severe withdrawal symptoms and delayed central nervous system organization. The long-term effects of maternal syphilis are still unclear, but preliminary data indicate a greater incidence of prematurity and later motor, sensory, and cognitive disabilities.

### Hormonal and Chemical and Imbalances

An inadequate hormonal or chemical environment in the thyroid patient, for example, can result in congenital hypothyrodism and cretinism in the infant, due to a lack of thyroxine in the mother's blood during the early months of pregnancy.

Diabetes in the expectant mother is a chronic chemical imbalance that may adversely affect later development in the child. The inadequate production of insulin prevents the proper metabolizing of sugar and other carbohydrates. Untreated diabetes can result in mental retardation, circulatory and respiratory problems in the infant, or even death.

## Rh Incompatibility

Rh incompatibility results from the incompatibility of blood types between mother and child. Although there is no direct link between the bloodstream of the infant and that of the mother, there may be some seepage of blood from the fetus to the mother during the later stages of pregnancy. If the expectant Rh negative mother is carrying her first Rh positive child, this seepage to the mother will cause her to produce antibodies in her blood. The production of antibodies generally has no effect on the first child. The time lag between the first and subsequent children, however, provides ample opportunity for the production of antibodies in the mother. These antibodies can have a devastating effect on future pregnancies, by destroying the fetal red corpuscles. *Erythroblastosis fetalis* is the name given to this condition, which is characterized by anemia and jaundice (Winchester, 1979).

Rh incompatibility occurs only in cases where the father is Rh positive and the mother is Rh negative. Routine blood tests and a rhogam injection immediately after birth of the first child will prevent the formation of antibodies. Rhogam is the gamma globulin component of blood obtained from an Rh negative person previously sensitized to the Rh factor. The rhogam neutralizes the Rh factor in the mother and prevents the buildup of antibodies by her (Espenschade and Eckert, 1980).

## Maternal Stress

Evidence from a growing body of research has raised concern over the effects of severe prolonged maternal emotional stress on the unborn child. Severe stress factors such as death of a loved one and marital problems have been associated with complications during pregnancy and fetal abnormalities (Davids et al., 1961). Although there is no direct link between the nervous system of the mother and the fetus, the mother's emotional state can influence development. It is hypothesized that because the nervous system and the endocrine system communicate through the blood, the emotional trauma experienced by the mother is transferred from the cerebral cortex to the thalamus and hypothalamus. The autonomic nervous system acts on the endocrine system, which empties into the bloodstream. The mother's bloodstream then transports the endocrine secretions to the placenta through which some are passed into the fetal bloodstream and finally to its nervous system (Montague, 1962). This hypothesis is speculative, but it is clear that prolonged maternal stress may have detrimental effects. Children born of emotionally stressed mothers are more prone to a variety of illnesses and physical problems throughout life (Bee, 1975).

## Toxoplasmosis

Besides all of the infections, diseases, and special conditions already discussed as high-risk considerations, expectant parents need to be aware of toxoplasmosis so that they can protect their unborn child against the offending protozoan. Toxoplasmosis is amazingly prevalent. It has been estimated that 1 in every 1000 infants and 1 in every 500 pregnant women are infected by it (Litch, 1978). Infected children may appear normal at birth and even until their twenties, when the toxoplasma cysts rupture, releasing thousands of parasites that attack the eyes, heart, other internal organs, and the central nervous system.

Toxoplasmosis is a more prevalent health problem than either rubella or PKU but its devastation to the unborn child has had little publicity. However, the parents of an unborn child can do some very specific things to protect their child from this infection. All beef, pork, and lamb should be cooked until well done because the protozoan cysts exist in the muscle of meat. Because the toxoplasma organisms are transmitted by cats, it is wise to avoid contact with cats during pregnancy.

The natural reservoir of the *Toxoplasma gondii* sporozoan is the mouse, and most cats come in contact with mice! The spores passed in the feces of infected cats can be inhaled or ingested. The symptoms of infection in humans are similar to the flu, or many times there are no symptoms at all. Persons who have been infected carry antibodies against toxoplasmosis. However, the fetus *does not* have the ability to make such antibodies and takes the effects of the infection with full force. About 10 percent of the 3000 infants infected with toxoplasmosis each year are severely brain damaged and suffer a variety of sensory and motor disabilities.

## BIRTH PROCESS FACTORS

The average length of intrauterine life is 279 days—from the day of conception to the day of birth. Two thirds of all expectant mothers give birth within 279 days plus or minus a two-week period. The beginning of labor is marked by the passage of blood and amniotic fluid from the ruptured amniotic sac through the vagina and the onset of labor pains. There are three distinguishable stages of labor. In the first stage the neck of the uterus (the cervix) dilates to about 4 cm in diameter. Dilation is responsible for labor pains and may last for only a few hours or up to several hours. Labor is generally longer with the first child (primiparas) than for subsequent children (multiparas). When the cervix reaches 2 cm, full labor begins. It is at this point that the amniotic sac breaks and the fluid flows out of the mother. Complete dilation marks the onset of the second stage of labor: the expulsion period. During this stage the baby, through the continued increase in uterine pressure, is forced down the birth canal. This phase takes an average of ninety minutes for the first child and about half as long for subsequent children. The third stage of labor begins after the baby has emerged and continues until after the umbilical cord and placenta (afterbirth) have been delivered. During any stage of the birth process a number of obstetrical medications and obstetrical procedures may influence the later development of the child.

## Obstetrical Medication

One of the most controversial issues today among obstetricians and ·infant researchers is the effects of obstetrical medication commonly used during the birth process. The paper published by Yvonne Brackbill (1979), the sensational journalistic attention that it received in the popular press and the subsequent rebuttal of her findings by many have done much to add fuel to this already heated debate. Basically, the argument is as follows: Because of the structural and functional immaturity of the nervous system at birth and because of the rapid absorption rate across the placenta, drugs given during the birth process will have an adverse effect on the newborn and its subsequent development. It is estimated, based on a variety of surveys, that 90 to 95 percent of all hospital births involve the use of some form of medication (Brackbill, 1979; Standley, 1974). Table 4.5 lists common types of predelivery, general, and local anesthetics used during delivery. These medications are used to initiate or augment labor (oxytoxics), relieve pain (analgesics), and relieve anxiety (sedatives).

The results of several studies point to a relationship between drug use during labor and later development. There is compelling evidence that muscular strength and motor coordination are impaired as measured on infant development scales (Brackbill, 1970; Conway and Brackbill, 1970). Muller et al. (1971) and Goldstein et al. (1976) have found a relationship between obstetrical drugs and lowered IQ

**Table 4.5   Function of Common Types of Predelivery and Delivery Drugs**

| Predelivery Drugs | Delivery Drugs |
|---|---|
| Oxytoxics | General anesthetics |
|   Induce labor |   Relieve fetal distress |
|   Augment labor |   Speed up delivery |
|   Increase uterine tonus |   Mother emotionally unsuited to |
| Sedatives |     remain awake |
|   Reduce anxiety |   Multiple births |
|   Reduce excitement | Local anesthetics |
|   Slow down labor |   Pain relief |
| |   Relaxation |

scores. Brackbill (1979) contends that obstetrical drug use has had a significant effect on lowering the IQ of most Americans. This is due to the increased risk of anoxia and delay in organization of the CNS. The extent of these influences is open to considerable debate and is dependent on a variety of factors, including type and combination, amount administered, and the time lag between administration and birth. It is safe at this point to say, however, that drugs taken during the birth process put the newborn at risk. The extent and certainty of this risk is not yet clear, but it seems reasonable to assume that a drug-free birth or at least the judicious use of drugs during labor would do much to reduce the risk of later developmental difficulties.

## Birth Entry

A variety of birth entry factors also have been shown to put the infant at risk. Among them are malpresentation, the use of forceps, and Caesarean section.

About 4 in every 100 babies are born buttocks first, or feet first (breech position), and 1 out of 100 are in a crosswise position (transverse presentation) (Travers, 1977). These presentations can sometimes be altered by the attending physician or midwife. The danger in malpresentation, as with drug-assisted labor and umbilical cord difficulties is anoxia. In fact, anoxia has been described as the major cause of perinatal death and has been implicated as the cause of mental retardation, learning disabilities, and cerebral palsy (Bonica, 1967).

Forceps are occasionally used to withdraw the baby from the birth canal. Today, the use of forceps is limited largely to emergency situations, but they were used routinely in obstetrics until the 1940s. Forceps are used to speed delivery when the mother is displaying uncontrollable pushing, when the infant has a weak heartbeat, when the umbilical cord emerges before the head and endangers the baby's oxygen supply, or when there is a premature separation of the placenta (Milinaire, 1974). Forceps have played and continue to play a vital role in obstetrics as a lifesaving device, but their overuse, and misuse, have had debilitating and lethal effects on both mothers and children.

A Caesarean section involves surgical delivery of the baby. The survey conducted by Jones (1976) based on over 72,000 births over a period of thirty-five years showed a definite increase in the number of Caesarean operations. The reasons for this seem to be associated with planning the exact delivery date, avoidance of pain (a general anesthetic is usually given), the advent of newer incision techniques leaving a smaller and less noticeable scar, and the desire to spare the fetus any distress. A Caesarean section is a major operation and in the past was considered only in cases of necessity in that it was performed due to malpresentation, fetal distress, and failed use of forceps. Recently, however, Caesarean section has become an operation of choice, but most obstetricians still recommend that it be used only when there are extenuating circumstances.

## Summary

A wide variety of factors have been shown to adversely influence the process of later development. There is a growing realization among many prospective parents that they *can* do something to reduce the chances of putting their offspring at risk. Many now realize that their choice of what they ingest in the way of nutrients, alcohol, tobacco, and other drugs can have an impact on the unborn child. Many are now sensitive to the possible harmful effects of caffeine, saccharin, overexposure to radiation and noxious chemicals, and obstetrical medication. As a result there has been a resurgence of interest in ''natural'' childbirth techniques, rooming-in, and home births, and a return to a more responsible attitude about giving birth. A greater number of mothers are asserting their rights for a drug-free pregnancy and are working knowledgeably with concerned obstetricians to produce the healthiest offspring possible.

The birth process can be an important beginning in the three-way bonding of mother, infant, and father. Because of this, parents should be granted the right to choose the method in which they wish to introduce their offspring into the world. The Lamaze (1970) and the Le Boyer (1975) methods of childbirth are two procedures from which prospective parents can choose. The Lamaze method centers on the mother and father. It is a conscious relaxation technique that incorporates rhythmical breathing to block the sensations of pain and a complete knowledge of what to expect during labor and delivery. The Le Boyer method focuses almost entirely on the infant. The aim is to simulate the conditions of the womb as closely as possible. Delivery occurs in a dimly lit room without loud noises. The baby is immediately immersed in a warm fluid solution and gradually, but gently, introduced into the world.

The prenatal period is too important to be left to chance. An ''intelligent'' pregnancy and delivery, although not a guarantee, can do much to reduce the risk involved to both mother and child.

## CHAPTER HIGHLIGHTS

1.  Growth and motor development begin at conception and are influenced by numerous factors.
2.  Malnourishment is a problem in many developed as well as developing countries and has been shown to have a negative impact on the unborn child.
3.  Children born to malnourished and undernourished mothers tend to be smaller, have a higher number of developmental difficulties, and have a higher mortality rate than children born to properly nourished mothers.
4.  Maternal malnutrition cuts across all socioeconomic classes, ethnic and racial backgrounds.
5.  Many nonprescription drugs routinely taken during pregnancy may have a negative effect on the developing fetus.

6. Several commonly prescribed drugs for special maternal conditions have a negative effect on the developing fetus.
7. Mind-altering drugs have been shown to have a negative effect on the development of the fetus and infant.
8. The dosage, duration, time during pregnancy, and genetic predisposition of the fetus determine whether the unborn child will be adversely affected by improper nutrition or chemical substances.
9. The regular use of alcohol and tobacco by the expectant mother has been shown to increase the risk of damage to the fetus.
10. The genetic inheritance of the fetus will control the upper and lower limits of its functioning.
11. Several chromosome-based factors may adversely affect the development of the fetus and infant.
12. Gene-linked abnormalities have been shown to adversely influence development.
13. A variety of maternal medical conditions may adversely influence development.
14. Maternal infections and the buildup of antibodies may adversely affect development.
15. Severe maternal stress has been associated with complications during pregnancy and fetal abnormalities.
16. The use of drugs and medication during the birth process has been shown to affect later development.
17. The use of certain birthing techniques and procedures has been shown to affect later development.
18. The mother- and father-to-be have an obligation to their unborn child to ensure its normal development by monitoring the factors over which they exercise some control.

## CRITICAL READINGS

Brackbill, Y.: "Obstetrical Medication and Infant Behavior," in J.D. Osofsky (ed.), *The Handbook of Infant Development*, New York: Wiley, 1979, pp. 76–125.

Le Boyer, *Birth Without Violence*, New York: Knopf, 1975.

Espenschade, A., and H. Eckert: *Motor Development*, Columbus, Ohio: Merrill, 1980, Chapter 2.

# Infant and Childhood Factors Affecting Development

The process of motor development is influenced by a number of biological and environmental factors operating both in isolation from and in combination with one another. The child who comes to us in the preschool or elementary school is the product of the interaction of these factors. The development and refinement of movement patterns and movement skills is influenced in complex ways. Both the process and product of the child's movement and physical performance are rooted in his or her unique genetic and experiential background. Any study of motor development would be incomplete without a discussion of several of these influencing factors. This chapter focuses on influences during infancy and childhood—biological trends in motor development, caregiver factors, and a variety of associated factors—that impact on the child's motor development.

## PREMATURITY

The normal birthweight of an infant is about 7 lb (about 3300 g). Formerly, any infant weighing under 2500 g (about 5½ lb) was classified as premature. Today, however, 2000g (4½ lb) is often used, unless there is evidence that the gestation period was less than thirty-seven weeks. The practice of labeling a newborn as premature based on gestation period or weight alone is no longer used for two reasons. First, it is often difficult to accurately determine the gestational age of the infant, and second, the highest mortality and morbidity rates are present for infants of the very lowest birthweight (Susser et al., 1972). As a result the terms *low birthweight* and *young for date* have emerged as more accurate indicators of prematurity in the true sense of the word (Kopp and Parmelee, 1979). Prematurity is of major concern because it is closely associated with physical and mental retardation and hyperactivity (Caputo and Mandell, 1970).

### Low-Birthweight Infants

Low-birthweight infants are those whose birthweight is clearly below the expected weight for their gestational age. Two standard deviations below the mean for a given gestational age is the generally accepted criterion for low birthweight. (Ounsted and Ounsted, 1973). Therefore, a low-birthweight infant may be one who is born at term (forty weeks) or preterm (thirty-seven weeks or under). Low-birthweight infants have experienced what Warkany et al. (1961) termed as "intrauterine growth retardation" and are generally called "small for date."

A variety of prenatal maternal factors have been implicated in low birthweight, including diet, drugs, smoking, infections, and disease (DeMyer, 1975). Other factors such as social class, multiple births, and geographic locale have been shown to influence birthweight (Ounsted and Ounsted, 1973). The long-term effects of low birthweight are directly related to the degree of intrauterine growth retardation and gestational age of the child. Kopp and Parmalee (1979) have stated:

> In summary, it is clear that the infant born with intrauterine growth retardation may have severe medical problems in the neonatal period. Reflexive and behavioral differences may occur in early life, possibly leading to disrupted patterns of parent-infant interaction. The overall outcome for intellectual functioning is relatively positive, even for pre-terms who were small-for-date. Yet, inevitable questions arise. Would the intelligence of this group of children have been higher if they had not been malnourished in utero? (p. 59)

## Young-for-Date Infants

Children born at the expected birthweight (less than 2 SD below the mean) for their gestational age but before full term (thirty-seven weeks or less) are called young-for-date or preterm infants. There is little agreement on the exact causes of preterm birth, but a number of factors have been shown to contribute to its likelihood. Factors such as drug use, smoking, maternal age, excessive weight gain, and adverse social and economic conditions have been shown to contribute to the incidence of young-for-date births (Susser et al., 1972). Until a few years ago the prognosis for young-for-date infants who were either small for date or of normal weight for date was bleak. Their morbidity and mortality rates were abnormally high. Drillien (1970) reported that as many as 40 percent showed evidence of neurological and intellectual damage. Recent advances in neonatal intensive care have, however, done much to reduce this unusually high rate of difficulties in some locations.

The preterm infant is still likely to have more learning difficulties, language and social interaction problems, and motor coordination problems than his or her full-term counterpart (Davies and Stewart, 1975). For some unknown reason, boys seem to be more severely affected than girls. The usual treatment of hospital-born premature infants is to put them in a sterile isolette, where temperature, humidity, and oxygen can be precisely controlled. It has been suggested that the absence of normal stimulation from the mother and the surrounding environment contributes to the retardation (Hasselmeyer, 1964). A study by Solkoff et al. (1969), although tentative, seems to verify this notion. The results of the two-treatment-group study of premature infants in which one group was given routine care and the other was given five extra minutes of handling per hour seem to support the need for early handling. The extra handling group performed better on two measures. The infants were more active and gained weight faster. Seven months later the handled group still performed better on tests of motor performance and appeared more active and healthier.

## DEVELOPMENTAL TRENDS

The unique genetic inheritance that accounts for our individuality can also account for our similarity in many ways. One of these similarities is the trend for human development to proceed in an orderly, predictable fashion. A number of biological trends affecting motor development seem to emerge from this predictable pattern of development.

### Developmental Direction

Developmental direction refers to the orderly, predictable sequence of physical development that proceeds from the head to the feet *(cephalocaudal)* and from the center of the body to its periphery *(proximodistal)*.

The cephalocaudal aspect of development refers specifically to the gradual progression of increased control over the musculature, moving from the head to the feet. It may be witnessed in the prenatal stages of fetal development as well as in later postnatal development. In the developing fetus, for example, the head forms first, and the arms form prior to the legs. Likewise, infants exhibit sequential control over the musculature of the head, neck, and trunk, prior to gaining control over the legs. Preschool children are often thought to be clumsy and to exhibit poor control over the lower extremities. This may be due to incomplete cephalocaudal development.

The second aspect of developmental direction, known as proximodistal development, refers specifically to the child's progression in control of the musculature from the center of the body to its most distant parts. The young child, for example, is able to control the muscles of the trunk and shoulder girdle prior to gaining control over the muscles of the wrist, hand, and fingers. This principle of development is utilized by teachers of primary grade children in the teaching of the less refined elements of manuscript writing prior to the introduction of the more complex and refined movements of cursive writing.

### Rate of Growth

The rate of growth for children follows a characteristic pattern that is universal for all children and resistant to external influence. Even the interruption of the normal pace of growth is compensated for by a still unexplained self-regulatory process that comes into operation to help the child catch up to his or her age-mates. For example, a severe illness may retard a child's gain in height and weight and movement ability, but on recovery from the illness there will be a tendency to catch up with the other children. The same phenomenon is seen with the low-birthweight infant. Despite this low birthweight, there is still a tendency to catch up to the characteristic growth rate of one's age-mates in a few years. Therefore, measures of height, weight, and motor development taken prior to age 2 are generally meaningless for predicting later growth and development.

The self-regulatory process of growth will compensate for *minor* deviations in the growth pattern, but it is unable to make up *major* deviations such as in the low-birthweight infant weighing under 3½ lb. In this case the child often suffers permanent deficits in height and weight, and in cognitive and motor abilities, and is unable to recoup these initial losses completely.

Restricted opportunity for movement and deprivation of experience have been shown repeatedly to interfere with children's abilities to perform motor tasks that are characteristic of their particular age level. The effects of this deprivation of sensory and motor experience can sometimes be overcome when nearly optimal conditions are established for a child (McGraw, 1939a). The extent to which the child will be able to catch up to his or her peers, however, depends on the duration and severity of deprivation and the age of the child.

## Differentiation and Integration

The coordinated and progressive intricate interweaving of neural mechanisms of opposing muscle systems into an increasingly mature relationship is characteristic of the developing child's motor behavior. There are two different but related processes associated with this increase of functional complexity, known as *differentiation* and *integration*. Differentiation is associated with the gradual progression from the gross globular (overall) movement patterns of infants to the more refined and functional movements of children as they mature. Integration refers to bringing various opposing muscle and sensory systems into coordinated interaction with one another. For example, the young child gradually progresses from ill-defined corralling movements when attempting to grasp an object to more mature and visually guided reaching and grasping behavior. This differentiation of movements of the arms, hands, and fingers, followed by integration of the use of the eyes with the movements of the hand to perform rudimentary eye-hand coordination tasks, is crucial to normal development.

There is little doubt that differentiation and integration operate simultaneously. The complex abilities of the adult cannot be explained merely in terms of a process of integration of simpler responses. What occurs, instead, is a constant interlacing of both differentiation and integration. The term *reciprocal interweaving* is sometimes used to describe this ever-expanding tapestry of movement behavior.

## Readiness

Thorndike, the "grandfather" of learning theory, first proposed the principle of readiness primarily in reference to emotional responses to actions or expected actions. According to his concept, readiness was dependent on the biological maturation model, which was popular at the turn of the century. Today's concept of readiness, however, is much broader and refers to readiness for learning. *Readiness* may be defined as conditions within the individual and the environment that make a particular task an appropriate one for an individual to master. The concept of readiness, as used today, extends beyond biological maturation and includes consideration of environmental factors that can be modified or manipulated to encourage or promote learning. Therefore, there are several related factors that in combination promote readiness. Physical and mental maturation, interacting with motivation, prerequisite learnings, and an enriching environment all influence readiness.

In recent years a great deal of attention has been focused on the concept of developing reading readiness with regard to the appropriate types of experiences in which preschool and primary grade children should be involved. Entire educational programs have been built around the notion that children must achieve a certain level of development before they are ready to pursue intellectual tasks such as reading and writing. Readiness training is a part of many preschool and primary grade educational programs. An integral part of these readiness programs in recent years has been the use of movement as a means of enhancing basic perceptual-motor qualities such as directional and temporal awareness and body and spatial awareness. The remedial and readiness programs of Frostig (1969), Getman (1952), and Kephart (1971) have been used to get children ready for learning. Each of these programs uses movement as an integral part of readiness training. Although it has not been documented that the inclusion of these perceptual-motor experiences have a *direct* effect on the attainment of specific skills necessary for success in school, it is safe to assume that they have at least an indirect influence through enhancement of the child's self-concept and the development of a more positive, "I can" attitude. The concept of readiness as it is used today, whether for the learning of cognitive skills or motor skills, is probably best summed up in Bruner's (1965) statement that "the foundation of any subject may be taught to anybody at any age in some form" (p. 12). In other words the burden of being "ready" is as much the teacher's responsibility as the child's. Readiness is a combination of maturational "ripeness," environmental openness, and teacher sensitivity.

## Critical Learning Periods

The concept of critical or sensitive periods is closely aligned to readiness and revolves around the observation that there are certain periods when an individual is more sensitive to certain kinds of stimulation. Normal development in later periods may be hindered if the child fails to receive the proper stimulation during a critical period. For example, inadequate nutrition, prolonged stress, inconsistent mothering, or a lack of appropriate learning experiences may have a more negative impact on development if introduced early in life rather than at a later age. The concept of critical periods also has a positive side. It suggests that appropriate treatment during a critical period tends to facilitate more positive forms of development at later stages than if the same treatment is introduced later.

One should recognize that the trend of the child to follow a critical period pattern is closely linked to the theory of developmental tasks and to a lesser degree linked to the milestone and age-stage views. Havighurst's (1972) theoretical framework of development is actually a critical period hypothesis, applied from the perspective of education.

The notion of critical periods of development has been so pervasive in education that an entirely new federally funded educational program was instituted based on this premise. Operation Head Start, begun in the 1960s, viewed the age period of 3 to 5 as critical to children's intellectual development. It was hypothesized that if given a "head start" through a carefully structured environment designed to develop school-oriented skills, deprived children would be able to begin school on a more nearly equal basis with their nondeprived counterparts. The results of Head Start programs did not entirely bear out the critical period hypothesis. This was probably due to the existence of more than one critical period for intellectual development. In addition, the age period of 3 to 5 may not be as critical as originally assumed. Current views of the critical period hypothesis reject the notion that there are highly specific time frames in which one must develop motor skills (Seefeldt, 1975). There are, however, broad periods during which development of certain skills is most easily accomplished.

It is safe to assume that there are *sensitive periods* for development. The point to be made is that care should be taken that critical or sensitive periods not be too narrowly defined. Failure to account for individual differences and for special environmental circumstances will lead one to conclude that a sensitive period is a universal point in time that may be described in terms of weeks, months, or a few years. Instead, a notion of sensitive periods as broad, general guidelines susceptible to modification should be adopted and adhered to.

## Individual Differences

The tendency of children to exhibit individual differences is crucial. Each child is a unique individual with his or her own timetable for development. This timetable is a combination of a particular individual's heredity and environmental influences, and although the sequence of appearance of developmental characteristics is predictable, the rate of appearance may be quite variable.

The "average" ages for the acquisition of all sorts of developmental tasks, ranging from learning how to walk (the major developmental task of infancy), to gaining bowel and bladder control (the first restrictions of a civilized society on the child) have been bandied about in the professional literature and the daily conversation of parents and teachers for years. It must be remembered that these average ages are just that and nothing more. They are merely approximations and are meant to serve as convenient indicators of developmentally appropriate behaviors. It is common to see deviations from the mean of as much as six months to one year in the appearance of numerous motor abilities. The tendency to exhibit individual differences is closely linked to the concept of readiness and helps to explain why some children are ready to learn new skills when others are not.

### Phylogeny and Ontogeny

Many of the rudimentary abilities of the infant and the fundamental movement abilities of the young child are considered to be phylogenetic. That is, they tend to appear somewhat automatically and in a predictable sequence within the maturing child. Phylogenetic skills are resistant to external environmental influences. Such abilities as the rudimentary manipulative tasks of reaching, grasping, and releasing objects, the stability tasks of gaining control of the gross musculature of the body, and the fundamental locomotor abilities of walking, jumping, and running are examples of phylogenetic skills. Ontogenetic behaviors, on the other hand, are those that depend primarily on learning and environmental opportunities. Such skills as swimming, bicycling, and ice skating are ontogenetic because they do not appear automatically within individuals but require a period of practice and experience and are influenced by the child's culture. The entire concept of phylogeny and ontogeny needs to be reevaluated in light of the fact that many skills heretofore considered phylogenetic can be influenced by environmental interaction (Bower et al., 1970; Bower, 1974).

Although there may be a biological tendency for the development of certain abilities due to phylogenetic processes, it is ludicrous to assume that maturation alone will account for motor development. The extent or level to which any voluntary movement ability is mastered depends, in part, on ontogeny or the environment. In other words, practice, instruction, and encouragement contribute significantly to motor skill development, particularly beyond the rudimentary movement phase. There seems to be little solid support for the notion that ontogeny recapitulates phylogeny, although some phylogenetic behaviors are present in humankind.

## PARENTAL FACTORS

Over the past several years there has been considerable speculation and research on the effects of parenting behaviors during infancy and early childhood as they influence the subsequent functioning of the child. Because of the extreme dependence of the human infant on its caregivers and because of the length of this period of dependence, a variety of parental care factors have been shown to influence later development. Among the most crucial are the effects of environmental stimulation and deprivation, the temperament of the child, and the bonding that occurs between parent and child during the early days of life.

## Bonding

The study of parent-to-infant attachment, or bonding, has its roots in the imprinting studies conducted by Lorenz (1935), Hess (1959), and others on birds, ducks, and other animals. Basically, these experiments with animals revealed that the degree to which the newborn would imprint on its mother was directly related to their contact time. This sensitive period for imprinting in animals has been shown to be very short. Klopper et al. (1964), for example, has shown that separation of a mother goat from her kid right after birth for little more than an hour will result in the mother's refusal to accept or nurse it.

Although human infants do not imprint in the narrow sense of the word as animals do, there is compelling evidence that there is a "sensitive" period in which parent-to-infant attachment occurs. If this sensitive period is missed, the parent and child fail to bond. This may result in later developmental difficulties, particularly in the affective development of the child.

In their excellent review of bonding, Kennell et al. (1979) stated:

> Perhaps the parent's attachment to a child is the strongest bond in the human species. The power of this attachment is so great that it enables the mother and father to make the unusual sacrifices necessary for the care of the infant. Early in life the infant becomes attached to one individual, most often it is the mother. The original mother-infant bond is the wellspring for all the infant's subsequent attachments and is the relationship through which the child develops a sense of himself. (p. 786)

The effects of long-term maternal separation on the motor, cognitive, and emotional aspects of the infant's development have been documented by Spitz (1945), Bolby (1958), and S. Freud (1962) on children evacuated from London during World War II. The results of these investigations, according to Kennell et al. (1979) "have dramatically altered infant care throughout the world" (p. 786).

Bonding, in essence, is a strong emotional attachment that endures over time, distance, hardship, and desirability. Recent research has shown that this emotional bond begins developing at birth and can fail to develop or be incompletely established with early separation (Kennell et al., 1974; Leifer et al., 1972; Robson, 1967; Winters, 1973). The leading factors contributing to initial separation are prematurity and low birthweight, which result in the incubation of the newborn; mild or severe neonatal problems at birth; and standard hospital operating procedures. Fortunately, the trend is now in favor of promoting early parental contact. Fathers are often permitted in the labor and delivery rooms and allowed to take a greater role in the child-rearing process. Rooming-in is on the increase in many maternity hospitals. Breastfeeding has gained renewed acceptance, and home births are on the rise. Giving birth at home—not always a recommended procedure—is dramatically different from the usual hospital routine. In the home birth, the mother is clearly in command. Instead of being a passive patient, she is an active participant in the birthing process, along with her husband and the midwife.

Early attachment between parent and child appears to be crucial to all aspects of the child's development. The reciprocal interaction between parent and child creates a mutually satisfying and rewarding bond, whose importance cannot be overemphasized.

## Stimulation and Deprivation

A great deal of study has been done over the years in an effort to determine the relative merits of stimulation and deprivation in the learning of a variety of skills. In fact, there has been considerable controversy among hereditarians and environmentalists over the issue during the past 100 years. Numerous textbooks have recorded the nature versus nurture debates, but little has been settled in the attempt to categorize the effects of each on development. The current trend has been to respect the individual importance of each and to recognize the fact that the influences of both maturation and experience are complexly intertwined.

Students of motor development have recognized the futility of debating the separate merits of maturation and experience and have instead concentrated their research and study on three major questions. The first of these questions deals with the approximate ages at which various skills can be learned most effectively. The research of Bayley (1935), Shirley (1931), and Wellman (1937) in the 1930s represents the first serious attempts to describe the age at which many of the rudimentary and fundamental movement abilities appear. Each of these researchers reported a somewhat different timetable for the appearance of numerous phylogenetic skills. They did, however, show amazing consistency in the order of appearance of these abilities. This factor illustrates the combined effect of both intrinsic, or maturationally determined, influences on behavior and extrinsic, or environmentally influenced, behaviors. Unfortunately, until recently, little has been done to more clearly ascertain the ages at which both phylogenetic and ontogenetic skills can be learned most effectively. The principle of readiness has been viewed as a cornerstone of our educational system, but little more than lip service has been paid to its importance, particularly with regard to developing movement abilities. We know that children can develop many movement abilities early in life, but we still do not know the best time to introduce specific skills. Only recently has this important question come under serious study. The excellent work being done at many colleges and universities represents a first step in answering many of the important questions concerning the age at which fundamental movement patterns can be effectively developed and refined in young children.

The second question being studied deals with the effects of special training on the learning of motor skills. A number of co-twin control studies have been conducted in an effort to ascertain the influence of special practice on early learning. The use of identical twins enables the researcher to ensure identical hereditary backgrounds and characteristics of the subjects. One twin is given advanced opportunities for practice, while the other is restricted from practicing the same skills over a prescribed length of time. The famous studies of Gesell and Thompson (1929), Hilgard (1932), and McGraw (1935) have all demonstrated the inability of early training to hasten development to an appreciable degree. However, it is important to note that follow-up studies of the co-twin control experiments of both Gesell and McGraw showed that the trained subjects exhibited greater confidence and assurance in the activities in which they had received special training. In other words, special attention and training may not have an influence on the quantity or rate of onset of the movement skills learned, but it may have an effect on the *quality* of performance of specific skills. Again, we see the complex interrelationship between maturation and experience.

Investigations by Gerber and Dean (1957) recorded the advanced development in Ugandan infants during the first days and months of life. The investigators concluded that the infants' motor superiority over infants raised in the United States was due, *in part*, to the enriched environmental stimulation that they received. They were carried on their mothers' back much of the time, were fed on demand, and were constantly the center of attention and affection. However, their advanced state at birth (that is, ability to hold head erect, early disappearance of certain reflexes, and so forth) suggests that a genetic factor may also have been the cause of their developmental superiority. Again, we see the relatedness of maturation and experience.

The third question being studied is the effect of limited or restricted opportunities for practice on the acquisition of motor skills. Studies of this nature have generally centered on experimentally induced environmental deprivation in animals. Only a few studies have been reported in which children have actually been observed in environments where unusual restrictions of movement or experience have existed.

An investigation conducted by Dennis (1960) examined infants reared at three separate institutions in Iran. The infants in two of the institutions were found to be severely retarded in their motor development. In the third there was little motor retardation. The discrepancy between institutions led Dennis to investigate the life styles of the children in each institution. The results of his investigation led to the conclusion that lack of handling, blandness of surroundings, and general lack of movement opportunity or experience were causes of motor retardation in the two institutions. Another investigation, by Dennis and Najarian (1957), revealed similar findings in a smaller number of crèche infants reared in Beirut, Lebanon. Both of these investigations lend support to the hypothesis that behavioral development cannot be fully accounted for by the maturation hypothesis.

Due to cultural mores, the humanistic virtues of most investigators, and concerned parents, there are few experiments in which the environmental circumstances of the infant or young child have been intentionally altered in an attempt to determine whether serious malfunctioning or atypical behavior will result from these practices. The general consensus of the research that exists is that severe restrictions and lack of experience can delay normal development. We need only to look as far as the school playground and observe the girls jumping rope expertly and the boys throwing and catching balls with great skill. When asked to reverse the activities, however, each tends to revert to more primitive patterns of movement. Factors within our culture, unfortunately, often predetermine the types of movement experiences in which boys and girls engage.

Dennis (1935) conducted an investigation in which fraternal twin infant girls were reared in a very sterile nursery environment (that is, they were intentionally given a minimal amount of motor and social stimulation). After fourteen months in this environment, their movement behavior was compared with normative data and was found to be retarded beyond the normal limits. Social development, however, was well within the limits of the standard norms, a factor that may suggest a greater need for motor than for social stimulation of the infant. This investigation, however, represents the only attempt at intentionally limiting the child's environment in order to study the possible consequences on development. Care should be taken in drawing any sweeping conclusions from a single investigation without collaborative support.

The child-rearing practices of the Hopi Indians were the subject of still another investigation by Dennis (1940). These Indians have traditionally restricted their infants' movement by binding them to a cradle board that the mother carries on her back. The infants spend nearly all of their time bound in the cradle board for their first three months of life. As they grow older, the number and length of freedom periods is gradually increased. Dennis observed that the movement abilities of these children were *not* retarded as might be expected from the results of the investigations just mentioned. It may be beneficial to consider that perhaps motor activity is not of crucial importance during the first months of life. Being bound securely to the cradle board and the rhythmical movements of the mother carrying the child may have simulated life in the womb. The close physical contact with the mother and an opportunity to begin utilizing perceptual modalities may have been crucial factors in these first months. One may also consider what the infant observed through his or her developing visual sense while bound to the cradle board. While on the board, the infant was generally on the mother's back in a position that permitted viewing of the many new and interesting sights that were going on all around. When not being carried about, the child was generally propped up by a nearby tree or in a corner and able to observe the mother going about her daily chores. In other words, the visual and motor stimulation of the Hopi Indian infants was of considerably higher quality than the sterile environments of the Iranian and Lebanese infants and the two girls investigated by Dennis. This study may point up the close identification of the visual modality with the motor dimension of behavior. It leads one to consider the interrelatedness of perceptual and motor functions and the importance of enriching stimulation.

It becomes impossible to make a case for either maturation or learning as the sole or even primary influence on development. The literature is overwhelmingly in favor of the interaction of one with the other. This compromise view of development is summed up by Carmichael, who, as early as 1925, recognized that "Heredity and environment are not antithetical, nor can they expediently be separated; for in all maturation there is learning: in all learning there is hereditary maturation" (p. 260).

Both maturation and learning play important roles in the acquisition of movement abilities. Although experience seems to have little influence on the sequence of their emergence, it does affect the time of appearance of certain movements and the extent of their development.

One of the greatest needs of children is for the opportunity to practice skills at a time when they are developmentally ready to benefit the most from such skills. Special practice prior to being ready maturationally is of dubious benefit. The key is to be able to accurately judge the time at which each individual is "ripe" for learning and then to provide a series of educationally sound and effective movement experiences. However, all indications are that young children are generally capable of more than we have suspected, and many of the traditional readiness signposts that we use in teaching may actually be incorrect. It is our job as educators to determine just what children are capable of and to provide ample opportunities for them to engage in a multitude of movement experiences.

## Temperament

Anyone who has been around young children for an extended period is quick to notice the differences in temperament (i.e., disposition) that exist. These individual differences in the responsiveness of children are probably caused by their unique environmental and experiential histories. It is interesting to note, however, that differences in temperament are observable even at birth. Persistent differences in newborns have been documented on a variety of physiological and perceptual-motor dimensions in newborns (Eisenberg, 1966). Differences in cardiac reactions and response intensity have also been observed, along with many other individual differences in reactions to environmental conditions (Lipton et al., 1961; Westman, 1973).

The temperaments of children have been classified in a number of ways. The method utilized by Chess and Thomas (1973) is a popular one. They classify children as (1) the easy child, (2) the difficult child, and (3) the slow-to-warm-up child. Chess and Thomas have observed children longitudinally, using a parental report system of data collection. Infants divided into "cuddler" and "noncuddler" classifications exhibited a variety of differences when viewed over time. Non-cuddlers were found to sit, stand, and crawl sooner than cuddlers. They were also found to sleep less and to protest more than those identified as cuddlers.

Although the research on the development of temperament is speculative, it seems safe to assume that because the temperament of the child from birth tends to remain consistent, that temperament will have an effect on how parents respond to the child (Osofsky and Conners, 1979). The hyperactive child, the chronic crier, or the fussy child may be inadvertently adversely influencing the nurturing responses of his or her caregivers. The ill-tempered child may receive less attention than the even-tempered child and, as a consequence, be slower to talk and slower to develop mature movement and socialization skills. The epidemic proportions of child battering in our culture may be attributable, in part, to the interaction between the ill-tempered child and the parent who in stressful situations is unable to cope with such a child. Infantile autism, a profound disorder, may even be related to the early interaction between some children's natural aloofness and parents who quickly become equally distant or "cold" to the child. Temperament is indeed an important factor influencing the developing child.

## Associated Factors

A number of other interesting environmental factors have been shown to have an impact on the development of children. The vast majority of research, however, has centered on the influence of these factors on cognitive and affective behavior, with relatively little emphasis on motor development. The parental factors influenced by social class, sex differences, birth order, and ethnic and cultural background have all been shown to have an impact on the motor development of infants and children. The reader is referred to the excellent reviews of these factors presented by Robert Malina (1980) in *A Textbook of Motor Development* and by John Leuko and Susan Greendorfer (1978) in *Psychology of Motor Behavior and Sport.*

Motor development is not a static process. It is not only the product of biological factors but is also influenced by a host of cultural or environmental factors. The social-cultural milieu of the child plays an important role in the direction and extent of motor development of the child. The interaction of environmental factors, biological trends, and the conditions of growth discussed in the following chapter modifies the course of motor development during infancy and childhood.

## Summary

The motor development of children represents *one* aspect of the total developmental process. It is intricately interrelated with both the cognitive and affective domains of human behavior and is influenced by a variety of factors. The importance of optimal motor development in children must not be minimized or thought of as being second in importance to the other developmental areas. The unity of humankind clearly demonstrates the integrated development of the mind and the body and the many subtle interrelationships of each. Trends in motor development emerge from the study of children as they grow. These trends illustrate the gradual progression from relatively simple levels of functioning to more complex levels. Each of these trends is affected by the influences of the child's experiences.

Biological and experiential factors influence the development of rudimentary, fundamental, and sport-related movement abilities. Developing the many movement abilities characteristic of the preschool and elementary school years contributes markedly to the physical development of children. The physical fitness and motor fitness of today's children are of great concern to many because of the frequent lack of opportunity and/or motivation to be physically active. The movement education program in the home, nursery school, or elementary school must provide many opportunities for large muscle activities and must strive to increase the child's level of motivation for vigorous activity. It must also, however, recognize that each child is unique in his or her development and will progress at a rate determined by both environmental and biological circumstances.

## CHAPTER HIGHLIGHTS

1. The infant weighing under 2500 g at birth (5½ lb) is *not* automatically classified as premature.
2. The term prematurity has given way to the terms low birthweight, and young for date, which more accurately describe the condition of the newborn.
3. A wide variety of maternal factors have been associated with prematurity.
4. Advanced hospital techniques and sophisticated intensive care procedures have done much to reduce the abnormally high mortality and morbidity rates for premature infants.
5. Development of muscular control proceeds from the center of the body to the periphery and from the head toward the feet.
6. The rate of growth of children follows a universal pattern.
7. The infant can recover from limited amounts of interruption in the normal growth process by a phenomenon called catch-up growth.
8. Restricted opportunity for practice and other forms of deprivation adversely influence the child's ability to perform motor tasks that are characteristic of the child's particular age.
9. Children gradually gain mastery over the intricate operation of their bodies through the process of differentiation and integration.
10. Readiness for learning involves the combination of biological and environmental processes into a congruent whole.
11. The environment may be manipulated or altered in order to promote readiness for learning.

12. Taking advantage of an individual's readiness requires maturational ripeness, environmental openness, and teacher sensitivity.
13. Some movement abilities are phylogenetic while others are ontogenetic.
14. There are broadly defined sensitive periods during which the child can learn a new task most efficiently.
15. The parent-child bond is probably the strongest of all bonds in nature.
16. Proper bonding may have a dramatic affect on parent-child interaction later in life.
17. Severe deprivation of experiences will have a debilitating effect on the individual. The degree to which this can be overcome depends on many factors.
18. Social class, sex, birth order, and ethnic group, all play a role in the child's motor development.

## CRITICAL READINGS

Kopp, C.B., and A.H. Parmelee: "Prenatal and Perinatal Influence on Infant Behavior," in J.D. Osofsky (ed.), *The Handbook of Infant Development,* New York: Wiley, 1979, Chapter 2.

Leuko, J.H., and S.L. Grundorfer: "Family Influences and Sex Differences In Children's Socialization into Sport. A Review," in D.M. Landers and R.W. Christina (eds.), *Psychology of Motor Behavior and Sport 1977,* Champaign, Ill.: Human Kinetics, 1978, pp. 434–447.

Malina, R.M.: "Environmentally Related Correlates of Motor Development In Performance During Infancy and Childhood," in C. Corbin (ed.), *A Textbook of Motor Development,* Dubuque, Iowa: W.C. Brown, 1980, Chapter 24.

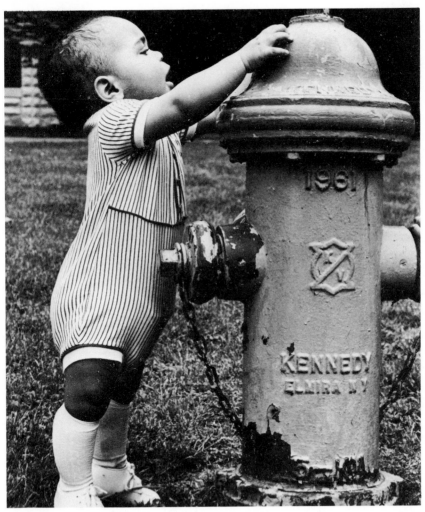

CHAPTER **6**

# Prenatal and Infant Growth

A wide variety of factors may affect the physical growth and motor development of children. Many prenatal, infant, and childhood influences were discussed in the previous two chapters. These chapters focused on factors that may have a negative affect on the process of development. This chapter will focus on the process of normal growth from conception through the period of infancy.

It is important for the student of motor development to have a reference point from which to view the normal growth process. The approach taken here provides that reference point from the standpoint of the mythically "average" child. In other words, heights, weights, and other growth statistics are presented in terms of averages. There may be considerable normal variation from these figures. This variation may be thought of as the result of the interaction between biological and environemntal processes on the child.

## PRENATAL GROWTH

Growth begins at the moment of conception and follows an orderly sequence throughout the prenatal period. Hooker's (1952) study of the motor responses of the fetus demonstrated that prenatal growth patterns are just as predictable during the fetal period as they are throughout infancy. The uniting of a mature sperm and ovum marks the beginning of the growth process. The ovum is one of the largest cells in the female body. It is about 0.004 in. in diameter and is just barely visible to the naked eye. The sperm, on the other hand is microscopic and one of the smallest cells in the male body. Fertilization occurs if one of the approximately 20 million sperm released from the male during intercourse meets and penetrates the ovum in the Fallopian tube. Once the sperm cell penetrates the outer membrane of the egg, fertilization occurs. The two cell nuclei lie side by sie for a few hours before they merge to form a *zygote* (the fertilized egg). It is at this instant that much of one's life is determined. The genetic inheritances of both mother and father are transferred to this single cell. The pattern for a variety of traits is now established, including eye and hair color, general body shape and complexion. During the germinal period, the zygote splits into two cells through mitosis. The two cells from four cells, and the four cells form eight. After three days the ovum has grown into thirty-two cells, and after four days it consists of about 90 cells. Because all cells have the same genetic setup *except* sex cells, the division of cells is not simultaneous, and stages in early embryonic life have been observed where there is an odd number of cells (Sundberg and Wirsen, 1977). After the first three or four days of mitotic cell division, the zygote travels down the Fallopian tube to the uterus, where it attaches itself to the uterine wall. This implantation process marks the true onset of pregnancy, although the days of pregnancy are counted from the first day of the last menstrual bleeding. The ovum is normally fertilized within a day of ovulation, near the fourteenth day of the cycle. Therefore, during the first two weeks of what is considered pregnancy, the woman is actually not pregnant. Implantation generally occurs by the end of the first week after fertilization.

### First Two Weeks

During the first few weeks (period of the zygote) the fertilized egg remains practically unchanged in size. It lives off its own yoke and receives little outside nourishment. By the end of the second week the zygote is only a small round disk about 0.01 in. wide. The situation for the zygote is especially precarious during this time. Although the mother-to-be may not be aware of being pregnant, her system will automatically attempt to slough off this foreign body, as it would any foreign body. Also, the expectant mother may continue to ingest a variety of chemical substances, drugs, alcohol, and tobacco that may prove damaging, if not lethal, to the zygote.

## First Two Months

By the end of the first month there is a definite formation of three layers of cells. The *ectoderm,* from which the sense organs and nervous system develop, begins to form. The *mesoderm* accounts for the formation of the muscular, skeletal, and circulatory systems. The *endoderm* eventually accounts for the formation of the digestive and glandular systems. Special cells form the *placenta,* through which nutritive substances will be carried and wastes removed. Another special layer of cells begins formation of the *amnion,* which will enclose the embryo except at the umbilical cord throughout the prenatal period.

By the end of the first month the embryo is about ¼ in. long and weighs about 1 oz. It is crescent shaped, with small bumps on its sides (limb buds). It has a tail and tiny ridges along the neck. These gill-like ridges mark the beginning of a primitive mouth opening, heart, face, and throat. By the end of the first month the embryo has a rudimentary circulatory system, and the heart begins to beat. Growth accelerates toward the end of the first month. The organism grows about ¼ in. each week. By the end of the second month the embryo is about 1½ in. long. The beginnings of the face, neck, fingers, and toes develop, and the embryo starts to take on a more human appearance. The limb buds lengthen, the muscles enlarge, and the sex organs begin to form. Brain development is rapid and is represented by a very large head in comparison to the rest of the body. The embryo is now firmly implanted in the uterine wall and receiving nourishment through the placenta and the umbilical cord. This marks the end of the embryonic period and the beginning of the fetal period of prenatal life.

## Third Through Sixth Month

The fetal period begins around the third month and continues until delivery. This is a critical time for the fetus, which is easily influenced by a variety of factors over which it has no control. During the third month the fetus continues to grow rapidly. It is about 3 in. long by the end of the third month. Sexual differentiation continues, buds for the teeth emerge, the stomach and kidneys begin to function, and the vocal cords appear. By the beginning of the fourth month the first reflex actions begin to be felt. The fetus opens and closes its mouth, swallows, clenches its fist, and can even reflexively suck its thumb. The growth rate during the fourth month is the most rapid for the fetus. During this period it doubles in length to about 6 or 8 in. and weighs about 4 oz. The hands are fully shaped, and the transparent cartilaginous skeleton begins to turn into bony tissue, starting in the middle of each skeletal bone and progressing toward the ends. The lower limbs, which had been lagging behind in their development, now catch up with the rest of the body. By the beginning of the fifth month the fetus has reached half of its birth length.

At the beginning of the fifth month the fetus is about 8 to 10 in. long and weighs about ½ lb. Skin, hair, and nails appear. The internal organs continue to grow and assume their proper anatomical positions. The entire body of the fetus is temporarily covered with a very fine soft hair called *lanugo*. The lanugo on the head and eyebrows becomes more marked by the end of the fifth month and is replaced by pigmented hair. The lanugo is generally shed before birth, although some may still remain. The larger size and cramped quarters of the rapidly developing fetus generally result in considerable reflexive movement during the fifth month.

By the sixth month the fetus is about 13 in. long and weighs over a pound. During this month the eyelids, which have been fused shut since the third month, reopen and are completed. The *vernix caseosa* forms from skin cells, and a fatty secretion protects the thin and delicate skin of the fetus. There is little in the way of subcutaneous fat at this point, and the fetus appears red and wrinkled and resembles a very old and frail individual. An infant born prematurely during the sixth month has a very poor chance of survival even with the most sophisticated technology available. Although it can cry weakly and move about, it cannot perform the more basic functions of spontaneous breathing and temperature regulation. By the end of the sixth month, the fetus weighs approximately 2 lb and is about 14 in. long. It is structurally complete but needs additional time for functional maturity of the various systems of the body.

## Seventh Through Ninth Month

From the seventh month to term the fetus triples its weight. A layer of adipose tissue begins to form under the skin and serves as both an insulator and food supplier. The lanugo hair is shed, along with much of the vernix fluid, and the nails often grow beyond the ends of the fingers and toes, necessitating an immediate manicure after birth to prevent scratching. During the seventh month the fetus is often quiet for long periods of time as if resting up for the "big event." The fetal brain becomes more active and takes increasing control over the body systems. Over 70 percent of fetuses born at the end of the seventh month survive, although most require special handling during the early months after birth (Rogers, 1977).

During the eighth and ninth months the fetus becomes more active. The cramped quarters result in frequent changes in position, kicking, and thrusting of the legs and arms. During these last two months the red coloration disappears as fatty deposits become more evenly distributed. The birth process is initiated by the placenta and contraction of the uterine musculature and not the fetus. At birth the normal term infant is about 18 to 20 in. long and weighs between 6 and 8 lb. Refer to Table 6.1 for a summary of development during the fetal period.

## INFANT GROWTH

The growth process during the first two years of life is truly amazing. The infant progresses from a tiny, helpless, horizontal, sedentary creature to a considerably larger, autonomous, vertical, active child. The physical growth of the infant has a very definite influence on its motor development. The size of the head, for example, will influence the child's developing balance abilities. Hand size will influence the mode of contact with different-size objects, and strength development will influence the onset of locomotion.

**Table 6.1   Highlights of the Prenatal Growth Period**

| Age | Length | Weight | Major Events |
|-----|--------|--------|--------------|
| Conception | 1 cell | Less than 1 g | Genetic inheritance determined |
| 1 week | 0.01 in. | less than 1 g | Germinal period, period of rapid cell differentiation |
| 2 weeks | 0.05 in. | 1.5 g | Implantation in the uterus |
| 1 month | 0.25 in. | 1 oz | Endoderm, mesoderm, and ectoderm formed |
| 2 months | 1.5 in. | 2 oz | Rapid growth period, begins to take on human form |
| 3 months | 3 in. | 3 oz | Sexual differentiation, stomach and kidney function, eyelids fuse shut |
| 4 months | 6 to 8 in. | 6 oz | Rapid growth period, first reflexive movements, bone formation begins |
| 5 months | 8 to 10 in. | 8 oz | Half birth height, internal organ completion, hair over entire body |
| 6 months | 15 in. | 1 to 2 lb | Eyes reopen, vernix caseosa forms, structurally complete but functionally immature |
| 7 months | 14 to 16 in. | 2 to 4 lb | Rapid weight gain, adipose tissue deposited |
| 8 months | 16 to 18 in. | 4 to 6 lb | Active period, fatty deposits distributed |
| 9 months | 18 to 20 in. | 6 to 8 lb | Uterine contractions, labor, and delivery |

## Neonatal Period (Birth to 4 Weeks)

The neonatal period is generally considered to comprise the first month of life. The typical full-term newborn is 18 to 20 in. long, but the head accounts for fully one fourth of that length. The large size when compared to the adult head size (one seventh of total length) makes it difficult to gain and maintain equilibrium. The remaining body length is taken up with a 4-to-3 ratio of trunk to lower-limb length. The eyes are about half their adult size, and the body is about one twentieth its eventual adult dimension (Figure 6.1)

There is considerable normal variation in the weight of newborns, which may be accounted for by a variety of environmental and hereditary factors. Birthweight is closely related to the socioeconomic and nutritional status of the mother (Eichorn, 1968; Meredith, 1952). The birthweight of male infants is about 4 percent higher than females. Optimal growth requires proper nutrition, a positive state of health, and a nurturing environment. It is interesting to note, however, that low-birthweight babies and young-for-date babies have a definite tendency to catch up to their age-mates if their retarded condition of development is not too severe. J.M. Tanner (1978), a physician who has devoted much time to the study of the growth characteristics of the infant, notes that an individual's ultimate growth seems to be determined early in life and may be amended under limited conditions if prematurity, illness, or malnutrition deflects the child from his or her normal growth curve. Growth will accelerate (or catch up) to the normal trajectory on resumption of an adequate diet or termination of the illness, and then slow down again when it reaches its goal (Figure 6.2). Therefore, under most conditions we see infants and children fitting into broadly determined ranges for height and weight, with little in the way of extremes at either end of the developmental continuum. It should be noted, however, that although the trajectory approximates the normal curve, low-birthweight children usually remain somewhat smaller than full-term children throughout life.

Figures 6.3 through 6.6 provide graphic representations of the changes in

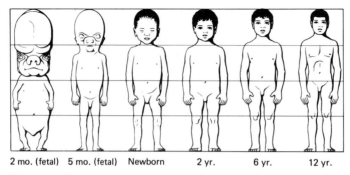

2 mo. (fetal)   5 mo. (fetal)   Newborn      2 yr.         6 yr.        12 yr.

**Figure 6.1.** *Changes in body form and proportion before and after birth.*

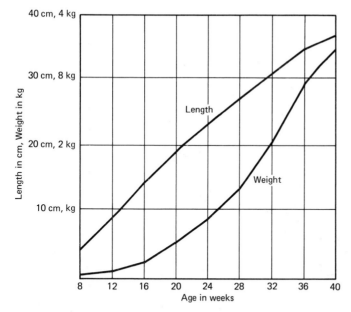

12. Sex distinguishable. Eyelids sealed shut. Buds for deciduous teeth. Vocal cords. Digestive tract. Kidneys, and liver secrete.

16. Head about one third of total length. Nose plugged. Lips visible. Fine hair on body. Pads on hands and feet. Skin dark red, loose, wrinkled.

20. Body axis straightens. Vernix caseosa covers skin as skin glands develop. Internal organs move toward mature positions.

24—28  Eyes open. Taste buds present. If born, can breathe, cry, and live for a few hours.

28—40  Fat deposited. Rapid brain growth. Nails develop. Permanent tooth. Testes descend. Becomes viable.

**Figure 6.2.** Summary of development during the fetal period. *(Source:* M. S. Smart and R. C. Smart: *Infants: Development and Relationships,* New York: Macmillan, 1973, p. 10. Used with permission.)

height and weight of both boys and girls from birth to age 3. These growth charts from the National Center for Health Statistics indicate by age percentiles the growth patterns of infants and young children.

## Early Infancy (4 Weeks to 1 Year)

During the first year of life there are rapid gains in both weight and length. During the first six months growth is mainly a process of "filling out," with only a slight change in body proportions. In fact, the "newborns" often pictured in advertise-

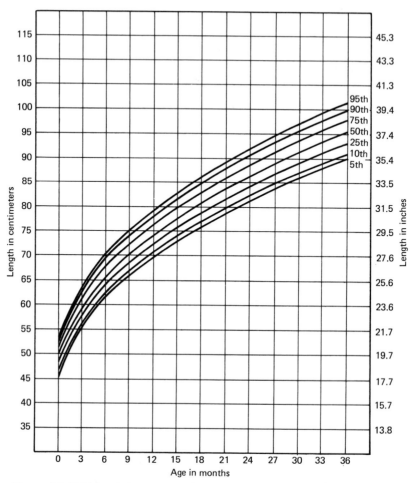

**Figure 6.3.** Girls' length by age percentiles: birth to 36 months. *(Source:* National Center for Health Statistics. U.S. Department of Health, Education and Welfare, HRA, 25, 3, June 22, 1976.)

ments are actually 2 or 3 months old, displaying the chubby look, not the reddish, wrinkled look of the actual newborn. Birthweight is doubled by the fifth month and almost tripled by the end of the first year. Length is not doubled until around the fourteenth month but increases to around 30 in. by the first birthday. After 6 months of age the thoracic region is larger than the head in normal children and increases with age. Infants suffering from malnutrition will have a weight deficit but will have a head size larger than the thorax (Dean, 1965).

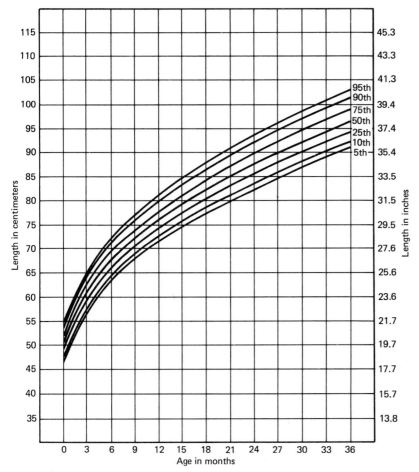

**Figure 6.4.** Boys' length by age percentiles: birth to 36 months. *(Source:* National Center for Health Statistics. U.S. Department of Health, Education and Welfare, HRA, 25, 3, June 22, 1976.)

## Later Infancy (1 Year to 2 Years)

Physical growth during the second year of life continues at a rapid pace but at a slower rate than the first year. By age 2 the height of the average boy is about 35 in. Girls are about 34 in. tall and weigh about 31 lb, whereas boys average 32 lb (National Center for Health Statistics, 1976). Height and weight have about a .60 correlation, showing a moderate degree of relationship between these two indices of physique. Because growth follows a directional trend (i.e., proximodistal and

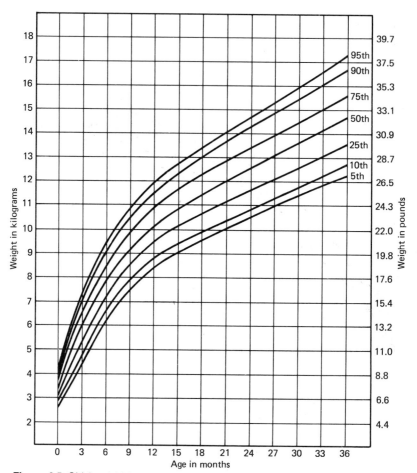

**Figure 6.5.** Girls' weight by age percentiles: birth to 36 months. *(Source:* National Center for Health Statistics. U.S. Department of Health, Education and Welfare, HRA, 25, 3, June 22, 1976.)

cephalocaudal), increase in size of the body parts is uneven. Upper arm growth proceeds lower arm growth and hand growth. Therefore, from infancy to puberty the greatest amount of growth takes place in the distal portions of the limbs. Head growth slows from infancy onward, trunk growth proceeds at a moderate rate, limb growth is faster, and growth of the hands and feet is most rapid.

### Summary

Throughout the prenatal period a variety of environmental factors may influence and dramatically alter later development. The relationship between the unborn child

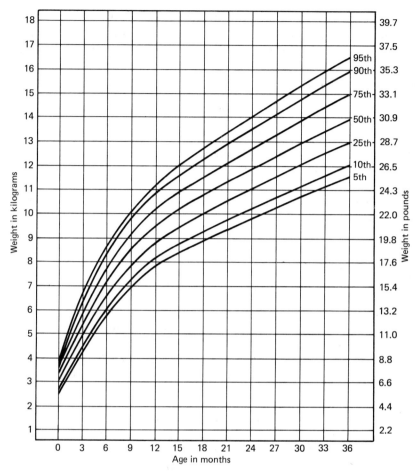

**Figure 6.6.** Boys' weight by age percentiles: birth to 36 months. *(Source:* National Center for Health Statistics. U.S. Department of Health, Education and Welfare, HRA, 25, 3, June 22, 1976.)

and the mother is essentially one of parasite and host. The fetus uses the mother to supply all of its vital needs, including the intake of oxygen and nutrients and the expulsion of carbon dioxide and other wastes. These nutrients are "screened" by the mother in that they are found in her bloodstream. As a result the condition and content of the circulatory systems of both mother and fetus are crucial to future growth and development.

The normal process of prenatal and infant growth is crucial to the motor development of the child at the preschool and elementary school level. The height, weight, physique, and maturational level of the child plays an important role in his or her acquisition and performance of fundamental and sport-related movement abilities. The prenatal period and infancy set the stage for what is to come in the development of the child's repertoire of movement and physical abilities.

## CHAPTER HIGHLIGHTS

1. Prenatal growth patterns are predictable and can be charted from the moment of conception.
2. The union of an ovum and a sperm marks the point of conception and the determination of one's genetic inheritance.
3. Implantation of the zygote in the uterine wall marks the true beginning of pregnancy.
4. The period of the zygote from conception to the fourth week is especially precarious because the expectant mother is often unaware that she is pregnant.
5. The period of the embryo marks the formation of the endoderm, mesoderm, and ectoderm, the three layers of cells that will eventually form the various systems of the body.
6. Growth proceeds at a more rapid pace by the end of the first month in utero.
7. The fetal period begins during the third month and is marked by the very first reflexive movements.
8. Growth is rapid during most of the fetal period, and there is considerable movement felt by the mother-to-be.
9. The fetus triples its weight from the seventh to the ninth month.
10. The seventh month is generally quiet, with increasing activity during the eighth and ninth months.
11. The head of the newborn makes up about one-fourth of its entire length. Other body parts are in less dramatic proportional deviation.
12. Birthweight is related to a variety of factors, including the nutritional status of the mother.
13. Early infancy is characterized by rapid growth in length and an increase in subcutaneous tissue.
14. Growth during later infancy is less rapid than during the first year.
15. Increases in body proportions are uneven and based on the principles of proximodistal and cephalocaudal development.

## CRITICAL READINGS

Caplan, F. (ed.): *The First Twelve Months of Life,* New York: Grosset & Dunlap, 1973.

Sundberg, I.A. and C. Wirser. *A Child Is Born: The Drama of Life Before Birth,* New York: Delacorte, 1977.

Tanner, J.M.: *Fetus into Man,* Cambridge, Mass.: Harvard University Press, 1978.

# CHAPTER 7

# Childhood Growth

The period of childhood marks a steady increase in height, weight, and muscle mass. Growth is not as rapid during this period as during infancy, and it shows a gradual deceleration throughout childhood until the adolescent growth spurt. Childhood is divided here into the early childhood period of 2 to 6 years of age and the later childhood period of 6 through 12 years of age. Figures 7.1 through 7.4 present height and weight growth charts for males and females from age 2 to age 18.

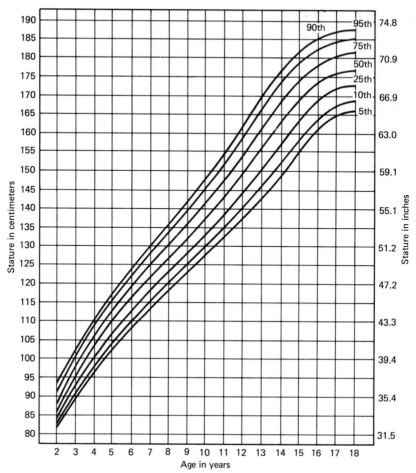

**Figure 7.1.** Boys' stature by age percentiles: ages 2 to 18 years. *(Source:* National Center for Health Statistics. U.S. Department of Health, Education and Welfare, HRA, 25, 3, June 22, 1976.)

## EARLY CHILDHOOD (2 to 6 YEARS)

During the early childhood years, growth in terms of height and weight is not as rapid as during infancy. The growth rate decelerates slowly. By 4 years of age, the child has doubled his or her birth length, which represents only about one half the gain experienced during the first two years of life. The total amount of weight gain from 2 through 5 years of age is less than the amount gained during the first year of life. The growth process slows down after the first two years but maintains a constant rate until puberty. The annual height gain from the early childhood period

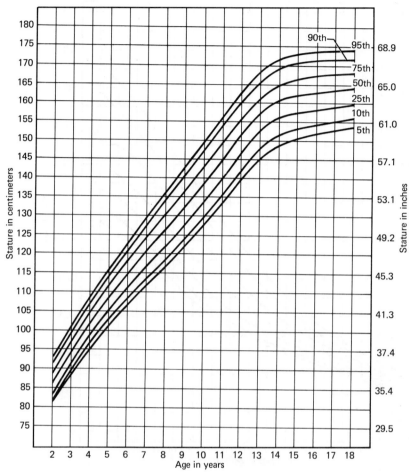

**Figure 7.2.** Girls' stature by age percentiles: ages 2 to 18 years. *(Source:* National Center for Health Statistics. U.S. Department of Health, Education and Welfare, HRA, 25, 3, June 26, 1976.)

to puberty is about 2 in. per year. Weight gains average 5 lb. per year. This, therefore, represents an ideal time for the child to develop and refine a wide variety of movement tasks ranging from the fundamental movements of early childhood to the sport skills of middle childhood.

Sex differences may be seen between boys and girls in terms of height and weight, but they are minimal. The physiques of male and female preschoolers are remarkably similar when viewed from a posterior position, with boys being slightly taller and heavier. Boys have more muscle and bone mass than girls, and both show a gradual decrease in fatty tissue as they progress through the early childhood period

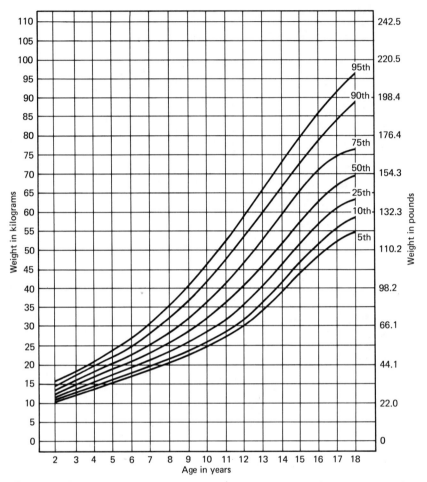

**Figure 7.3.** Boys' weight by age percentiles: ages 2 to 18 years. *(Source:* National Center for Health Statistics. U.S. Department of Health, Education and Welfare, HRA, 25, 3, June 22, 1976.)

(Smart and Smart, 1973a). The proportion of muscle tissue remains fairly constant throughout early childhood at about 25 percent of total body weight (Espenschade and Eckert, 1980).

Body proportions change markedly during early childhood because of the various growth rates of the body. The chest gradually becomes larger than the abdomen, and the stomach gradually protrudes less. By the time preschoolers reach the first grade, their body proportions more closely resemble those of older children in the elementary school.

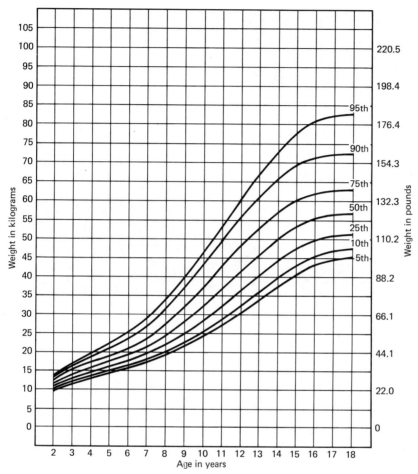

**Figure 7.4.** Girls' weight by age percentiles: ages 2 to 18 years. *(Source:* National Center for Health Statistics. U.S. Department of Health, Education and Welfare, HRA, 25, 3, June 22, 1976.)

Bone growth during early childhood is dynamic, and the skeletal system is particularly vulnerable to malnutrition, fatigue, and illness (Brain and Moslay, 1968). The bones ossify at a rapid rate during early childhood and have been shown to be retarded by as much as three years in growth in deprived children (Scrimshaw, 1967).

Smart and Smart (1973a) report that the brain is about 75 per cent of its adult weight by age 3, and almost 90 percent by age 6. The midbrain is almost fully developed at birth, but it is not until age 4 that the cerebral cortex is completely developed.

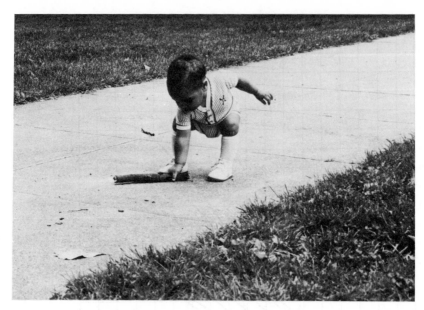

Growth is rapid during the first two years of life but decelerates during the early childhood period.

The development of myelin around the neurons (myelination) permits the transmission of nerve impulses and is not complete at birth. At birth many nerves lack myelin, but with advancing age greater amounts of myelin are laid down along nerve fibers. Myelination is largely complete by the end of the early childhood period, thus allowing for the complete transference of nerve impulses throughout the nervous system. It is interesting to note that increased complexity in the child's movement patterns are possible following myelination of the cerebellum. Also, Espenschade and Eckert (1980) state that "myelination of the corpus callosum, which joins the two hemispheres of the brain, is a precursor to the development of optimal alternate arm-leg action in such things as the throw and the kick" (p. 129). Therefore, as the cortex matures and becomes progressively organized, the child is able to perform at higher levels both motorically and cognitively.

The sensory apparatus is still developing during the preschool years. The eyeball does not reach its full size until about 12 years of age. The macula of the retina is not completely developed until the sixth year, and the young child is generally farsighted. Preschool children have more taste buds than adults. They are generously distributed throughout the insides of the throat and cheeks as well as on the tongue, causing greater sensitivity to taste. Because of the shorter eustachian tube connecting the middle ear with the throat, the child is also more sensitive to infections of the ear.

## LATER CHILDHOOD (6 to 12 YEARS)

The period of childhood from the sixth through the eleventh years of life is typified by a slow but steady increase in height and weight and progress toward greater organization of the sensory and motor systems. Changes in body build are slight during these years. Childhood is more a time of lengthening out and filling out prior to the prepubertal growth spurt that occurs around the eleventh year for girls and the thirteenth year for boys. Although these years are characterized by slow, steady growth, the child makes rapid gains in learning and functions at increasingly mature levels in the performance of games and sports. This period of slow growth in height and weight gives the child time to get used to his or her body and is an important factor in the typically dramatic improvement seen in coordination and motor control during the childhood years. The gradual change in size and the close relationship maintained between bone and tissue development may be an important factor in increased levels of functioning.

Differences between the growth patterns of boys and girls are minimal during the middle years. Both have greater limb growth than trunk growth, but boys tend to have longer legs, arms, and standing height during childhood. Likewise, girls tend to have greater hip width and thigh size during this period. There is relatively little difference in physique or weight exhibited until the onset of the preadolescent period (Figures 7.5 and 7.6). Therefore, in most cases, girls and boys should be able to participate together in activities.

During early adolescence, girls tend to be taller than boys because of girls' earlier entrance into puberty. It is not until around age 14 that boys catch up to and begin to surpass girls in height. Between ages 12 and 14, girls also tend to weigh more than boys, but boys catch up and surpass girls after that. Because of the frequent lag of six months or so in corresponding weight gain to increases in height, there is a filling-out period during adolescence. Gains in height cease long before the normal gain in weight that is associated with adolescence. Muscle mass is increasing steadily to about one quarter of the body weight by the end of childhood, readying the adolescent for intense practice and participation in sport.

During childhood there is very slow growth in brain size. The size of the skull remains nearly the same although there is a broadening and a lengthening of the head toward the end of childhood.

Perceptual abilities during childhood are becoming increasingly refined. The sensorimotor apparatus is working in ever greater harmony so that by the end of this period the child can perform numerous sophisticated skills. Striking of a pitched ball, for example, improves with age and practice due to the improved visual acuity, tracking abilities, reaction and movement time, and sensorimotor integration. A key to maximum development of more mature growth patterns in the child is utilization. In other words, if the child has, through the normal process of maturation, improved perceptual abilities, they must be experimented with and integrated more com-

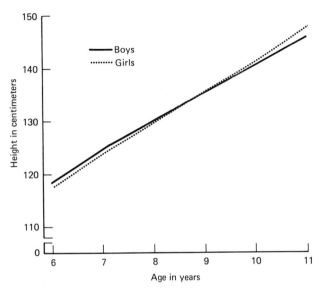

**Figure 7.5.** Mean height of U.S. children by age and sex. *(Source:* U.S. Department of Health, Education and Welfare, DHEW Publication No.—HSM—73-1605, January 1973.)

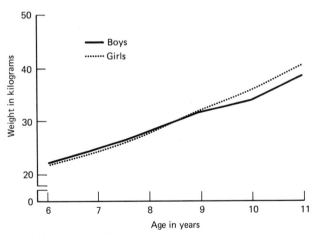

**Figure 7.6.** Mean weight of U.S. children by age and sex. *(Source:* U.S. Department of Health, Education and Welfare, DHEW Publication No.—HSM—73-1605, January 1973.)

pletely with the motor structures through practice. Failure to have the opportunity for practice, instruction, and encouragement during this period will prevent many individuals from acquiring the perceptual and motor information needed to perform skillful movement activities.

## FACTORS AFFECTING CHILD GROWTH

Growth is not an independent process. Although heredity sets the limits of growth, environmental factors play an important role in the extent to which these limits are reached. The degree to which these factors affect motor development is not clear and needs further study. Nutrition, as well as exercise and physical activity, has been shown to be a major factor affecting growth.

### Nutrition

The potentially harmful effects of poor nutrition during the prenatal period were highlighted in Chapter 4. Barness (1975) noted that among the factors influencing physical development during the prenatal period, nutrition "probably represents the most important single factor" (p. 345). Numerous investigations have also provided clear evidence that dietary deficiencies can have a very harmful effect on growth during infancy and childhood. The extent of growth retardation obviously depends on the severity, duration, and time of onset of undernourishment. For example, if severe chronic malnutrition occurs during the first four years of life, there is little hope of catching up to one's age-mates in terms of mental development, because the critical brain growth period has passed.

The physical growth process can be interrupted through malnutrition at any time between infancy and adolescence. Malnutrition may serve also as a mediating condition for certain diseases that affect physical growth. For example, lack of vitamin D in a diet can result in rickets, vitamin B-12 deficiencies may cause pellagra, and chronic lack of vitamin C results in scurvy. All are relatively rare in our modern society, but the effects of kwashiorkor, a debilitating disease, are seen in many parts of the world where there is a general lack of food and good nutrition. In the child with kwashiorkor, growth retardation can be expected as well as a large, puffed belly, sores on the body, and diarrhea.

Studies indicate that children suffering from chronic malnutrition, particularly during infancy and early childhood, never completely catch up to the growth norms for their age level (Behar, 1968; Eichenwald and Frye, 1969; Kallen, 1973). Evidence of this is shown in developing nations where adult height and weight norms are considerably lower than for industrialized nations. Nutritional status is linked to income level. The results of the National Nutrition Survey as reported by Eichorn (1968) indicate that in the United States "growth retardation was found in all ethnic groups and in all states, but the prevalence varied with sex, ethnic origin, and income level'' (p. 266).

Popular opinion has it that children of low-income families most generally have a poor diet simply because food of low nutritional value is purchased. This simply is not true. The results of the Preschool Nutrition Survey (Owen et al., 1974) indicated that the "feeding style" of low-income families is important. The quantity of food available to all members is less in low-income families, and there is a tendency toward greater permissiveness in the eating habits of children by low-income parents. The survey revealed that the quantity of food available increased with income level, and permissiveness about eating decreased.

Dietary excesses also represent nutritional factors affecting the growth of children. Among affluent countries, obesity is a major problem. Recent research (Oscai, 1974; Oscai et al., 1974; Eichorn, 1979) has proposed an interesting hypothesis linking obesity and its intractability to dietary habits during infancy and the preadolescent period. The causes of childhood obesity and its influences on motor development are discussed further in Chapter 13. There is considerable concern among professionals over the high consumption of refined starches and sugars by children. The constant barrage of television commercials loudly extolling one junk food or another, the "fast food" addiction of millions, and the use of edibles as a reinforcer for good behavior all may have an effect on the nutritional status of children. What is not known, however, is where the critical point between adequate and inadequate nutrition lies. The individual nature of the child, with his or her own unique biochemical composition, makes it difficult to pinpoint where adequate nutrition ends and malnutrition begins. It seems, however, to be a critical question that needs further exploration. The welfare of a vast number of children hinges, in part, on the answer to this question.

## Exercise and Injury

One of the principles of physical activity is the principle of use and disuse. Basically, this principle revolves around the notion that a muscle that is used will hypertrophy (i.e., increase in size) and a muscle that is not used will atrophy (i.e., decrease in size). Anyone who has had a limb placed in a cast for several weeks knows about atrophy. In children, activity definitely promotes muscle development. Although the number of muscle fibers does not increase, the size of the fibers does increase. Muscles respond and adapt to increased amounts of stress. Maturation alone will not account for increases in muscle mass. An environment that promotes vigorous physical activity on the part of the child will do much to promote muscle development. Active children have less body fat in proportion to lean body mass. They do not have more muscle fibers; they simply have more muscle mass per fiber.

Although it is doubtful that permanent changes can be made in an individual's physique, it is certain that modifications within limits can be made. A popular method of classification of physiques was developed by Sheldon et al. (1940). His much-used system classifies individuals on the basis of fat, muscle, and bone length. An *endomorphic physique* is one that is soft and rounded in physical features (pear shape). The *mesomorphic physique* is well muscled, with broad shoulders, narrow waist, and thick chest (V shape). The *ectomorphic physique* is characterized by a tall, thin, lean look (angular shape). Within each classification a person is rated on a scale of 1 to 7, with 1 representing the least amount of a characteristic, 4 being average, and 7, the most of a characteristic. Therefore, the three-number sequence of 1-7-1 would represent a person very low on endomorphy, very high on mesomorphy, and very low on ectomorphy. A 2-3-6 would typify a person low on endomorphy, with some mesomorphic characteristics, and high on ectomorphy (perhaps a high jumper, or middle distance runner). Sheldon et al. (1954) found that males could typically be classified at the middle of the scale (i.e., 3-4-4 or 4-4-3) and females rated higher in endomorphy and lower in mesomorphy (i.e., 5-3-3).

Although physical activity generally has positive effects on the growth of children, it may have some negative effects if carried to the extreme (D. Clarke, 1974). Seefeldt and Gould (1980) indicate that several studies have reported reduced growth rate in both height and weight of young athletes involved in moderate to intensive training programs, but that the controls in these investigations were weak at best. D. Clarke (1974) and Tipton and Tcheng (1970) did, however, report retarded growth in the height and weight of wrestlers. This was probably due to the unusually strenuous nature of training for this sport. Considerably more research needs to be conducted on the beneficial limits of strenuous physical activity. The critical point separating harmful and beneficial activity is not clear. The rapid rise of youth sport and the intensity of training that often accompanies it leave many unanswered questions. It seems reasonable to assume, however, that strenuous activity carried out over an extended period of time may result in injury to muscle and bone tissue of the child. "Swimmer's shoulder," "tennis elbow," and "runner's knees" are but a few of the ailments plaguing children who have exceeded their developmental limits (Gilliam, 1981). Care must be taken to supervise the exercise and activity programs of children. The potential benefits to the growth process are great, but the limits of the individual must be carefully considered.

Little evidence exists on the direct effects of exercise on bone growth. Bone growth is a hormonal process and is little affected by activity levels. Exercise does, however, increase bone width and promote mineralization, which make for stronger, less brittle bones. Larson (1973) indicates that stress within the limits of the particular individual is beneficial to the bones. Chronic inactivity, on the other hand, has harmful effects on bone growth and may result in growth retardation (Krogman, 1972).

In summary, activity stimulates bone and muscle development and helps retard the depositing of fat. The vast majority of physical activity and athletic programs engaged in by children, other than the most strenuous forms of training such as marathon running, wrestling, and other heavy strength and endurance activities, have beneficial effects on growth. Injury, whether acute or chronic, may have negative effects depending on its severity and location.

## Illness and Climate

A number of other factors have been associated with influencing the growth process. Such environmental factors as illness and disease, climate, emotions, and handicapping conditions have all been shown to influence the growth of the child (Krogman, 1972; Malina, 1980).

The standard childhood illnesses (chicken pox, colds, measles, and mumps) do not have a marked effect on the growth of the child. The extent to which illnesses and diseases may retard growth is dependent on the duration, severity, and timing. Krogman (1972) has reported that ''there is some reason to use age three years as a cut-off point: before the age of three years the registry of health damage may be more marked and rebound may be slower'' (p. 144). Often, the interaction of malnutrition and illnesses in the child makes it difficult to accurately determine the specific cause of growth retardation. The combination of conditions, however, puts the child at risk and greatly enhances the probability of measurable growth deficits.

A great deal of literature has reported the differences in height, weight, and onset of adolescence between individuals of varying climates (Krogman, 1972). The interacting effects of nutrition and health as well as possible genetic differences (e.g., when comparing black Africans with white Americans) make it impossible to demonstrate a direct causal relationship between climate and physical growth. The available data suggest that American children born and raised in the tropics have more linear physiques, but grow and mature at a slower rate than American children raised in a more temperate climate (Mills, 1942). Malina (1980) reported that Eskimos show prolonged growth and are delayed in obtaining adult height. They also tend to have a more stocky physique and to mature earlier than individuals raised in the tropics.

## Secular Trends

A secular trend is the tendency for children to be both taller and heavier, age for age, and to mature at an earlier age than children several generations ago. The trend for secular increases is not universal. Increases in growth, maturation and physical performance levels have been demonstrated in most developed countries. Developing nations throughout the world, however, have not demonstrated secular increases and in some cases have even shown decreases in stature (Gangirly, 1977). There may be many reasons for this, but it is largely a reflection of the little improvement in life style and nutritional habits from one generation to another.

Malina (1978) reported that secular changes in length and weight are slight at birth but become progressively more pronounced until puberty, when there is again a lessening of differences. The largest differences in height and weight are found from age 11 to 15 (the pubertal years) and are apparent across all socioeconomic classes and races in developed countries.

Children today mature more rapidly than they did 100 years ago. The age at menarche, for example, has decreased in European populations from an estimated range of 15.5 to 17.4 years to between 12.5 and 14 years (Eveleth and Tanner, 1976). Although secular trends in the maturation of boys are no doubt present, maturity data for them are lacking. It may be noted, however, that the average age at which the voice begins to change for members of boys' choirs today is considerably lower (about 13 years) than that estimated for boys performing in choirs over a 100 years ago (about 18 years) (Daw, 1974).

Malina (1978) reported that the secular trend in size and maturation in the United States and many other developed nations has stopped. There has been little indication of secular trends in height, weight, and maturation in the past twenty years. This is probably due largely to the elimination of growth-inhibiting factors and a peaking of improved nutritional and health conditions.

**Summary**

Growth during childhood decelerates from the rapid pace characteristic of the first two years. This slow but steady increase in height and weight during childhood provides the child with an opportunity to coordinate perceptual and motor information. The child has time to lengthen out, fill out, and gain control over his or her world. Numerous factors, however, can interrupt the normal growth process. Nutritional deficiencies and excesses can severely affect the growth process and have a lasting negative impact on the child, depending on the severity and duration of poor nutrition. Severe and prolonged illness has also been shown to interrupt the growth process.

Physical exercise has a positive influence on the growth process. Little evidence exists to support the claim that physical activity can be harmful to children, except in cases of extreme training requirements. Climatic factors have also been shown to accelerate or decelerate growth in children. North American children today are taller and heavier than their counterparts of 100 years ago. Definite secular trends can be seen in many but not all cultures. Differences in life style and dietary circumstances play an important role in the presence or absence of secular trends.

## CHAPTER HIGHLIGHTS

1.  Growth rates decelerate slowly during the early childhood period, with average annual gains in height and weight of 2 in. and 5 lb, respectively.
2.  Birth length is doubled by age 4.
3.  Minimal sex differences are seen in children during the early childhood years, but boys tend to be taller, heavier, and have slightly more muscle mass.

4.  Body proportions change markedly during early childhood, and myelination is completed.
5.  The pace of growth is slow but steady during late childhood. It is a time of lengthening out and filling out prior to puberty.
6.  Boys and girls are similar in their growth patterns. Limb growth is greater than trunk growth.
7.  Girls generally enter puberty earlier than boys and as a result are often taller and heavier than their male counterparts during early adolescence.
8.  Perceptual and motor abilities are refined during childhood.
9.  Dietary deficiencies and excesses can have a serious impact on the growth patterns of children.
10. Active children have less body fat in proportion to lean body mass.
11. Body types have been classified as endomorphic, mesomorphic, and ectomorphic.
12. Physical activity generally has positive effects on growth except in cases of extreme exertion.
13. The critical line between beneficial and harmful physical activity is not clear.
14. Exercise promotes bone mineralization and tends to increase bone width. Little evidence exists, however, to support the contention that it promotes growth in bone length.
15. Illnesses may negatively affect growth, depending on the time of onset, duration, and severity.
16. Research suggests that individuals born and raised in tropical climates have more linear physiques and grow and mature more slowly than North American children.
17. Research suggests that individuals born and raised in artic climates have more rounded physiques and grow at a slower rate over a more extended period of time than North American children.
18. North American children today become taller, heavier, and mature at an earlier age than children 100 years ago.
19. Secular trends are not universal and primarily reflect changes in life style and nutritional habits.

## CRITICAL READINGS

Fishbein, H.D.: *Evolution, Development, and Children's Learning,* Pacific Palisades, California: Goodyear, 1976, (Chapters 1 and 2).

Krogman, W.M.: *Child Growth,* Ann Arbor: University of Michigan Press, 1972.

Malina, R.: *Growth and Development: The First Twenty Years,* Minneapolis, Minn.: Burgess, 1975.

Morley, D., and M. Woodland: *See How They Grow—Monitoring Child Growth for Appropriate Health Care in Developing Countries,* New York: Oxford University Press, 1979, (Chapters 1, 8 and 9).

# 8

# General Growth and Development Characteristics of Childhood

Growth and development are such complex processes with so many interrelated aspects that it is virtually impossible to deal with the child as a whole through the written word. Perhaps it would be best to stop and reflect at this point on the typical or "average" preschool and elementary school child. In this chapter we will take a brief look at the general growth, motor development, cognitive, and affective characteristics of the average child during early childhood and later childhood in an effort to form a more complete picture of the whole child as he or she actually comes to us in the classroom or gymnasium. Although no two children are exactly alike and the individuality of the learner should always be maintained, certain general characteristics do emerge.

## EARLY CHILDHOOD (2 to 6 YEARS)

Play is what young children do when they are not eating, sleeping, or complying with the wishes of adults. Play occupies most of their waking hours, and it may literally be viewed as the child's equivalent of work as performed by adults. Children's play serves as the primary mode by which they learn about their bodies and its movement capabilities. It also serves as an important facilitator of cognitive and affective growth in the young child, as well as an important means of developing both fine and gross motor skills.

Preschool children are actively involved in enhancing their cognitive abilities in a variety of ways. These early years are a period of important cognitive development that have been termed the preoperational thought phase by Piaget. For it is during this time that children develop cognitive functions that will eventually result in logical thinking and concept formulation. Young children are not capable of thinking from any point of view other than their own. They are extremely egocentric and view almost everything in terms of themselves. For preschoolers, their perceptions dominate their thinking, and what is experienced at a given moment in time has great influence on them. During this preconceptual phase of cognitive development, seeing is, literally, believing. In the thinking and logic of preschool children, their conclusions need no justification. Even if they did, the children would be unable to reconstruct their thoughts and show others how they arrived at their conclusions. Play serves as a vital means by which higher cognitive structures are gradually developed. It provides a multitude of settings and variables for promoting cognitive growth.

Affective development is also dramatic during the preschool years. During this period children are involved in the two crucial social-emotional tasks of developing a sense of autonomy and a sense of initiative. Autonomy is expressed through a growing sense of independence, which may be seen in children's delight in the use of the word *no* to almost any direct question. The answer will be often be no to a question such as "Do you want to play outside?" even though they clearly would like to. This may be viewed as an expression of a new-found sense of independence and an ability to manipulate some factors in the environment rather than always as an expression of sheer disobedience. A way in which to avoid this natural autonomous reaction to a question is to alter it to form a positive statement such as "Let's go play outdoors." In this way, the child is not confronted with a direct yes-or-no choice. Care must be taken, however, to give children abundant situations in which an expression of their autonomy is reasonable and proper.

Young children's expanding sense of initiative is seen through their curious

. Children now engage in new experiences, such
throwing objects, for their own sake and for the
hat they are capable of doing. Failure to develop
sense of autonomy leads to feelings of shame,
. Establishment of stable self-concept is crucial to
preschoolers because it has an effect on both
ons.

y, preschoolers are developing a wide variety of
ative, and stability abilities. If they have a stable
in control over their musculature is a smooth one.
red movements of the 2-to-3-year-old gradually
r, and often reckless abandon of the 4-and-5-year-
tions make it possible for them to jump from "great
ns," leap over "raging rivers," and run "faster"
d beasts."
e are rapidly expanding their horizons. They are
eveloping their abilities, and testing their limits as
ly and others around them. In short, young children
i in many complex and wondrous ways. Care must be
taken, however, to understand their developmental characteristics and their limitations as well as their potentials. Only in this way can we effectively structure
movement experiences for them that truly reflect their needs and interests and are
within their level of ability.

The following developmental characteristics represent a synthesis of research
findings from a wide variety of sources and are presented here to provide a more
complete view of the total child during the preschool years.

## Growth and Motor Development Characteristics

1. Boys and girls range from about 33 to 47 in. in height and 25 to 53 lb.
2. Perceptual-motor abilities are rapidly developing, but confusion often
   exists in body, directional, temporal, and spatial awareness.
3. Good bladder and bowel control are generally established by the end of
   this period, but accidents sometimes still occur.
4. Children during this period are rapidly developing fundamental movement abilities in a variety of motor skills. Bilateral movements such as
   skipping, however, often present more difficulty than unilateral movements.
5. Children are active and energetic and would often rather run than walk,
   but they still need frequent short rest periods.
6. Motor abilities are developed to the point that the children are beginning
   to learn how to dress themselves, although they may need help
   straightening and fastening articles of clothing.

7. The body functions and processes become well regulated. A state of physiological homeostasis (stability) becomes well established.

8. The body builds of both boys and girls are remarkably similar. A back view of boys and girls reveals no readily observable structural differences.

9. Fine motor control is not established, although gross motor control is developing rapidly.

10. The eyes are not generally ready for extended periods of close work due to farsightedness, which is characteristic of both preschool and primary grade children. Also, binocular vision is often not completely established.

## Cognitive Development Characteristics

1. There is constantly increasing ability to express thoughts and ideas verbally.

2. A fantastic imagination enables imitation of both actions and symbols with little concern for accuracy or the proper sequencing of events.

3. There is continuous investigation and discovery of new symbols that have a primarily personal reference.

4. The "how" and "why" of the child's actions are learned through almost constant play.

5. There is a preoperational thought phase of development, resulting in a period of transition from self-satifying behavior to fundamental socialized behavior.

## Affective Development Characteristics

1. During this phase children are egocentric and assume that everyone thinks the way they do. As a result, they often seem to be quarrelsome and exhibit difficulty in sharing and getting along with others.

2. They are often fearful of new situations, shy, self-conscious, and unwilling to leave the security of that which is familiar.

3. They are learning to distinguish right from wrong and are beginning to develop a conscience.

4. Two- and 4-year-old children are often seen to be unusual and irregular in their behavior, while those who are 3 and 5 are often viewed as stable and conforming in their behavior.

5. Their self-concepts are rapidly developing. Wise guidance, success-oriented experiences, and positive reinforcement are especially important during these years.

## Implications for the Motor Development Program

1. Plenty of opportunity for gross motor play must be offered in both undirected and directed settings.

2. The movement experiences of the preschooler should involve primarily movement exploration and problem-solving activities in order to maximize the child's creativity and desire to explore.

3. The movement education program should include plenty of positive reinforcement in order to encourage the establishment of a positive self-concept and to reduce the fear of failure.

4. Stress should be placed on developing a variety of fundamental locomotor, manipulative, and stability abilitites, progressing from the simple to the complex as the children become "ready" for them.

5. Interests and abilities of boys and girls are similar, with no need for separate activities during this period.

6. Plenty of activities designed specifically to enhance perceptual-motor functioning are necessary.

7. Advantage should be taken of the child's great imagination through the use of a variety of activities, including drama and imagery.

8. Because of their often awkward and inefficient movements, be sure to gear movement experiences to their maturity level.

9. Provide a wide variety of activities that require object handling and eye-hand coordination.

10. Begin to incorporate bilateral activities such as skipping, and galloping and hopping, with alternate foot leading, after unilateral movements have been fairly well established.

11. Encourage the children to take an active part in the movement education program by "showing" and "telling" others what they can do in order to help overcome tendencies to be shy and self-conscious.

12. Activity should stress arm, shoulder, and upper body involvement.

13. Mechanically correct execution in a wide variety of fundamental movements is the primary goal, without emphasis on standards of performance.

14. Do not stress coordination in conjunction with speed and agility.

15. Poor habits of posture are beginning. Reinforce good posture with positive statements.

16. Provide convenient access to toilet facilities and encourage the children to accept this responsibility on their own.

17. Provide for individual differences and allow for children to progress at their own individual rate.

18. Establish standards for acceptable behavior and abide by them. Provide wise guidance in the establishment of a sense of doing what is right and proper instead of what is wrong and unacceptable.

**19.** The motor development program should be prescriptive and based on each individual's readiness level.

**20.** A multisensory approach should be utilized by the instructor, that is, one in which a wide variety of experiences are incorporated, using several sensory modalities.

## LATER CHILDHOOD (6 to 12 Years)

Children in the elementary grades are generally happy, stable, eager, and able to assume responsibilities. They are able to cope with new situations and are anxious to learn more about themselves and their expanding world. Primary grade children take the first big step into their expanding world when they enter first grade. For many, first grade represents the first separation from the home for a regularly scheduled, extended block of time. It is the first step out of the secure play environment of the home and into the world of adults. Entering a school represents the first time that many children are placed in a group situation in which they are not the center of attention. It is a time when sharing, concern for others, and respect for the rights and responsibilities of others are established. Kindergarten is a readiness time in which to begin making the gradual transition from an egocentric, home-centered play world to the group-oriented world of adult concepts and logic. In the first grade, the first formal demands for cognitive understanding are made. The major milestone of the first- and second-grader is learning how to read at a reasonable level. The 6-year-old is generally developmentally ready for the important task of "breaking the code" and learns to read. The child is also involved in developing the first real understanding of time and money and numerous other cognitive concepts. By the second grade, children should be well on their way to meeting and surmounting the ever-broadening array of cognitive, affective, and psychomotor tasks that are placed before them.

The following is a listing of the general developmental characteristics of the child from age 6 to age 12. It is presented here in order to provide a more complete view of the total child and represents a synthesis of current research.

### Growth and Motor Development Characteristics

**1.** Boys and girls range from about 44 to 60 in. in height and 44 to 90 lb.

**2.** Growth is slow especially from age 8 to the end of this period. There is a slow but steady pace of increments, unlike the more rapid gains in height and weight during the preschool years.

**3.** The body begins to lengthen out with an annual gain of only 2 to 3 in. and an annual weight gain of only 3 to 6 lb.

**4.** The cephalocaudal (head to toe) and proximodistal (center to periphery) principles of development are now quite evident, in which the large muscles of the body are considerably better developed than the small muscles.

5.  Girls are generally about a year ahead of boys in physiological development, and separate interests begin to develop toward the end of this period.

6.  Hand preference is firmly established with about 90 percent preferring the right hand and about 10 percent preferring the left.

7.  Reaction time is quite slow, causing difficulty with eye-hand and eye-foot coordination at the beginning of this period. By the end they are generally well established.

8.  Both boys and girls are full of energy but often possess a low endurance level and tire easily. Responsiveness to training, however, is great.

9.  The visual perceptual mechanisms are fully established. Such perceptual qualities are figure-ground perception, speed of vision, perceptual constancy, and spatial relationships are generally well established by the end of this period.

10.  Children are often farsighted during this period and are not ready for extended periods of close work.

11.  Fundamental movement abilities *should* be well defined by the beginning of this period. Locomotor abilities are developed to the extent that children are able to gallop, skip, jump, and climb in a mature pattern.

12.  Stability abilities are both static and dynamic. Balancing abilities are improved.

13.  Basic skills necessary for successful play become well developed.

14.  Activities involving the eyes and limbs develop slowly. Such activities as catching, kicking, striking, and throwing require considerable practice in order for mastery to occur.

15.  This period marks a transition from refining fundamental movement abilities to the establishment of transitional movement skills in lead-up games and athletic skills.

## Cognitive Development Characteristics

1.  Attention span is generally short at the beginning of this period but gradually lengthens. However, boys and girls of this age will often spend hours on activities that are of great interest to them.

2.  They are eager to learn and to please adults but need assistance and guidance in decision making.

3.  Children have good imaginations and display extremely creative minds; however, self-consciousness seems to become a factor again toward the end of this period.

4.  They are often interested in songs, television, movies, rhythmic games, and gymnastic activities.

5. They are not capable of abstract thinking and deal best with concrete examples and situations during the beginning of this period. More abstract cognitive abilities are evident by the end of this period.
6. Children are intellectually curious and anxious to know "why."

## Affective Development Characteristics

1. Interests of boys and girls are similar at the beginning of this period but soon begin to diverge.
2. The child is self-centered and plays poorly in large groups for extended periods of time during the primary years, although small group situations are handled well.
3. The child is often aggressive, boastful, self-critical, overreactive, and accepts defeat and winning poorly.
4. There is an inconsistent level of maturity; the child is often less mature at home than in school, due to parental influence.
5. The child is responsive to authority, "fair" punishment, discipline, and reinforcement.
6. Children are adventurous and eager to be involved with a friend or group of friends in "dangerous" or "secret" activities.
7. The child's self-concept is becoming firmly established.

## Implications for the Motor Development Program

1. There should be opportunities for children to refine fundemantal movement abilities in the areas of locomotion, manipulation, and stability to a point where they are fluid and efficient.
2. Children need to be helped in making the transition from the fundamental movement phase to the sport-related movement phase.
3. The assurance of being accepted and valued as a human being is important to children in order to know they have a stable and secure place in their school environment as well as in the home.
4. Abundant opportunities for encouragement and positive reinforcement from adults are necessary in order to promote continued development of a positive self-concept.
5. Opportunities and encouragement to explore and experiment through movement with their bodies and objects in their environment enhance perceptual-motor efficiency.
6. There should be exposure to experiences in which progressively greater amounts of responsibility are introduced to help promote self-reliance.
7. Adjustment to the rougher ways of the school playground and neighborhood without being rough or crude themselves is an important social skill to be learned.

8.  Opportunities for gradual introduction to group and team activities should be provided at the proper time.

9.  Storyplays, imaginary, and mimetic activities may be effectively incorporated into the program during the primary years because of the child's vivid imagination.

10. Activities that incorporate the use of music and rhythmics are enjoyable at this level and are valuable in enhancing fundamental movement abilities, creativity, and a basic understanding of the components of music and rhythm.

11. Children at this level learn best through active participation. Integration of academic concepts with movement activities provides an effective avenue for reinforcing academic concepts in science, mathematics, social studies, and the language arts.

12. Activities that involve climbing and hanging are beneficial to development of the upper torso and should be included in the program.

13. Discuss play situations involving such topics as taking turns, fair play, cheating, and sportsmanship as a means of establishing a more complete sense of right or wrong.

14. Interests in sports are beginning to develop toward the end of this period. Introduce basic athletic skills and simple lead-up games.

15. Begin to stress accuracy, form, and skill in the performance of movement skills.

16. Encourage children to "think" before engaging in an activity. Help them recognize potential hazards as a means of reducing their often reckless behavior.

17. Encourage small-group activities followed by larger-group activities and team sport experience.

18. Posture is important. Activities need to stress proper body alignment.

19. Use of rhythmic activities to refine coordination is desirable.

20. Specialized movement skills begin to be developed and refined toward the end of this period. Plenty of opportunity for practice, encouragement, and selective instruction is important.

21. Opportunities should be provided for participation in youth sport activities that are developmentally appropriate and geared to the needs and interests of children.

## Summary

Several developmental specialists have closely studied the phenomena of human behavior and have constructed a variety of theoretical models of the developmental process. Each of these theories reflects the originator's particular interest in certain aspects of development. As a result none paints a complete picture of the developmental process.

Study of the many models of growth and development, along with careful observation and daily contact with children, enables one to compile a set of developmental characteristics in the psychomotor, affective, and cognitive domains that typify the mythical "average" child. By no means should any of these characteristics be considered to be universal; one may easily call to mind a number of children who do not exhibit one or more of these characteristics at any given age. Careful study of the developmental characteristics typical of children at varying ages enables us to formulate programs that meet the needs, interests, and developmental capabilities of the greatest number of children. It does not guarantee that each child will exactly fit into a predescribed mold. This important fact is recognized by teachers who make room for individual differences through individualized instruction whenever possible.

## CHAPTER HIGHLIGHTS

1.  Human growth and development are complex interrelated processes.
2.  The early childhood period ranges from age 2 through age 5.
3.  The later childhood period ranges from age 6 through age 12.
4.  Numerous characteristics of children including cognitive, affective, growth and motor developmental can be readily observed.
5.  Typical characteristics of behavior provide important implications for planning and organizing educational programs.
6.  The successful teacher of children is aware of the developmental characteristics of children and pays close attention to these characteristics when planning a sound educational program.

## CRITICAL READINGS

Erikson, E.: *Childhood and Society,* New York: Norton, 1963.
Havighurst, R., and E. Levine: *Society and Education,* Reading, Mass.: Allyn and Bacon, 1979.
Zaichkowsky, L. B., et al.: *Growth and Development: The Child and Physical Activity,* St. Louis, Mo.: Mosby, 1980.

# PHASES AND STAGES
# OF MOTOR
# DEVELOPMENT

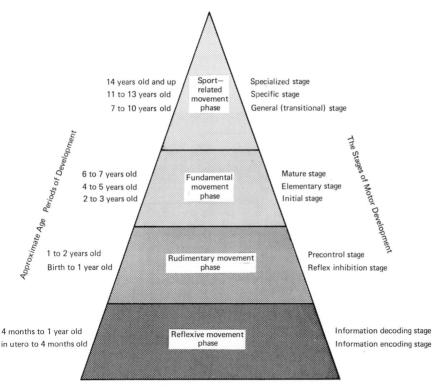

| | | |
|---|---|---|
| 14 years old and up | Sport—related movement phase | Specialized stage |
| 11 to 13 years old | | Specific stage |
| 7 to 10 years old | | General (transitional) stage |
| 6 to 7 years old | Fundamental movement phase | Mature stage |
| 4 to 5 years old | | Elementary stage |
| 2 to 3 years old | | Initial stage |
| 1 to 2 years old | Rudimentary movement phase | Precontrol stage |
| Birth to 1 year old | | Reflex inhibition stage |
| 4 months to 1 year old | Reflexive movement phase | Information decoding stage |
| in utero to 4 months old | | Information encoding stage |

Approximate Age Periods of Development

The Stages of Motor Development

The Phases of Motor Development

# Reflexive Movement

Reflex movements are evidenced in all fetuses, neonates, and infants to a greater or lesser degree, depending on their age and neurological makeup. Reflex movements are involuntary reactions of the body to various forms of external stimulation. They are subcortical in that they are controlled by the lower brain center, which is also responsible for numerous involuntary life-sustaining processes, such as breathing. Voluntary motor control in the normal child is a function of the mature cerebral cortex. Movements that are consciously controlled result from nerve impulses transmitted from the cerebral cortex along afferent (motor) neurons. In the developing fetus and newborn infant, the cortex, more specifically, the motor area of the cortex, is generally considered to be nonfunctional (Wyke, 1975). Thus movement is thought to be largely of a reflexive or involuntary nature.

Many early reflexes are related to infant survival (primitive reflexes), while others are precursors of voluntary movements that will appear between the ninth and fifteenth months after birth (postural reflexes). Reflexive walking, swimming, crawling, and climbing movements were reported by Shirley (1931), McGraw (1939b), and Ames (1937). These reflexes are inhibited prior to the appearance of their voluntary counterparts, but their mere presence is an indication of how deeply locomotor activities are rooted within the nervous system. The investigations by Hooker (1952) lend further support to the influence of genetics on motor behavior. He indicated that the voluntary movements of the postnatal period develop in the same sequence in which they are elicited as reflexes during fetal life.

From about the fourth month of fetal life until about the fourth month of infancy, movement is controlled largely, but not entirely, by involuntary reactions to changes in pressure, sight, sound, and tactile stimulation. These stimuli and resultant responses form the basis for the *information gathering stage* of the reflexive movement phase. Reflexes, at this point in the child's life, serve as his or her primary information gathering device for information storage in the developing cortex. As higher brain centers gain greater control of the sensorimotor apparatus, the memory trace that has been established through repeated performance of various postural reflex actions enables the infant to process information more efficiently (Hebb, 1949). This *information processing stage* parallels Piaget's first three stages within his sensorimotor phase of development, namely, the use of reflexes, primary circular reactions, and secondary circular reactions.

## REFLEXIVE BEHAVIOR AND VOLUNTARY MOVEMENT

As the primitive developmental reflexes are examined, two of their main functions are revealed to be nourishment seeking and protection. It is within these categories that primitive reflexes relate to the movement patterns of the lower primates. The palmar and plantar grasping reflexes, for example, have been related to arboreal primates, as have the various righting reflexes that have frequently been associated with the amphibious behavior of the lower life forms. The swimming reflex, which occurs during the second week after birth, provides what appears to be a fascinating link with the past. A coordinated swimming movement is elicited in the infant when held in or over water. One's creative mind may play with each of the reflexes and fit its occurrence into a lower order of life.

Several reflexes exist during early infancy that resemble later voluntary movements. These postural reflexes, as they are sometimes called, have been a topic of considerable debate over the past several years. It has been hypothesized and demonstrated that these reflex movements form the basis for later voluntary movement (McGraw, 1954; Thelen, 1980; Zelazo, 1976). As the cortex gradually matures, it assumes control over the postural reflexes of walking, climbing, swimming, and the like. In fact, Zelazo (1976) questions the dualistic position of the anatomists in favor of a hierarchical view, stating:

> Indeed, current behavioral and neurological research with infants challenges the validity and generality of the hypothesized independence between early reflexive and later instrumental behavior. An alternative hypothesis holds that the newborn's reflexes do not disappear but retain their identity within a hierarchy of controlled behavior. (p. 88)

Anatomists and neurologists, on the other hand, argue that there is a recognizable gap of up to several months between the inhibition of a postural reflex and the onset of voluntary movement (Kessen et al., 1970; Prechtl and Beintema, 1964; Titchner, 1909; Wyke, 1975). This time lag, they contend, clearly indicates that there is no direct link between postural reflexes and later voluntary movement. Cratty (1979) sums up the controversy by stating, "There seems to be no direct connection in time between these reflexive movements and the infant's later attempts to assume, voluntarily, an upright position to walk, to swim, and to climb" (p. 56).

From these statements, and the research of the anatomists, it appears that there is no basis for assuming that the infant's first reflexive movements prepare him or her for later voluntary movement in any *direct* way. We know, however, that the results of early reflexive activity of the infant are internalized and that this information is stored for future use when attempting similar voluntary movements when neurologically ready (Zelazo, 1976). This accounts for at least an *indirect* link between the infant's postural reflexes and later voluntary movement. Because of this, it becomes important for those interested in the study of movement to have a clearer understanding of the very first forms of movement behavior.

As the cortex develops, it inhibits some of the functions of the subcortical layers and assumes ever-increasing neuromuscular control. The cortex joins in its ability to store information that is received by way of efferent (sensory) neurons. This phenomenon is evidenced in the phasing-out of reflex behaviors and the assumption of voluntary movements by the infant. Concurrent formation of myelin or nerve fibers prepares the body for the mature neuromuscular state. Movements become more localized as functional neural pathways serve isolated regions of the body with greater precision and accuracy.

The transition from subcortical neuromuscular control of a postural reflex to voluntary control usually involves a period of inactivity or inhibition. This might manifest itself as a weak or totally absent reflex response during the interim period of change to a higher level of functioning. In many cases progressive development of the cortex will cause the substitution of one reflex for another. As an example, the body righting reflex appears as the neck righting reflex is inhibited.

## DIAGNOSING CENTRAL NERVOUS SYSTEM DISORDERS

It is common procedure for the pediatrician to attempt to elicit primitive and postural reflexes in the neonate and young infant. If a reflex is absent, irregular, or uneven in strength, neurological dysfunction is suspected. The failure of normal reflexive movements to develop or the prolonged continuation of various reflexes beyond their normal period may also cause the physician to suspect neurological impairment.

The use of developmental reflexes as a tool for diagnosing central nervous system damage has been widespread. Over the years, scientists have compiled an approximate timetable for the appearance and inhibition of neonatal and infant behaviors. Prechtl and Beintema (1964), for example, have noted that the resting posture of the newborn is the flexed position. The flexors, in fact, are dominant over the extensors in the early part of life. Shortly, however, cortical control permits the normal neonate to raise its head from the prone position. Prechtl notes that:

> an absence of the head-lifting response at the third day or later was highly correlated with other signs of neurological abnormalities. We may conclude therefore that normal babies are able to lift their chins when they are in the prone position. (p. 83)

Several other meaningful examples of this principle exist. The *doll-eye* movements of the neonate permit it to maintain constancy of the retinal image. When the head is tilted back, the eyes look down toward the chin, and when the head is tilted forward, the eyes look up toward the forehead. This response is almost always seen in premature infants and during the first day of life in the normal neonate, after which it is replaced by voluntary eye movements. Perseveration of this reflex could indicate delayed cortical maturation.

One means of diagnosing possible central nervous system disorders, therefore, is through perseverating reflexes. It must be noted that complete absence of a reflex is usually less significant than a reflex that remains too long. Other evidence of possible damage may be reflected in a reflex that is too strong or too weak. A reflex that elicits a stronger response on one side of the body than on the other may also indicate central nervous system dysfunction. An asymmetrical tonic neck reflex, for example, which shows full arm extension on one side of the body and only weak extensor tone when the other side is stimulated may also provide evidence of damage.

## PRIMITIVE REFLEXES

Primitive reflexes are closely associated with the obtainment of nourishment and the protection of the infant. They first appear during fetal life and persist well into the first year. The following is a partial list of the numerous primitive reflexes exhibited by the fetus and the neonate. Their approximate times of appearance and inhibition are found in Table 9.1

### Moro and Startle Reflexes

The Moro and startle reflexes may be elicited in the infant by placing it in a supine position and tapping it on the abdomen, or by producing a feeling of insecurity of support (for instance, allowing the head to drop sharply backward a short distance). It may even be self-induced by a loud noise or the infant's own cough or sneeze. In the Moro reflex, there is a sudden extension and bowing of the arms and spreading of the fingers. The legs and toes perform the same actions, but less vigorously. The limbs then return to a normal flexed position against the body. The startle reflex is similar in all ways to the Moro reflex except that it involves flexion of the limbs without prior extension (Figure 9.1).

The Moro reflex is normally present at birth and during the first three months of life. The Moro reflex has been one of the most widely used tools in the neurological examination of the young infant (Bench et al., 1972). The reaction is most pronounced during the infant's first few weeks. The intensity of the response gradually decreases until it is finally characterized by a simple jerking motion of the body in response to the stimulus (startle reflex). Persistence of the reflex beyond the sixth month may be an indication of neurological dysfunction. An asymmetrical Moro reflex may indicate Erb's palsy or an injury to a limb.

### Search and Sucking Reflexes

The search and sucking reflexes enable the newborn to obtain nourishment from its mother. Stimulation of the cheek (search reflex) will result in the infant's turning its head toward the source of stimulation. Stimulation of the area above or below the lips will cause a sucking motion (sucking reflex) in an attempt to ingest nourishment.

Both of these reflexes are present in all normal newborns. The search reflex may persist beyond the first year of life; the sucking movement generally disappears as a reflex by the end of the third month but persists as a voluntary response.

**Table 9.1  Developmental Sequence for Appearance and Inhibition of Selected Primitive Reflex Behaviors**

| Reflex | | | | | | | Month | | | | | | |
|---|---|---|---|---|---|---|---|---|---|---|---|---|---|
| | 0 | 1 | 2 | 3 | 4 | 5 | 6 | 7 | 8 | 9 | 10 | 11 | 12 |
| Moro | X | X | X | X | X | X | X | | | | | | |
| Startle | X | X | X | X | | | | X | X | X | X | X | X |
| Search | X | X | X | X | X | X | X | X | X | X | X | X | X |
| Sucking | X | X | X | X | | | | | | | | | |
| Palmar-mental | X | X | X | | | | | | | | | | |
| Palmar-mandibular | X | X | X | X | | | | | | | | | |
| Palmar grasp | X | X | X | X | | | | | | | | | |
| Babinski | X | X | X | X | | | | | | | | | |
| Plantar grasp | X | X | X | X | X | X | X | X | X | X | X | X | X |
| Tonic neck | X | X | X | X | X | X | X | | | | | | |

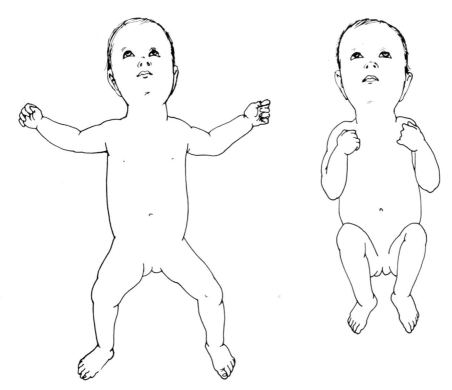

**Figure 9.1.** The Moro reflex.

## Hand-Mouth Reflexes

Two hand-mouth reflexes are found in the newborn and relate to the neonate's ancestry. The *palmar-mental reflex,* elicited by scratching the base of the palm, causes contraction of the chin muscles, which lift the chin up. This reflex has been observed in newborns but disappears early in life.

The *palmar-mandibular reflex,* or Babkin reflex, as it is sometimes called, is elicited by applying pressure to the palms of both hands. The responses usually include mouth opening, closing of eyes, and flexing the head forward. This reflex begins decreasing during the first month after birth and usually is not visible after the third month (von Bernuth and Prechtl, 1968).

## Palmar Grasping Reflex

During the first two months of life, the infant usually has its hands closed tightly. Upon stimulation of the palm, the hand will close strongly around the object without use of the thumb. The grip tightens when force is exerted against the encircling fingers. The grip is often so strong that the infant is able to support his or her own weight when suspended. (See Figure 9.2) Also, the grip with the left hand is generally stronger than the right. Grasping is also increased during sucking (von Bernuth and Prechtl, 1968).

The grasping reflex is normally present at birth and persists during the first four months of life. The intensity of the response tends to increase during the first month and slowly diminishes after that. Weak grasping or persistence of the reflex after the first year may be a sign of delay in motor development or of hemiplegia, if it occurs on only one side.

## Babinski and Plantar Grasp Reflexes

In the newborn the Babinski reflex is elicited by a stroke on the sole of the foot. The pressure causes an extension of the toes. As the neuromuscular system matures, the Babinski reflex gives way to the plantar reflex, which is a contraction of the toes upon stimulation of the sole of the foot (Figure 9.3).

The Babinski reflex is normally present at birth but gives way to the plantar grasp reflex around the fourth month which may persist until about the twelfth month. The plantar grasp reflex may be most easily elicited by pressing the thumbs against the ball of the infant's foot. Persistence of the Babinski reflex beyond the sixth month may be an indication of a developmental lag.

## Asymmetrical and Symmetrical Tonic Neck Reflexes

To elicit an asymmetrical tonic neck reflex, the infant is placed in a supine position, and the neck is turned so that the head is facing toward either side. The arms assume a position similar to the fencer's "on guard." That is, the arm extends on the side of the body that is facing the head and the other arm assumes an acute flexed position.

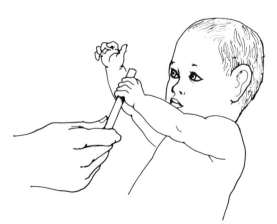

**Figure 9.2.** The palmar grasp reflex.

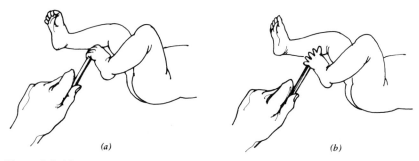

**Figure 9.3.** *(a)* The plantar grasp reflex. *(b)* Babinski reflex.

The lower limbs assume a position similar to the arms. The symmetrical tonic neck reflex may be elicited from a supported sitting position. Extension of the head and neck will produce extension of the arm and flexion of the legs. If the head and neck are flexed, the arms flex and the legs extend (Figure 9.4).

Both tonic neck reflexes may be observed in most premature infants, but they are not an obligatory response in newborns (that is, they do not occur each time the infant's head is turned). However, the 3- or 4-month-old infant assumes the asymmetrical position about 50 percent of the time and then this response gradually fades away (Mehlman, 1940). Persistence beyond the sixth month may be an indication of lack of control over lower brain centers by higher ones (Fiorentino, 1963).

Swartz and Allen (1975) indicate that vestiges of the asymmetical tonic neck reflex are apparent in some children and that this reflex can affect head position in the breaststroke of young swimmers. They further contend that reflexes do not totally disappear but are "integrated into the central nervous system largely through inhibition" (p. 311). If these reflexes are not properly inhibited, they may result in inadequate muscle tone, lack of independent movement of the head and extremities, midline problems, and difficulty in learning swimming strokes (Swartz and Allen, 1975).

## POSTURAL REFLEXES

Postural reflexes are those that resemble later voluntary movements. Postural reflexes automatically provide for maintenance of an upright position of the individual in relation to his or her environment (Twitchell, 1965). They are found in all normal infants during the early months of life and may, in a few cases, persist through the first year. The following sections discuss postural reflexes that are of particular interest to the student of motor development. These reflexes are associated with later voluntary movement behavior and should be carefully studied by all concerned with the development of voluntary patterns of movement. The approximate times of appearance and inhibition of these reflexes are found in Table 9.2.

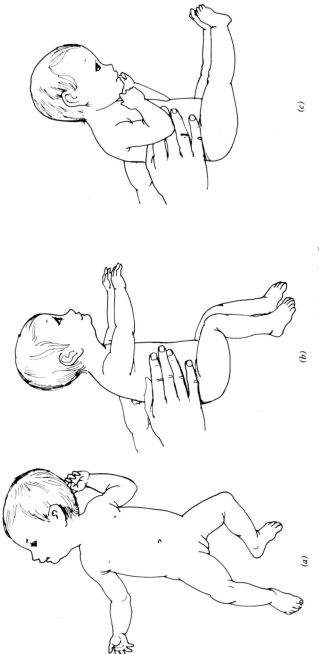

**Figure 9.4.** (a) The asymmetrical tonic neck reflex. (b) The symmetrical tonic neck reflex.

Table 9.2 Developmental Sequence for Appearance and Inhibition of Selected Postural Reflex Behaviors

| Reflex | Month | | | | | | | | | | | | |
|---|---|---|---|---|---|---|---|---|---|---|---|---|---|
| | 0 | 1 | 2 | 3 | 4 | 5 | 6 | 7 | 8 | 9 | 10 | 11 | 12 |
| Labyrinthine righting | | | X | X | X | X | X | X | X | X | X | X | X |
| Pull-up | | | | X | X | X | X | X | X | X | X | X | X |
| Parachute and propping | | | | | X | X | X | X | X | X | X | X | X |
| Neck and body righting | | | X | X | X | X | X | | | | | | |
| Crawling | X | X | X | X | X | | | | | | | | |
| Stepping | X | X | X | X | X | | | | | | | | |
| Swimming | X | X | X | X | | | | | | | | | |

## Labyrinthine Righting Reflex

The labyrinthine righting reflex may be elicited when the infant is held in an upright position and is tilted forward, backward, or to the side. The child will respond by attempting to maintain the upright position of the head by moving it in the direction opposite to the one in which its trunk is moved (Figure 9.5). Impulses arising in the otoliths of the labyrinth cause the head to be maintained in proper alignment to the environment even when other sensory channels (vision, touch) are excluded (Twitchell, 1965).

The labyrinthine righting reflex makes its first appearance around the second month and becomes stronger around the middle of the first year (Fiorentino 1963). It is a major factor in the infant's obtaining and maintaining an upright head and body posture, and contributes to the infant's forward movement around the end of the first year.

## Pull-Up Reflex

The pull-up reflex of the arms is an involuntary attempt on the part of the infant to maintain an upright positon. When the infant is in an upright sitting position and held by one or both hands, it will flex its arms in an attempt to remain upright when tipped backward. It will do the same thing when tipped forward. The reflexive pull-up reaction of the arms usually appears around the third or fourth month and often continues through the first year (Figure 9.6).

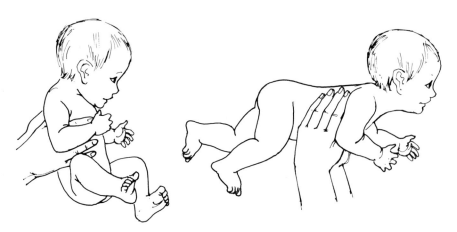

**Figure 9.5.** The labyrinthine righting reflex.

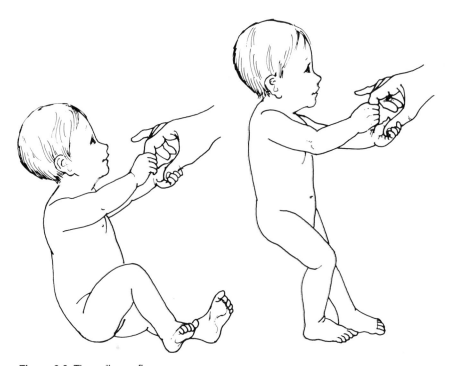

**Figure 9.6.** The pull-up reflex.

## Parachute and Propping Reflexes

Parachute and propping reactions are protective movements of the limbs in the direction of the displacing force. These reflexive movements occur in response to a sudden displacing force or when balance can no longer be maintained. Protective reflexes are dependent on visual stimulation and thus do not occur in the dark and may, in fact, be a form of a startle reflex.

The forward parachute reaction may be observed when the infant is held vertically in the air and then tilted toward the ground in an apparent attempt to cushion the anticipated fall. The downward parachute reactions may be observed when the baby is held in an upright position and rapidly lowered toward the ground. The lower limbs extend, tense, and abduct. Propping reflexes may be elicited by pushing the infant off balance from a sitting position either forward or backward (Figure 9.7).

The forward and downward parachute reactions begin to occur around the fourth month. The sideways propping reaction is first elicited around the sixth month. The backward reaction is first seen between the tenth and twelfth months.

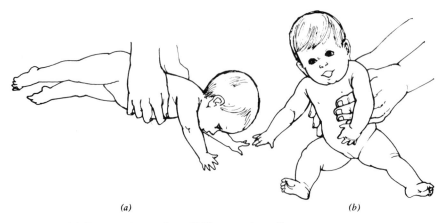

*(a)*                                                    *(b)*

**Figure 9.7.** *(a)* The parachute reflex. *(b)* The propping reflex.

Each of these reactions tends to persist beyond the first year and are necessary before the infant can learn to walk.

## Neck and Body Righting Reflexes

When the infant is placed in a prone position with the head turned to one side, the remainder of the body moves reflexively in the same direction. First the hips and legs turn into alignment, followed by the trunk. The reverse occurs from a side-lying position, with the legs and trunk turned in one direction, the head will turn reflexively in the same direction and right the body in a prone position (Twitchell, 1965) (Figure 9.8).

The neck and body righting reflexes disappear around the sixth month (Fiorentino, 1963). This reflex forms the basis for the voluntary rolling that occurs from the fifth month onward.

## Crawling Reflex

The crawling reflex can be seen when the infant is placed in a prone position and pressure is applied to the soles of one foot. It will reflexively crawl, using both its upper and lower limbs. Pressure on the soles of both feet will elicit a return in pressure by the infant. Pressure on the sole of one foot will produce returned pressure and an extensor thrust of the opposite leg (von Bernuth and Prechtl, 1968).

The crawling reflex is generally present at birth and disappears around the third or fourth month. There is a lag between reflexive crawling and voluntary crawling, which appears around the seventh month (Figure 9.9).

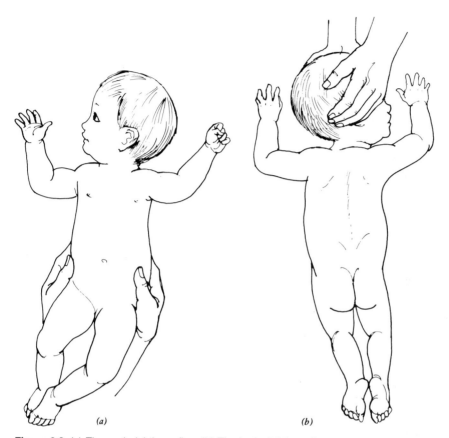

**Figure 9.8.** *(a)* The neck righting reflex. *(b)* The body righting reflex.

## Primary Stepping Reflex

When the infant is held erect, with its body weight placed forward on a flat surface, it will respond by "walking" forward. This walking movement involves the legs only. The primary stepping reflex is normally present during the first six weeks and disappears by the fifth month (Figure 9.10).

Zelazo (1972) studied the effects of early and persistent practice of the primary stepping reflex on the onset of voluntary walking behavior. The results of this investigation revealed that the age of independent walking was accelerated through conditioning of the stepping reflex in the experimental group; the control group did not show accelerated development. The implications of this important finding are enormous, but further research is necessary before it can be unequivocally stated

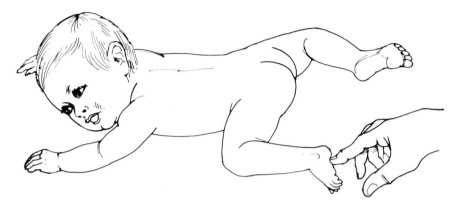

**Figure 9.9.** The crawling reflex.

that perpetuating a reflex through persistent exercise will accelerate the onset of voluntary behavior.

## Swimming Reflex

When placed in a prone position in or over water, the infant will exhibit rhythmical extensor and flexor swimming movements of the arms and legs. The movements are well organized and appear more advanced than any of the other locomotor reflexes. McGraw (1939b) filmed reflexive swimming movements in the human infant as early as the eleventh day of life. These involuntary movements generally disappear by the fifth month. McGraw discovered that a breath-holding reflex is elicited when the infant's face is placed in the water and that the swimming movements are more pronounced from this position. McGraw (1954) has since speculated on the theory that the infant's swimming reflex is a precursor to walking. She states: "Basically the neuromuscular mechanisms which mediate the reflexive swimming movements may be essentially the same as those activated in the reflexive crawling and stepping movements of the infant" (p. 360).

It is interesting to speculate on the relationship between the crawling, stepping, and swimming reflexes. Gordon (1981) makes this perceptive statement: "If the swimming reflex is a pattern from which later swimming or walking can build, its practice offers a legitimate reason for the existence of infant swim programs" (p. 48).

## Summary

Primitive reflexes, which are under the control of subcortical brain layers, are observed in the fetus from about the eighteenth week of gestation. Generally,

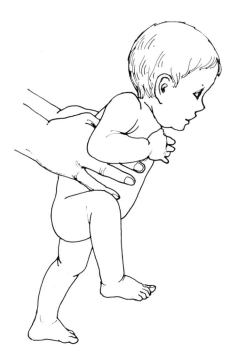

**Figure 9.10.** The primary stepping reflex.

reflexes serve the double function of helping the neonate to secure nourishment and protection. Many of the movements, however, are more closely related to functions in lower primates, indicating a possible phylogenetic link of the human with other forms of life.

As neurological development proceeds in the normal fetus, and later in the normal neonate, reflexes appear and disappear on a fairly standard, though informal, schedule. The presence of a primitive or postural reflex is evidence of subcortical control over some neuromuscular functions. This is indicated through voluntary control of a movement by the infant, reflecting operations at the cortical level. The function of the subcortex is not completely inhibited. Throughout life, it maintains control over such activities as coughing, sneezing, and yawning, as well as over the involuntary life processes. The cortex mediates more purposive behavior, whereas subcortical behavior is limited and stereotyped.

Although it is impossible to determine whether there is a direct relationship between reflexive behavior and later voluntary movement, it is safe to assume that there is at least an indirect link. This link is associated with the ability of the developing cortex to store information received from the sensory end-organs regarding the actual performance of the involuntary movement. The neonate, for example, is able to observe its involuntary stepping or grasping behavior and receives appropriate tactual and kinesthetic information. This information is stored in the association area of the cortex and may aid the infant in the performance of later voluntary stepping or grasping.

Examination of reflex movements in the infant has provided physicians with a primary means of diagnosing central nervous system damage. Neurological dysfunction may be suspected when any of the following four conditions appear (Egan et al., 1969).

1. Perseveration of a reflex beyond the age at which it should have been inhibited by cortical control.
2. Complete absence of a reflex (this is often a less accurate indicator than the others).
3. Unequal reflex responses bilaterally.
4. A response that is too strong or too weak.

## CHAPTER HIGHLIGHTS

1. Reflexive activity is the first form of movement engaged in by the fetus and the newborn.
2. Some reflexes are related to the performance of later voluntary movements.
3. Reflexive movements are subcortically controlled and are present in all fetuses and newborns.
4. The cerebral cortex of the newborn is not fully developed, and reflexive movements are predominant over the crude, ill-defined voluntary movements of the neonate.
5. Neonatal voluntary movements may develop in the same sequence in which they can be elicited as reflexes.
6. Reflex actions serve as the primary information gathering source for the young infant.
7. Changes in pressure, sight, sound, and tactile stimulation produce primitive and postural reflexes.
8. Primitive reflexes are nourishment-seeking and protective actions.
9. Postural reflexes resemble later voluntary movements.
10. Reflexive behaviors are observed in the early diagnosis of central nervous system disorder.
11. Reflexes appear and are inhibited on a standard schedule, indicating increased cortical control over movement.
12. Many reflexes are inhibited as higher brain centers take over.
13. The subcortex plays an important role throughout life by sustaining the involuntary life processes and controlling such behavior as coughing, sneezing, and yawning.
14. Early and regular stimulation of a postural reflex may hasten onset of the corresponding voluntary movement.

## CRITICAL READINGS

Easton, T.A.: "On the Normal Use of Reflexes," *American Scientist* 60, 591–599, 1972.

Kessen, W., et al.: "Human Infancy: A Bibliography and Guide," in P.H. Mussen (ed.), *Manual of Child Psychology*, New York: Wiley, 1970, pp. 311–329.

Wyke, B.: "The Neurological Basis of Movement: A Developmental Review," in K.S. Holt (ed.), *Movement and Child Development*, London: William Heinemann Medical Books, 1975, pp. 19–33.

Zelazo, P.: "From Reflexive to Instrumental Behavior," in L.P. Lipsett (ed.), *Developmental Psychobiology: The Significance of Infancy*, Hillsdale, N.J.: Lawrence Erlbaum, 1976, pp. 87–103.

# 10

# Rudimentary Movement

Preschool and elementary school children are products of a specific genetic structure and all of the experiences that they have ever had since conception.

Children are not a tabulae rasae, ready to be molded and shaped to our whims or a precut pattern. Current research is making it abundantly clear that infants are able to process a great deal more information that we had ever suspected (Horwitz, 1968; White and Held, 1966). Infants think and they use movement as a purposeful, though initially imprecise, way of gaining information about their environment (Bruner, 1969). Each child is an individual and no two individuals will respond in exactly the same manner. The child's hereditary and experiential backgrounds have a profound effect on the development of movement abilities. It is important that we study the child, beginning with the early movement experiences of infancy, in order to gain a better understanding of the development that has taken place before he or she ever enters the nursery or elementary school. It is also important to study infant motor development in order to gain a better understanding of the developmental concept of how mankind learns to move.

Gaining control over one's musculature, learning to cope with the force of gravity, and controlled movement through space are the major developmental tasks facing the infant. During the neonatal period, movement is random, ill defined, and primarily reflexive. As higher brain centers take over, however, these reflexes are gradually inhibited. The *reflex inhibition stage* is a period stretching throughout most of the first year of life. The infant gradually moves toward controlled rudimentary movement that represents a monumental accomplishment in suppressing reflexes and integrating the sensory and motor apparatuses.

As the primitive and postural reflexes of the previous phase begin to fade, higher brain centers take over many of the skeletal muscle functions of lower brain centers. The reflex inhibition stage essentially begins at birth. From the moment of birth the newborn is bombarded by sight, sound, smell, tactile, and kinesthetic stimulation. The task is to bring order to this sensory stimulation. Initial reflexive responses are gradually inhibited throughout the first year until around the first birthday, when the infant can be seen to have made remarkable progress and to have brought a semblance of order out of apparent chaos.

The period from about 12 months to between 18 and 24 months represents a time for practice and mastery of the many rudimentary tasks initiated during the first year. The infant brings his or her movements under control during this preinitial stage. The *preinitial stage* spans roughly the period between the first and second birthdays. During this stage the infant begins to gain greater control and precision in movement. Differentiation and integration of sensory and motor processes become more highly developed.

Changes in the nervous system are rapid during this period. The brain of the 2-year-old, according to Kessen et al. (1970), "is hardly discriminable in histological characterisistics from the adult brain" (p. 290). Myelination in neural development is largely completed by the end of the first year, rendering the child ready for development and refinement of a vast array of complex stability, locomotor, and manipulative tasks (Espenschade and Eckert, 1980). The infant makes crude but purposeful attempts at a variety of fundamental movements. These early attempts should be encouraged, and a home environment that stimulates their practice may prove beneficial in hastening their mature development. During this stage, however, the infant is primarily involved in gaining control and mastery over the rudimentary stability, locomotor, and manipulative tasks that will be discussed in this chapter.

## STUDY OF INFANT MOTOR DEVELOPMENT

Study of the rudimentary movement abilities of infancy received its impetus in the 1930s and 1940s, when a wealth of information was obtained from the observations of child psychologists. Many of these studies have become classics and have withstood the test of time because of their careful controls and thoroughness. The works of Halverson, Shirley, Bayley, and Gesell are particularly noteworthy.

The work by Halverson (1937) is probably the best ever completed on the sequence of emergence of voluntary grasping behavior during infancy. Through film analysis of infants from 16 to 52 weeks of age, he described three distinct stages of approach toward a cube, and the development of the use of fingers-thumb opposition in grasping behavior.

Shirley's (1931) extensive study of twenty-five infants from birth to age 2 enabled her to describe a sequential developmental progression of activities leading to upright posture and a walking gait. Shirley noted that "each separate stage was a fundamental step in development and that every baby advanced from stage to stage in the same order" (p. 98). She also noted that although the sequence was fixed, individual differences were expressed in differences in the rates of development between infants.

Bayley (1935) conducted an extensive study similar to that of Shirley. As a result of her observations of infants, Bayley was able to describe a developmental series of emerging locomotor abilities progressing from reflexive crawling to walking down a flight of stairs using an alternate foot pattern. Based on this information Bayley was able to develop a cumulative scale of infant motor development that has been widely used as a diagnostic tool to determine an infant's developmental status.

Gesell (1945) conducted extensive studies of infant motor development. He viewed posture (i.e., stability) as the basis of all forms of movement. Therefore, according to Gesell, any form of locomotion or infant manipulation is actually a closely related series of sequential postural adjustments.

The sequence of motor development is predetermined by innate biological factors that cut across all social, cultural, ethnic, and racial boundries. This common base of motor development during the early years of life has caused many to speculate that some voluntary movements (particularly locomotor movements) are phylogenetic (Eckert 1973), and that because these movements are maturationally based, they are not actually under voluntary developmental control (Helle-brandt et al., 1961). This has often led to the erroneous assumption that infants and particularly young children acquire their movement abilities at about the same chronological age solely by the action of maturation and with little dependence on experience. The fact is that although the sequence of skill acquisition is invariant during infancy and childhood, the rate of acquisition differs from child to child because of his or her experiential base (Frankenburg and Dodds, 1967; Sinclair, 1973).

From the moment of birth the infant is in a constant struggle to gain mastery over the environment in order to survive. During the earliest stages of development, the infant's primary interaction with the environment is through the medium of movement. There are three primary categories of movement that the infant must begin to master for survival as well as for effective and efficient interaction with the world. First, the infant must establish and maintain the relationship of the body to the force of gravity in order to obtain an upright sitting posture and an erect standing posture (stability). Second, the child must develop basic locomotor abilities in order to move through the environment (locomotion). Third, the infant must develop the rudimentary abilities of reach, grasp, and release in order that meaningful contact with objects may be made (manipulation).

The establishment of rudimentary abilities in the infant forms the building blocks for more extensive development of the fundamental movement patterns in early childhood and the sport-related movement skills of later childhood and adolescence. These so-called rudimentary movement abilities are highly involved tasks for the infant. The importance of their development must not be overlooked or minimized. The question that arises is: Can factors in the environment enhance the development of those movement abilities? The answer is an unqualified yes. They are not genetically determined to the point where they are not susceptible to modification. Early enrichment does seem to influence later development, but further information is needed about timing, degree, and duration.

## STABILITY

The infant is involved in a constant struggle against the force of gravity in the attempts to obtain and maintain an upright posture. Establishing control over the musculature in opposition to gravity is a process that follows a predictable sequence in all infants. The events leading to an erect standing posture begin with gaining control over the head and neck and proceed down to the trunk and the legs. Operation of the cephalocaudal trend of development is apparent in the infant's sequential progress from a lying position to a sitting posture and eventually to an erect standing posture. Table 10.1 provides a summary of the developmental sequence and the approximate age of onset of rudimentary stability abilities.

**Table 10.1  Developmental Sequence and Approximate Age of Onset of Rudimentary Stability Abilities**

| | | |
|---|---|---|
| Control of head and neck | Turns to one side | Birth |
| | Turns to both sides | 1 week |
| | Held with support | First month |
| | Chin off contact surface | Second month |
| | Good prone control | Third month |
| | Good supine control | Fifth month |
| Control of trunk | Lifts head and chest | Second month |
| | Attempts supine to prone position | Third month |
| | Success in supine to prone roll | Sixth month |
| | Prone to supine roll | Eight month |
| Sitting | Sits with support | Third month |
| | Sits with self-support | Sixth month |
| | Sits alone | Eighth month |
| Standing | Stands with support | Sixth month |
| | Supports with hand holds | Tenth month |
| | Pulls to supported stand | Eleventh month |
| | Stands alone | Twelfth month |

## Control of the Head and the Neck

At birth the infant has no control over the head and neck muscles. If held erect at the trunk, the head will drop forward. Around the end of the first month, control is gained over these muscles, and the infant is able to hold the head erect when supported at the base of the neck. By the end of the first month, the infant should be able to lift the chin off the crib when lying in a prone position. By the fifth month the infant should be able to lift the head off the crib when lying in a supine position.

## Control of the Trunk

After infants have gained mastery of the head and neck muscles, they begin to gain control of the muscles in the thoracic and lumbar regions of the trunk. The development of trunk control begins around the second month of life. Control of the trunk muscles may be observed by holding the infant off the ground by the waist and noting the ability to make postural adjustments necessary to maintain an erect position.

By the end of the second month, infants should be capable of lifting the chest off the floor when placed in a prone position. After infants are able to lift the chest, they begin to draw the knees up toward the chest and then kick them out suddenly as if swimming. This usually occurs by the sixth month. Another indication of gaining control over the muscles of the trunk is the ability to turn over from a supine to a prone position. This is generally accomplished around the sixth month and is easily done by flexing the hips and stretching the legs out at right angles to the trunk. Mastery of the roll from a prone to a supine position comes somewhat later.

## Sitting

Sitting alone is an accomplishment that requires complete control over the entire trunk. The infant of 4 months is generally able to sit with support. This support comes in the lumbar region. The infant has control over the upper trunk but not the

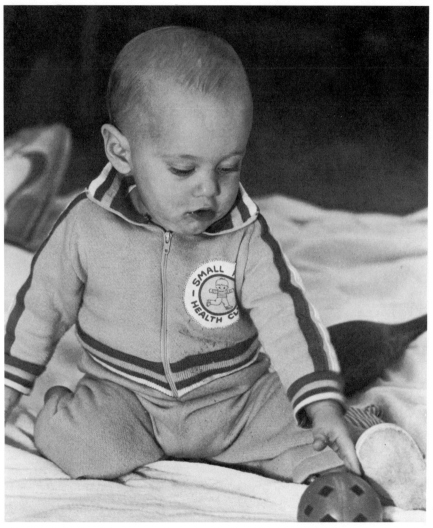

The infant is capable of sitting without support around the seventh month.

lower portion. During the next month or two the infant gradually gains control over the lower trunk. The first efforts at sitting alone are characterized by an exaggerated forward lean. This is an attempt to gain added support for the lumbar region. Gradually, the ability to sit erect with a limited amount of support develops. By the seventh month the infant is generally able to sit alone completely unsupported. At this juncture he or she has now gained control over the upper half of the body. At the same time that infant is learning to sit alone, he or she is developing control over the arms and hands: a further example of the cephalocaudal and proximodistal principles of development in operation (Figure 10.1).

## Standing

Achievement of an erect standing posture represents a developmental milestone in the infant's quest for stability. It is an indication that control over the musculature has been gained to the extent that the force of gravity can no longer place such demanding restraints on movement. The infant is now on the verge of achieving upright locomotion (walking), a feat that is heralded by parents and pediatricians alike as the child's most spectacular task of motor development.

The infant's first voluntary attempts at standing occur around the fifth month. When held under the armpits and brought in contact with a supporting surface, the infant will voluntarily extend at the hip, straighten and tense the muscles of the legs, and maintain a standing position with considerable outside support. Around the ninth or tenth month the infant is able to stand beside furniture and support himself

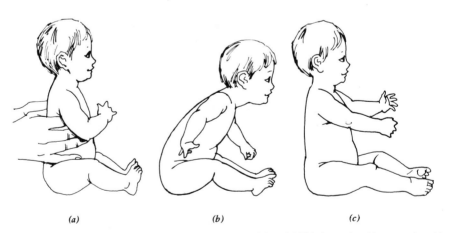

(a)                              (b)                              (c)

**Figure 10.1.** Three stages in achieving independent sitting. *(a)* Third month: with support—wide base of support; adult holding lumbar area. *(b)* Sixth month: unaided—exaggerated forward lean. *(c)* Eighth month: unaided—good control of lumbar region; narrower base of support; back straight.

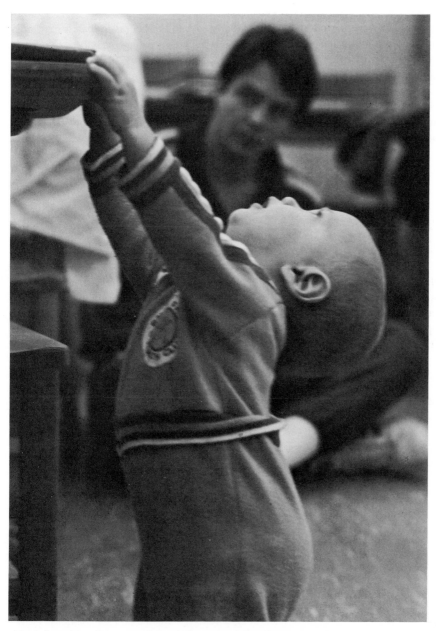

The infant can pull to a standing position around the eleventh month.

for a considerable period of time. Gradually, the infant begins to lean less heavily on the supporting object and can often be seen testing balance completely unsupported for a brief instant. Between the eleventh and twelfth months the infant learns to pull to a stand by first getting to the knees and then pushing with the legs while upward extended arms pull down. Standing alone for extended periods of time generally accompanies walking alone and does not appear separately in most babies. The onset of an erect standing posture normally occurs somewhere between 11 and 13 months (Figure 10.2).

At this point the infant has gained considerable control over the musculature. He is able to accomplish the difficult task of rising from a lying position to a standing position completely unaided.

## LOCOMOTION

The infant's movement through space is dependent on emerging abilities to cope with the force of gravity. Locomotion does not develop independently of stability; it relies heavily on it. The infant will not be able to move about freely until the rudimentary developmental tasks of stability (presented in the previous section) are mastered. Following are discussions of the most frequent forms of locomotion engaged in by the infant while learning how to cope with the force of gravity. These forms of locomotion are also summarized in Table 10.2.

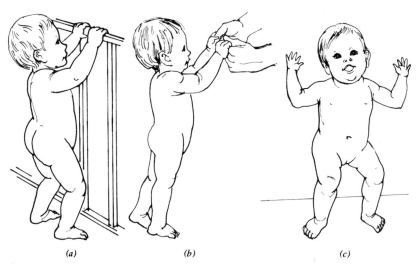

*(a)*                    *(b)*                    *(c)*

**Figure 10.2.** Three stages of gaining a standing posture. *(a)* Sixth month. *(b)* Tenth month. *(c)* Twelfth month.

**Table 10.2   Developmental Sequence and Approximate Age of Onset of Rudimentary Locomotor Abilities**

| | | |
|---|---|---|
| Horizontal movements | Scooting | Third month |
| | Crawling | Sixth month |
| | Creeping | Ninth month |
| | Walk on all-fours | Eleventh month |
| Upright gait | Walks with support | Sixth month |
| | Walks with handholds | Tenth month |
| | Walks with lead | Eleventh month |
| | Walks alone (hands high) | Twelfth month |
| | Walks alone (hands low) | Thirteenth month |

## Crawling

The crawling movements of the infant are the first attempts at purposive locomotion. Crawling evolves as the infant gains control of the muscles of the head, neck, and trunk. While in a prone position, the infant may reach for an object in front of her. In doing so, she raises her head and chest off the floor. On coming back down, the outstretched arms pull the back toward the feet. The result of this combined effort is a slight sliding movement forward (Figure 10.3). The legs are usually not used in these early attempts at crawling. Crawling generally appears in the infant around the sixth month. It may range in appearance, however, from the fourth to the twelfth month. Its onset and duration are highly variable and depend on the child's vigor, the nature of the supporting surface, and external motivation (Cratty 1979).

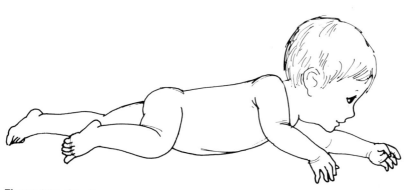

**Figure 10.3.** Crawling.

## Creeping

Creeping evolves from crawling and often develops into a highly efficient form of locomotion for the infant. Creeping differs from crawling in that the legs and arms are used in opposition to one another. The basic creeping posture is a hands-and-knees position. The infant's first attempts at creeping are characterized by very deliberate movements of one limb at a time. As the infant's proficiency increases, movements become synchronous and more rapid. Most efficient creepers utilize a contralateral pattern (right arm and left leg), but about 20 percent utilize a homolateral pattern (Cratty, 1979) (Figure 10.4).

There has been considerable speculation in the past decade concerning the importance of creeping in the infant's motor development and the "proper" method of creeping. The neurological organization rationale of Carl Delacato (1966a) has placed considerable importance on proper creeping and crawling techniques as a necessary stage in achieving cortical hemispherical dominance. Dominance of one side of the cortex is necessary, according to Delacato, for proper neurological organization. Faulty organization, it is hypothesized, will lead to motor, perceptual, and language problems in the child and adult. This hypothesis has come under considerable attack by neurologists, pediatricians, and researchers in the area of child development. Careful evaluation of the pros and cons of Delacato's rationale is necessary before making any definite conclusions.

## Upright Gait

The achievement of upright locomotion depends on the achievement of stability in the infant. The infant must first be able to control the body in a stand position before

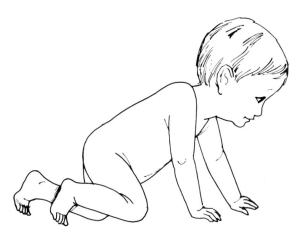

**Figure 10.4.** Creeping.

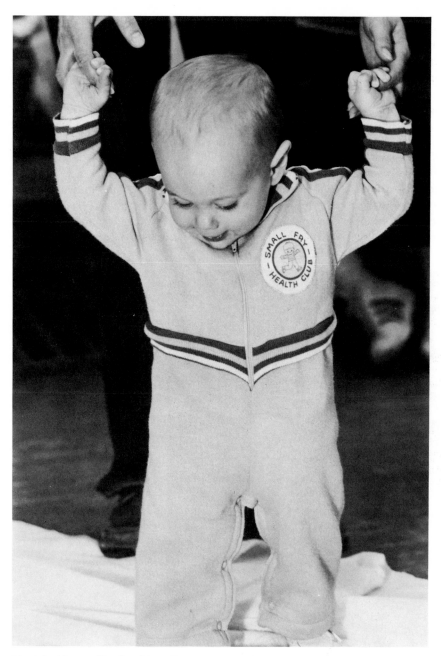

The infant is capable of walking with support around the tenth month.

attention can be turned to the dynamic postural shifts required of upright locomotion. The infant's first attempts at independent walking generally occur somewhere between the tenth and fifteenth months and are characterized by a wide base of support, the feet turned outward, and the knees slightly flexed. These first walking movements are not synchronous and fluid. They are irregular, hesitant, and are not accompanied by reciprocal arm movements. In fact, they only vaguely resemble the mature walking pattern of early childhood. The advent of walking and other forms of upright locomotion is influenced primarily by maturation but may also be influenced by environmental factors. A child cannot move through space until developmentally ready. Special training before being ready is not likely to accelerate learning. If, however, the child's nervous system and musculature are developed to the point of readiness, we may expect to witness slight acceleration in the advent of upright locomotion when the infant receives the benefit of additional environmental supports (that is, encouragement of parents and assistance of parents

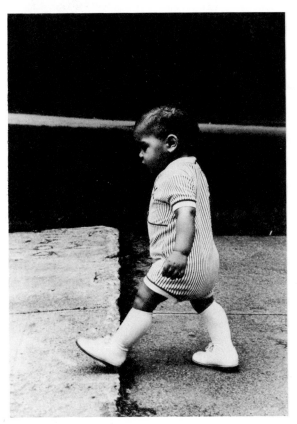

The walking pattern of the infant matures rapidly and resembles, in many ways, the initial pattern at the fundamental movement phase.

and furniture handholds). Physique, heredity, and environmental factors interact to determine the onset of independent walking in the child.

Shirley (1931) has identified four stages that the infant passes through in learning how to walk unaided. These are: ''(a) an early period of stepping in which slight forward progress is made (3−6 months); (b) a period of standing with help (6−10 months); (c) a period of walking when led (9−12 months); (d) a period of walking alone (12−15 months)'' (p. 18). As the infant passes through each of these stages and progresses toward a mature walking pattern, several changes occur. First, the speed of walking accelerates and length of the step increases. Second, the width of the step increases until independent walking is well established, and then decreases slightly. Third, the eversion of the foot gradually decreases until the feet are pointing straight ahead. Fourth, the upright walking gait gradually smooths out, the length of the step becomes regular, and the movements of the body become synchronous. See page 181 for a stroboscopic representation of the initial walking pattern.

## MANIPULATION

As with stability and locomotion, the manipulative abilities of the infant evolve through a series of stages. In this section, the most basic aspects of manipulation— reach, grasp, and release—will be considered. As with the sections on stability and locomotion, the manipulative abilities of the infant may be susceptible to early appearance even though the process is influenced greatly by maturation. If the child is maturationally ready, he will benefit from early opportunities to practice and perfect rudimentary manipulative abilities. Mussen et al. (1969) have pointed out:

> The child can be helped to master skills earlier than he ordinarily would through enrichment, but the timing of the enrichment is important. It is almost as bad to present enriching experiences before the child is ready to use them effectively as it is to deprive the child of these stimulations entirely. (p. 178)

The following are the three general steps in which the infant engages during the acquisition of rudimentary manipulative abilities. Shortly after independent walking has been achieved, the toddler will experiment with walking sideways and backward (Eckert, 1973) and on the tiptoes (Bayley, 1935). Table 10.3 provides a summary of the developmental sequence and approximate age of onset of rudimentary manipulative abilities.

### Reaching

During the first four months of life, the infant does not make definite reaching movements toward objects, although she may attend closely to them visually and make globular encircling motions in the general direction of the object (Bower,

**Table 10.3   Developmental Sequence and Approximate Age of Onset of Rudimentary Manipulative Abilities**

| | | |
|---|---|---|
| Reaching | Globular ineffective | First to third month |
| | Definite corralling | Fourth month |
| | Controlled | Sixth month |
| Grasping | Reflexive | Birth |
| | Voluntary | Third month |
| | Two-hand palmar grasp | Third month |
| | One-hand palmar grasp | Fifth month |
| | Pincer grasp | Ninth month |
| | Controlled grasping | Fourteenth month |
| | Eats without assistance | Eighteenth month |
| Releasing | Basic | Twelfth to fourteenth month |
| | Controlled | Eighteenth month |

1970). Around the fourth month the infant begins to make the fine eye and hand adjustments necessary for contact with the object. Often the infant can be observed making alternating glances between the two. The movements are slow and awkward, involving primarily the shoulder and elbow. Later the wrist and the hand become more directly involved. By the end of the fifth month, the child's aim is nearly perfect, and she is now able to reach for and make tactual contact with objects in the environment. This accomplishment is necessary before being able to actually take hold of the object and grasp it in the hand.

## Grasping

The newborn will grasp an object when it is placed in the palm of the hand. This action is entirely reflexive, however, until about the fourth month. Voluntary grasping must wait until the sensorimotor mechanism has developed to the extent that efficient reaching and meaningful contact can take place. Halverson (1937) has identified several stages in the development of prehension. Briefly, they are: (1) The 4-month-old infant makes no real voluntary effort at tactual contact with objects. (2) The infant of 5 months is capable of reaching for and making contact with the object. He is able to grasp the object with tthe entire hand but not firmly. (3) The child's movements are gradually refined so that by the seventh month the palm and fingers are coordinated. The child is still unable to effectively use the thumb and fingers. (4) By the ninth month the child begins use of the forefinger in grasping. By 10 months reaching and grasping are coordinated into one continuous movement. (5) Efficient use of the thumb and forefinger comes into play at around 12 months. (6) By the time the child is 14 months old, its prehension abilities are very much like those of adults.

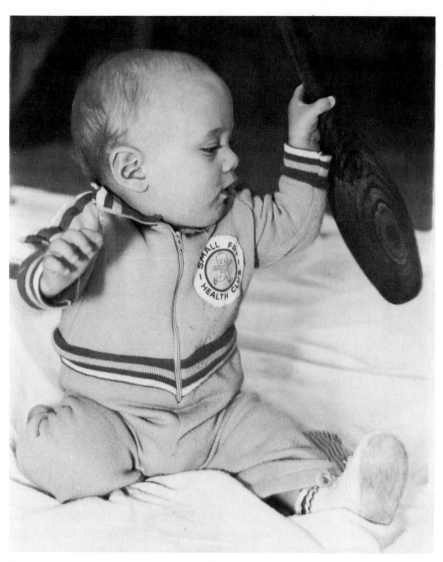

Basic grasping is mastered by the fourteenth month.

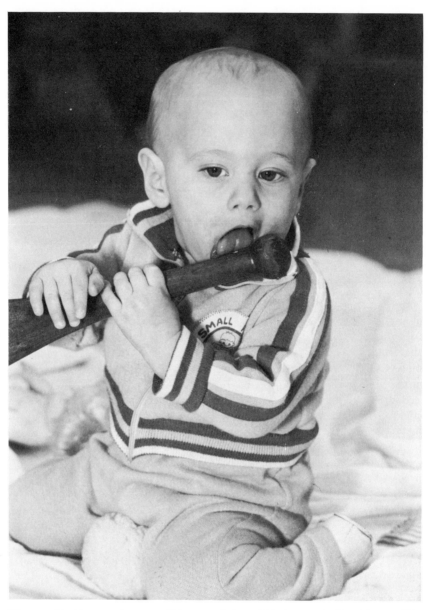

Once an object is securely grasped it is generally brought to the mouth. (Reminiscent of Freud's oral stage).

The developmental progression of reaching and grasping is complex. Landreth (1958) stated that six component coordinates appear to be involved in the development of prehension. Espenschade and Eckert (1980) have neatly summed up these six developmental acts in the following statement:

> These acts involve transitions and include: (1) the transition from visually locating an object to attempting to reach for the object. Other transitions involve: (2) simple eye-hand coordination, to progressive independence of visual effort with its ultimate expression in activities such as piano playing and typing; (3) initial maximal involvement of body musculature to a minimum involvement and greater economy of effort; (4) proximal large muscle activity of the arms and shoulders to distal fine muscle activity of the fingers; (5) early crude raking movements in manipulating objects with the hands to the later pincer-like precision of control with the opposing thumb and forefinger; and (6) initial bilateral reaching and manipulation to ultimate use of the preferred hand. (pp. 114–115)

## Releasing

The frantic shaking of a rattle is a familiar sight when observing a 6-month-old infant at play. This is a learning activity that is generally accompanied by a great deal of smiling, babbling,and obvious glee. Sometimes, however, the same infant may be observed shaking the rattle with obvious frustration and apparent rage. The reason for this shift in moods may be attributed to the fact that at 6 months of age the infant has yet to master the art of releasing an object from grasp. The child has succeeded in reaching for and grasping the handle of the rattle but is not maturationally able to command the flexor muscles of the fingers to relax their grip on the object on command. Learning to fill a bottle with stones, building a block tower, hurling a ball, and turning the pages of a book are seemingly simple examples of the young child's attempt to cope with the problem of release. But when compared with earlier attempts at reaching and grasping, these are indeed remarkable advances. By the time the child is 14 months old, she has mastered the rudimentary elements of releasing objects from her grasp. The 18-month-old has well-coordinated control of all aspects of reach, grasp, and release (Halverson, 1937).

As the infant's mastery of the rudimentary abilities of manipulation (reach, grasp, and release) are developing, the reasons for handling objects are revised. Instead of learning to manipulate objects simply to touch, feel, or mouth them, the child now becomes involved in the process of manipulating objects in order to learn more about the world in which he lives. The manipulation of objects becomes directed by appropriate perceptions in order to achieve meaningful goals (Figure 10.5).

The development of locomotor, stability, and manipulative movement abilities in infants is influenced by both maturation and learning. These two facets of

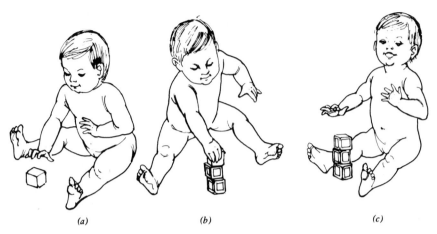

**Figure 10.5.** *(a)* Reach. *(b)* Grasp. *(c)* Release.

development are interrelated, and it is through this interaction that the infant develops and refines rudimentary movement abilities. These movement abilities are necessary steppingstones to the development of fundamental movement patterns and sport-related movement abilities.

## Summary

During infancy the child's primary concerns are with self-gratification. Primitive reflexes serve the infant well in meeting basic survival needs, but as the child develops, other needs emerge. Among them is the characteristic need to "know." The principle of cephalocaudal and proximodistal development governs activity as control is gained first over head and trunk and then over the limbs. Sitting enables the infant to more effectively use the arms for exploration. Manipulative skills including mouthing allow use of the sensorimotor mechanism to gain information. Movements become the symbols of the child's thought process because language is limited.

The motor activities of the human infant are genetically determined, and the order of the developmental sequence is fixed. The only room for variation is in the rate of development. Neuromuscular maturation must occur in order that the infant may progress to movements characteristic of the next higher developmental level. Several environmental factors determine this rate. Environments that provide stimulation and opportunities for exploration encourage early acquisition of fundamental movement patterns. Crawling, for example, is often the outgrowth of an ocular following pattern, while standing and upright gait are encouraged by the presence of handholds in the child's environment.

The argument as to the relative roles of maturation and learning in the development of movement abilities during the first year continues. Increasing support from motor programming theories and natural history studies suggests that during infancy maturation may be the overriding factor affecting development. However, even the best genetic specimen will not thrive or develop optimally in an unfavorable environment.

## CHAPTER HIGHLIGHTS

1.   The first two years of life are important determiners of future functioning.
2.   The developing movement abilities of the infant are highly involved and complicated tasks that require ever-greater movement control.
3.   Developing the rudimentary movement abilities of infancy is a process regulated by both maturation and experience.
4.   Maturation determines the sequential emergence of movement abilities.
5.   The rate of appearance of rudimentary movement abilities is influenced by factors within the environment.
6.   The sequence of emergence of stability, locomotor, and manipulative abilities in infancy is predictable and, in general, resistant to change.
7.   The extent of the development of rudimentary movement abilities is influenced by opportunities for practice.
8.   Rudimentary stability abilities are the most basic of the three forms of rudimentary movements. Their development is essential to the proper development of locomotor and manipulative abilities.
9.   The development of rudimentary locomotor movement abilities provides the infant with the means for exploring his or her environment.
10.  The development of rudimentary manipulative abilities provides the infant with the means for the first meaningful contact with objects in the environment.

## CRITICAL READINGS

Bailey, R.A., and E.C. Burton: *The Dynamic Self: Activities To Enhance Infant Development,* St. Louis: Mosby, 1982, Chapter 1, 2.
Bruner, J.S.: "Processes of Growth in Infancy," in A. Ambrose (ed.), *Stimulation in Early Infancy,* New York: Academic Press, 1969, pp. 205–225.
Hagstron, J., and J. Morrill: *Games Babies Play,* New York: A&W Visual Library, 1979.
Horwitz, F.: "Infant Learning and Development: Retrospect and Prospect," *Merrill-Palmer Quarterly,* 14, 101–120, 1968.
Murray, J.L.: *Infaquatics: Teaching Kids To Swim,* West Point, N.Y.: Leisure Press, 1980, pp. 10–84.
Ridenour, M.V.: "Programs to Optimize Infant Motor Development," in M.V. Ridenour (ed.), *Motor Development: Issues and Applications,* Princeton, N.J.: Princeton, 1978, pp. 39–61.

# CHAPTER 11

# Fundamental Movement

As children approach their second birthday, a marked change can be observed in how they relate to their environment. By the end of the second year, they have mastered the rudimentary movement abilities that are developed during infancy. These movement abilities form the basis on which the child develops or refines the fundamental movement patterns of early childhood and the sport-related movement skills of childhood and adolescence. Children are no longer immobilized by their basic inability to move about freely or by the confines of their crib or playpen. They are now able to explore the movement potentials of their bodies as they move through space (locomotion). They no longer have to maintain a relentless struggle against the force of gravity but are gaining increased control over their musculature in opposition to gravity (stability). They no longer have to be content with the crude and ineffective reaching, grasping, and releasing of objects characteristic of infancy but are rapidly developing the ability to make controlled and precise contact with objects in their environment (manipulation).

    Preschool and primary grade children are involved in the process of developing and refining fundamental movement abilities in a wide variety of stability, locomotor, and manipulative movements. This means that they should be involved in a series of coordinated and developmentally sound experiences that are designed to enhance knowledge of the body and its potential for movement. Movement pattern development is not specifically concerned with developing high degrees of skill in a limited number of movement situations, but rather with developing acceptable levels of proficiency and efficient body mechanics in a wide variety of movement situations. A fundamental movement involves the basic elements of that particular movement only. It does not include such things as the individual's style or personal peculiarities in performance. It does not emphasize the combining of a variety of fundamental movements into complex skills such as the lay-up shot in basketball or a floor exercise routine in gymnastics. Each movement pattern is first considered in relative isolation from all others, and then linked with others into a variety of combinations. The locomotor movements of running, jumping, and leaping, or the manipulative movements of throwing, catching, kicking, and trapping, are examples of fundamental movement abilities that are first dealt with separately by the child. They are then gradually combined in a variety of ways and elaborated upon to become sport skills. The basic elements of a fundamental movement should be the same for all children.

The development of fundamental movement abilities is basic to the motor development of children. A wide variety of movement experiences provide them with a wealth of information on which to base their perceptions of themselves and the world about them.

## DEVELOPMENTAL SEQUENCE OF FUNDAMENTAL MOVEMENTS

With the renewed interest in the study of motor development that began in the 1960s, several scales appeared that illustrated a relationship between age and motor performance. Johnson (1962) using a large sample of boys and girls from grades one through six, found that the mean scores on a variety of motor performance items showed a definite upward trend until the fifth grade. Cratty and Martin (1969) presented age-related sequences of acquisition for a variety of locomotor, manipulative, and perceptual abilities of 365 children ranging in age from 4 to 12 years. Williams' (1970) summary of the movement abilities of children between 3 and 6 years old revealed more advanced forms of movement with increases in age. Sinclair (1973) studied the motor development of 2- to six-year-old children. The results of her longitudinal film analysis of twenty-five movement tests at six-month intervals lent further support to the basic assumption that movement is a developing process during the early childhood years.

These normative studies of motor development are interesting and informative about the quantity or outcome of movement in that they tell "how far," "how fast," and "how many." They failed, however, to provide information about the *qualitative* changes that occur as the child progresses toward more mature form. As a result, a number of investigators, all using film and computer techniques to analyze the intraskill aspects of a variety of fundamental movement patterns, began to collect data leading to a stage concept of motor development during early childhood. Wild (1938) Halverson and Roberton (1966, 1979), Seefeldt (1972), Seefeldt and Haubenstricker (1976), and several others conducted important investigations into the intraskill sequences of a variety of fundamental movement tasks. Out of these investigations have come three popular methods of charting the stage classification of children in actual observational settings (see Chapter 19). The systems devised by Roberton (1978c), McClenaghan and Gallahue (1978b), and Seefeldt and Haubenstricker (1976) have been used successfully in observational assessment with young children. The Roberton method expands the stage theory to an analysis of the separate components of movement within a given pattern. The Seefeldt method assigns an overall stage classification score (stage 1 through stage 5), and the McClenaghan-Gallahue method provides opportunities for both, depending on the needs, interests, and abilities of the observer. Their method recognizes the differential rates of development within fundamental movement patterns as well as the need for an easy-to-apply tool for daily teaching situations.

In their book *Fundamental Movement: A Developmental and Remedial Approach,* McClenaghan and Gallahue (1978a) outline three stages within the fundamental movement phase of development as follows:

Initial Stage:
: Characterized by the child's first observable attempts at the movement pattern. Many of the components of a refined pattern, such as the preparatory action, and follow-through are missing.

Elementary Stage:
: A transitional stage in the child's movement development. Coordination and performance improve, and the child gains more control over his movements. More components of the mature pattern are integrated into the movement, although they are performed incorrectly.

Mature Stage:
: The integration of all the component movements into a well-coordinated, purposeful act. The movement resembles the motor pattern of a skilled adult [in terms of control and quality, but it is lacking in terms of movement performance as measured quantitatively*]. (p. 78, used with permission.)

Not all movement patterns fit precisely into an arbitrary three-stage progression. The developmental aspects of some movements may be more completely described in a four-, six-, or even an eight-stage sequence, depending on the specific pattern and the level of sophistication of the observer. The three-stage approach is used in the following sections because it accurately and adequately fits the developmental sequence of most movement patterns and provides the basis for a reliable, easy-to-use, observational assessment instrument.

## FUNDAMENTAL LOCOMOTOR MOVEMENTS

Locomotion is a fundamental aspect of learning to move effectively and efficiently within one's environment. It involves projection of the body into external space by altering its location relative to fixed points on the surface. Activities such as walking, running, jumping, hopping, sliding, and skipping are considered fundamental locomotor movements. Performance of these movements must be suffi-

---

*Author's addition.

ciently flexible so that they can be altered as the requirements of the environment demand without deflecting attention from the purpose of the act. The child must be able to: (1) use any one of a number of types of movements to reach the goal; (2) shift from one type of movement to another when the situation demands it; and (3) alter each movement as the conditions of the environment change. Throughout this process of alteration and modification, attention must not be diverted from the goal. For example, the locomotor pattern of walking may be used singularly, or it may be used in conjunction with manipulative or stability movements. As a result, the pattern of walking is elaborated upon with the inclusion of object handling such as bouncing a ball while walking on a balance beam. Development and refinement of the following locomotor patterns in children is essential since it is through these movements that they explore the world about them.

## Walking

Walking has often been defined as the process of continually losing and regaining balance while moving forward in an upright position. The walking pattern has been extensively studied in infants, children, and adults. The onset of walking behavior in the infant depends primarily on maturation but is also influenced by environmental factors such as the availability of handholds. Burnett and Johnson (1971) have indicated that the average age for achieving independent walking is 12½ months, with a range of from 9 to 17 months. Once independent walking has been achieved, the child progresses rapidly to the elementary, and mature stages. Several researchers have indicated that the mature walking pattern is achieved sometime between the fourth and the seventh year (Espenschade and Eckert, 1980; Grieve and Gaer, 1966; Guttridge, 1939; Saunders et al., 1953; Wickstrom, 1977). Many subtle changes continue to occur in the walking pattern, but they are not observable through unaided visual assessment. Sophisticated film analysis and electromyography techniques must be used in order to detect progress in walking skill beyond this point (Wickstrom, 1977). Gad-Elmawla's 1980 dissertation is used as the basis for description of the following developmental sequence in the walking pattern.

### Developmental Sequence

1. Initial stage.
   (a) Difficulty maintaining upright posture.
   (b) Unpredictable loss of balance.
   (c) Rigid, halting leg action.
   (d) Short steps.
   (e) Flat-footed contact.
   (f) Toes turn outward.
   (g) Wide base of support.

    **(h)**   Flexed knee at contact followed by quick leg extension.

    **(i)**   Arms held up for balance.

**2.**  Elementary stage.

    **(a)**   Gradual smoothing out of pattern.

    **(b)**   Step length increased.

    **(c)**   Heel-toe contact.

    **(d)**   Arms down to the sides, with limited swing.

    **(e)**   Base of support within the lateral dimensions of the trunk.

    **(f)**   Out-toeing reduced or eliminated.

    **(g)**   Increased pelvic tilt.

    **(h)**   Apparent vertical lift.

**3.**  Mature stage.

    **(a)**   Reflexive arm swing.

    **(b)**   Narrow base of support.

    **(c)**   Relaxed elongated gait.

    **(d)**   Little vertical lift.

    **(e)**   Definite heel-toe contact.

### Visual Description

**1.**  Initial stage.

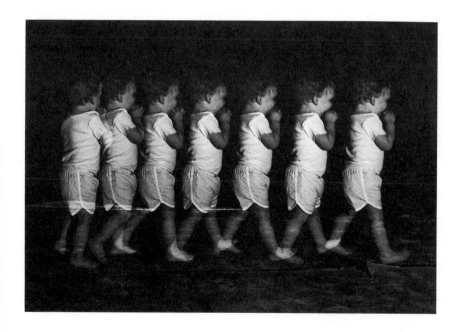

**2.** Elementary stage.

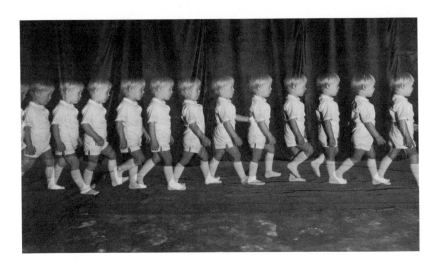

**3.** Mature stage.

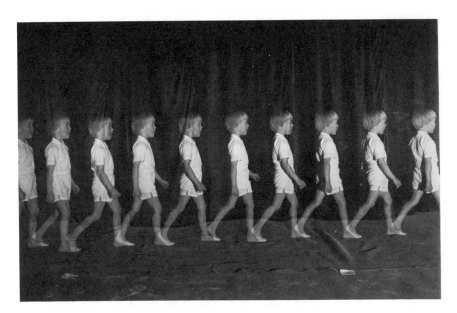

**Common Problems**

1. Walking on the toes.
2. Walking with the toes turned in (''pigeon-toed'').
3. Walking with the toes turned outward (''duck-footed'').
4. Poor rhythmical coordination and alteration of arms and legs.
5. Poor posture and body alignment.
6. Excessive vertical lift.
7. Wide base of support.

## Running

Running is an exaggerated form of walking. It differs principally from the walk in that there is a brief flight phase during each step, in which the body is out of contact with the supporting surface. The flight phase is first seen around the second birthday. Prior to that the run appears as a fast walk with one foot always in contact with the supporting surface. The initial stage of the running pattern does *not* depend on mature walking (Broer and Zernicke, 1979). Many young children begin to run prior to mastery of the mature walking pattern. The mature running pattern is fundamental to successful participation in a variety of sport-related activities. The running pattern has been extensively studied by a number of investigators (Seefeldt et al., 1972; Wickstrom, 1977). The developmental sequence enumerated by McClenaghan (1976), based on film analysis, is used here.

**Developmental Sequence**

1. Initial stage.
   (a) Leg swing is short, limited.
   (b) The stride is stiff and uneven.
   (c) No observable flight phase.
   (d) Incomplete extension of support leg.
   (e) Stiff, short swing, with varying degrees of elbow flexion.
   (f) The arms tend to swing outward horizontally.
   (g) Swinging leg rotates outward from the hip.
   (h) Swinging foot toes outward.
   (i) Wide base of support.
2. Elementary stage.
   (a) Length of stride, arm swing, and speed increase.
   (b) Limited but observable flight phase.
   (c) Support leg extends more completely at takeoff.
   (d) Arm swing increases.
   (e) Horizontal arm swing is reduced on the backswing.

      **(f)**   Swinging foot crosses the midline at the height of the recovery to the rear.

  **3.**  Mature stage.

      **(a)**   Length of stride is at its maximum; speed of stride is fast.

      **(b)**   Definite flight phase.

      **(c)**   Support leg extends completely.

      **(d)**   Recovery thigh is parallel to the ground.

      **(e)**   Arms swing vertically in opposition to the legs.

      **(f)**   Arms are bent at approximate right angles.

      **(g)**   There is little rotary action of the recovery leg and foot.

**Visual Description**

  **1.**  Initial stage.

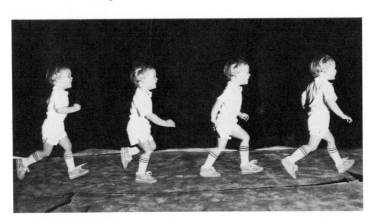

  **2.**  Elementary stage.

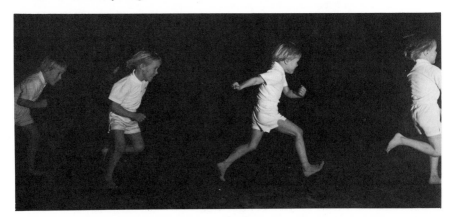

**3.** Mature stage.

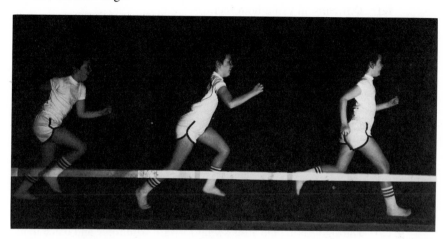

**Common Problems**

1. Inhibited or exaggerated arm swing.
2. Arms crossing the midline of the body.
3. Improper foot placement.
4. Exaggerated forward trunk lean.
5. Arms flopping at the sides or held out for balance.
6. Twisting of the trunk.
7. Arhythmical action.
8. Landing flat-footed.
9. Flipping the foot or lower leg in or out.


## Horizontal Jumping

The jump for distance or standing long jump as it is commonly called is an explosive movement requiring coordinated performance of all parts of the body. The take off and landing is with both feet. The developmental sequence proposed by McClenaghan (1976), based on film analysis, is used here.

**Developmental Sequence**

1. Initial stage.
   (a) Limited swing; the arms do not initiate the jumping action.
   (b) During flight, the arms move in a sideward-downward or rearward-upward to maintain balance.
   (c) The trunk moves in a vertical direction; little emphasis on length of jump.

(d) Preparatory crouch is inconsistent in terms of leg flexion.

(e) Difficulty in using both feet.

(f) Extension of the ankles, knees, and hips at takeoff is limited.

(g) Body weight falls backward at landing.

2. Elementary stage.

(a) Arms initiate jumping action.

(b) Arms remain toward the front of the body during the preparatory crouch.

(c) Arms move out to side to maintain balance during flight.

(d) Preparatory crouch is deeper and more consistent.

(e) Extension of the knees and hips is more complete at takeoff.

(f) Hips are flexed during flight, and the thighs are held in a flexed position.

3. Mature stage.

(a) Arms move high and to the rear during the preparatory crouch.

(b) During takeoff, the arms swing forward with force and reach high.

(c) Arms are held high throughout the jumping action.

(d) Trunk is propelled at approximately a 45° angle.

(e) Major emphasis is on horizontal distance.

(f) Preparatory crouch is deep and consistent.

(g) Complete extension of ankles, knees, and hips at takeoff.

(h) Thighs are held parallel to ground during flight; lower leg hangs vertically.

(i) Body weight is forward at landing.

## Visual Description

1. Initial stage.

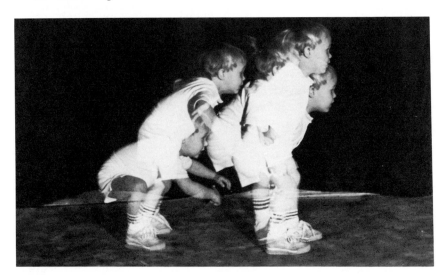

**2.**   Elementary stage.

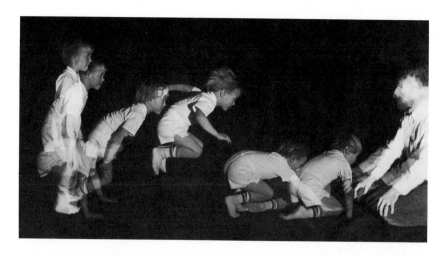

**3.**   Mature stage.

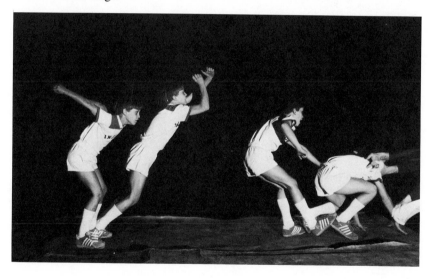

## Common Problems

**1.**   Improper use of the arms (that is, failure to use the arm opposite to the propelling leg in a down-up-down swing as the leg flexes, extends, and flexes again).

**2.**   Twisting or jerking of the body.

**3.**   Inability to perform either a one-foot or a two-foot takeoff.

4.  Poor preliminary crouch.
5.  Restricted movements of the arms or legs.
6.  Poor angle of takeoff.
7.  Failure to extend fully on takeoff.
8.  Failure to extend the legs forward on landing.
9.  Falling backward on landing.

## Vertical Jumping

Jumping for height, or vertical jump, has been studied by several investigators in recent years (Martin and Stull, 1969; Myers et al., 1977; Poe, 1976). The jump for height involves projecting the body vertically into the air from a one- or two-foot takeoff with a landing on both feet. The developmental sequence proposed by Myers et al. (1977), based on film analysis, is presented here.

### Developmental Sequence

1.  Initial stage.
    (a)  Inconsistent preparatory crouch.
    (b)  Difficulty in taking off with both feet.
    (c)  Poor body extension on takeoff.
    (d)  Little or no head lift.
    (e)  Arms are not coordinated with the trunk and leg action.
    (f)  Little height is achieved.
2.  Elementary stage.
    (a)  Knee flexion exceeds 90° angle on preparatory crouch.
    (b)  Exaggerated forward lean during crouch.
    (c)  Two-foot take-off.
    (d)  Entire body does not fully extend during the flight phase.
    (e)  Arms attempt to aid in flight (but often unequally) and to aid balance.
    (f)  Noticeable horizontal displacement on landing.
3.  Mature stage.
    (a)  Preparatory crouch with knee flexion from 60 to 90°.
    (b)  Forceful extension at the hips, knees, and ankles.
    (c)  Simultaneous coordinated upward arm lift.
    (d)  Upward head tilt with eyes focused on the target.
    (e)  Full body extension.
    (f)  Elevation of the reaching arm by shoulder girdle tilt combined with downward thrust of nonreaching arm at the peak of flight.
    (g)  Controlled landing very close to the point of takeoff.

## Visual Description

1. Initial stage.

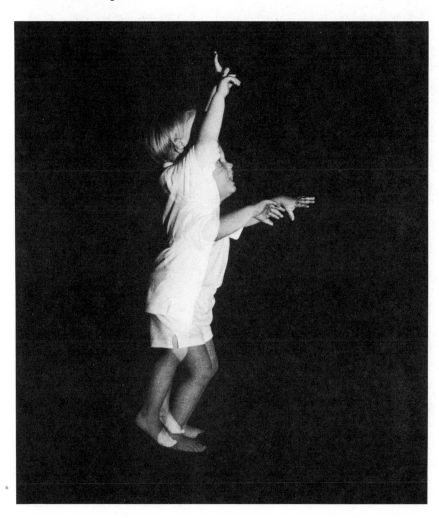

**2.** Elementary stage.

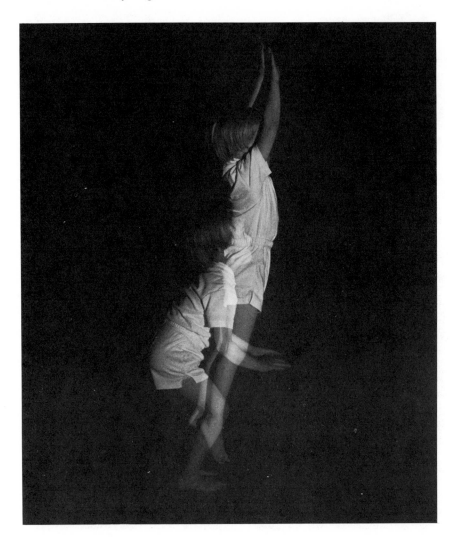

**3.** Mature stage

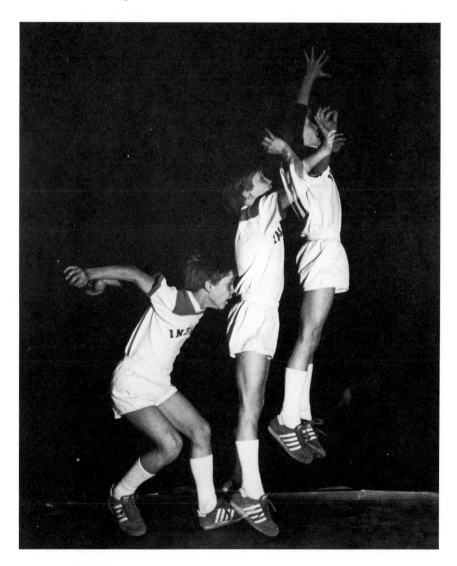

**Common Problems**

1. Failure to get airborne.
2. Failure to take off with both feet simultaneously.
3. Failure to crouch at about a 90° angle.
4. Failure to extend the body, legs, and arms forcefully.

5. Poor coordination of the leg and arm actions.
6. Swinging of the arms backward or to the side for balance.
7. Failure to lead with the eyes and the head.
8. One-foot landing.
9. Inhibited or exaggerated flexion of the hip and knee on landing.
10. Marked horizontal displacement on landing.

## Jumping from a Height

The movements involved in jumping from a low height are somewhat similar to those found in the jump for distance and the jump for height particularly at the initial stage. The jump from a low height has been studied by a few investigators (Bayley, 1935; McCaskill and Wellman, 1938) and has concentrated on the takeoff, flight phase, and landing aspects of the pattern. The description of stages that follows is based on my observation of numerous children and subject to refinement and verification.

### Developmental Sequence

1. Initial stage.
   (a) One foot leads on takeoff.
   (b) No flight phase.
   (c) Lead foot contacts lower surface prior to trailing foot leaving upper surface.
   (d) Exaggerated use of arms for balance.
2. Elementary stage.
   (a) Two-foot takeoff with one-foot lead.
   (b) Flight phase, but lacks control.
   (c) Arms used ineffectively for balance.
   (d) One-foot landing followed by immediate landing of trailing foot.
   (e) Inhibited or exaggerated flexion at knees and hip upon landing.
3. Mature stage.
   (a) Two-foot takeoff.
   (b) Controlled flight phase.
   (c) Both arms used efficiently out to the sides to control balance as needed.
   (d) Feet contact lower surface simultaneously, with toes touching first.
   (e) Feet land shoulder width apart.
   (f) Flexion at the knees and hip congruent with height of the jump.

**Visual Description**

1. Initial stage.

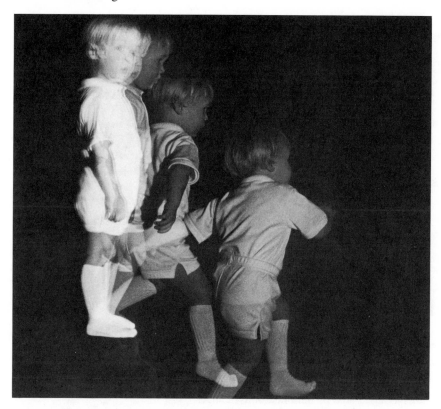

2. Elementary stage.

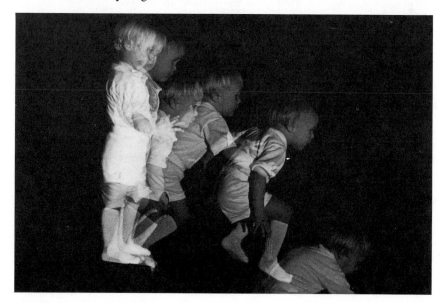

3. Mature stage.

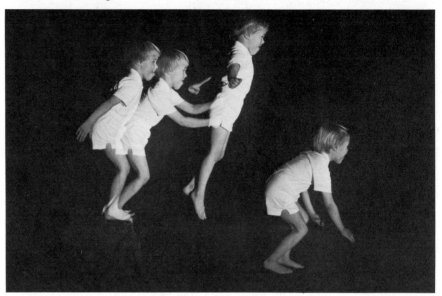

## Common Problems

   1. Inability to take off with both feet.
   2. Twisting the body to one side on takeoff.
   3. Exaggerated or inhibited body lean.
   4. Failure to coordinate the use of both arms in the air.
   5. "Tying" one arm to the side while using the other.
   6. Failure to land simultaneously on both feet.
   7. Landing flat-footed.
   8. Failure to flex the knees sufficiently to absorb impact of landing.
   9. Landing out of control.

## Hopping

Hopping is similar to the jump for distance and the vertical jump but both the takeoff and the landing are on the same foot. The hop has been studied by Seefeldt and Haubenstricker (1976). Their four-stage developmental sequence is summarized here and condensed into three stages.

### Developmental Sequence

   1. Initial stage.
      (a) Nonsupporting leg is flexed 90° or less.
      (b) Nonsupporting thigh is roughly parallel to the contact surface.

    **(c)** Body upright.

    **(d)** Arms flexed at elbows and held slightly to the side.

    **(e)** Little height or distance generated in a single hop.

    **(f)** Balance lost easily.

    **(g)** Limited to one or two hops.

**2.** Elementary stage.

    **(a)** Nonsupporting leg flexed.

    **(b)** Nonsupporting thigh at 45° angle to contact surface.

    **(c)** Slight forward lean, with the trunk flexed at the hip.

    **(d)** Nonsupporting thigh flexes and extends at the hip to produce greater force.

    **(e)** Force is absorbed on landing by flexing at the hip and by the supporting knee.

    **(f)** Arms move vigorously up and down bilaterally.

    **(g)** Balance poorly controlled.

    **(h)** Generally limited in the number of consecutive hops that can be performed.

**3.** Mature stage.

    **(a)** Nonsupporting leg flexed at 90° or less.

    **(b)** Nonsupporting thigh lifts with vertical thrust of supporting foot.

    **(c)** Greater body lean.

    **(d)** Rhythmical action of nonsupporting leg (pendulum swing aiding in force production.

    **(e)** Arms move together in rhythmical fashion, lifting as the supporting foot leaves the contact surface.

    **(f)** Arms not needed for balance but used for greater force production.

## Visual Description

**1.** Initial stage.

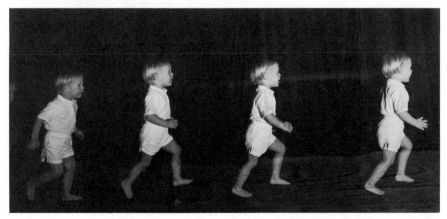

**2.** Elementary stage.

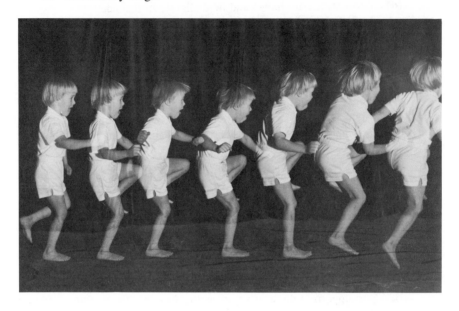

**3.** Mature stage.

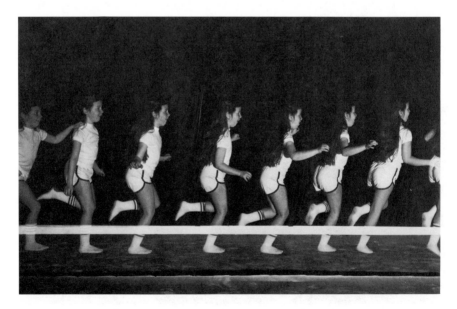

**Common Problems**

1.   Hopping flat-footed.
2.   Exaggerated movements of the arms.
3.   Exaggerated movement of the nonsupporting leg.
4.   Exaggerated forward lean.
5.   Inability to maintain balance for five or more consecutive hops.
6.   Lack of rhythmical fluidity of movement.
7.   Inability to hop effectively on both the left foot and the right foot.
8.   Inability to alternate hopping feet in a smooth, continuous manner.
9.   "Tying" one arm to the side of the body.

## Galloping and Sliding

Galloping and sliding involve the combination of two fundamental movements, the step and the hop, with the same foot always leading in the direction of movement. The movement is called a gallop when moving forward or backward, and a slide when progressing sideward. Sapp (1980) has described a developmental sequence for galloping that may also be applied to sliding.

**Developmental Sequence**

1.   Initial stage.
     (a)   Arhythmical at a fast pace.
     (b)   Often reverts to a run.
     (c)   Trail leg fails to remain behind and often contacts surface in front of the lead leg.
     (d)   45° flexion of trail leg during flight phase.
     (e)   Contact in a heel-toe combination.
     (f)   Arms of little use in balance or force production.
2.   Elementary stage.
     (a)   Moderate tempo.
     (b)   Appears choppy and stiff.
     (c)   Trail leg may lead during flight but lands adjacent to or behind the lead leg.
     (d)   Exaggerated vertical lift.
     (e)   Feet contact in a heel-toe, or toe-toe, combination.
     (f)   Arms slightly out to the side to aid balance.
3.   Mature stage.
     (a)   Moderate tempo.
     (b)   Smooth, rhythmical action.
     (c)   Trail leg lands adjacent to or behind lead leg.
     (d)   Both legs flexed at 45° angle during flight.

(e)  Low flight pattern.
(f)  Heel-toe contact combination.
(g)  Arms not needed for balance; may be used for other purposes.

**Visual Description**

1. Initial stage.

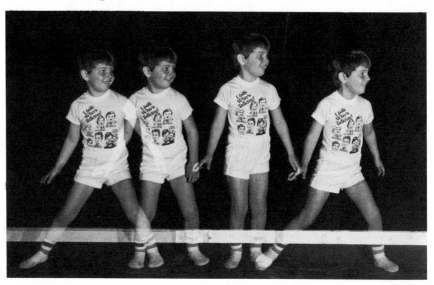

2. Elementary stage.

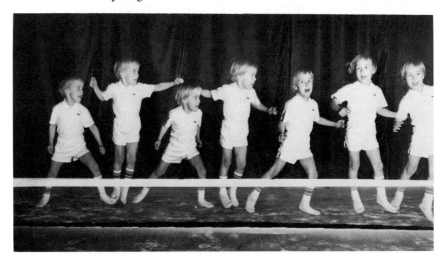

**3.** Mature stage.

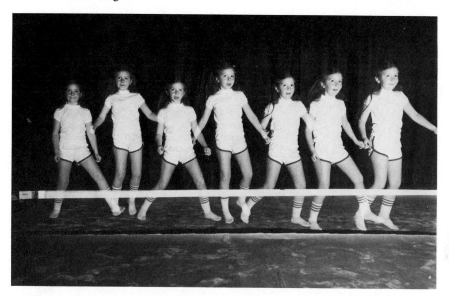

## Common Problems

**1.** Choppy movements.
**2.** Keeping the legs too straight.
**3.** Exaggerated forward trunk lean.
**4.** Overstepping with the trailing leg.
**5.** Too much elevation on the hop.
**6.** Inability to perform both forward and backward.
**7.** Inability to lead with the nondominant foot.
**8.** Inability to perform to both the left and the right.
**9.** Undue concentration on the task.

## Leaping

The leap is similar to the run in that there is a transference of weight from one foot to the other, but the loss of contact with the surface is sustained, with greater elevation and distance covered than in the run. Leaping involves using greater amounts of force in order to produce more height and to cover a greater distance than a run. Biomechanic studies have been conducted on the hurdle event in track, but there is a dearth of information about the developmental aspects of the leaping pattern. The description of stages that follows is based on my observational assessment of numerous children and is subject to refinement and verification.

**Developmental Sequence**

1. Initial stage.
   (a) Child appears confused in attempts.
   (b) Inability to push off and gain distance and elevation.
   (c) Each "attempt" looks merely like another running step.
   (d) Inconsistent use of takeoff leg.
   (e) Arms ineffective.
2. Elementary stage.
   (a) Appears to be thinking through the action.
   (b) Attempt looks like an elongated run.
   (c) Little elevation above the supporting surface.
   (d) Little forward trunk lean.
   (e) Stiff appearance in the trunk.
   (f) Incomplete extension of legs during flight.
   (g) Arms used for balance, not as aid in force production.
3. Mature stage.
   (a) Relaxed rhythmical action.
   (b) Forceful extension of takeoff leg.
   (c) Good summation of horizontal and vertical forces.
   (d) Definite forward trunk lean.
   (e) Definite arm apposition.
   (f) Full extension of legs during flight.

**Visual Description**

1. Initial stage.

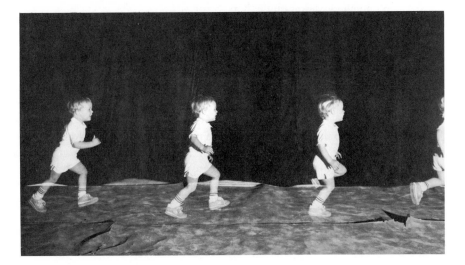

**2.**  Elementary stage.

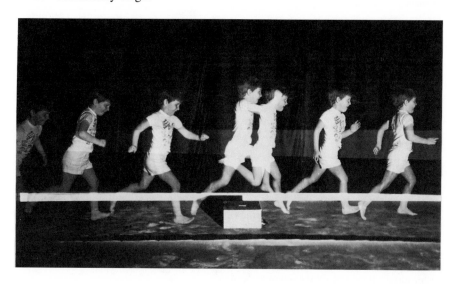

**3.**  Mature stage.

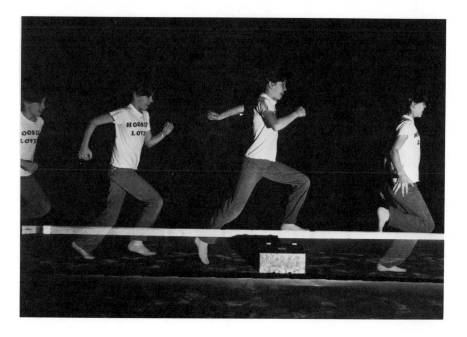

### Common Problems

1. Failure to use the arms in opposition to the legs.
2. Inability to perform the one-foot takeoff and land on the opposite foot.
3. Restricted movements of the arms or legs.
4. Lack of spring and elevation in the push-off.
5. Landing flat-footed.
6. Exaggerated or inhibited body lean.
7. Failure to stretch and reach with the legs.

## Skipping

The skipping action puts two fundamental movement patterns, the step and the hop, together into a combined pattern of movement. Seefeldt and Haubenstricker (1976) as well as Halverson and Roberton (1979) have studied the skipping pattern and reported a three stage developmental sequence which serves as the basis of the following description. The skip is a continuous flow of the step and hop involving rhythmical alteration of the leading foot.

### Developmental Sequence

1. Initial stage.
   - (a) "One-footed skip."
   - (b) Deliberate step-hop action.
   - (c) Double hop or step sometimes occurs.
   - (d) Exaggerated stepping action.
   - (e) Arms of little use.
   - (f) Action appears segmented.
2. Elementary stage.
   - (a) Step and hop coordinated effectively.
   - (b) Rhythmical use of arms to aid momentum.
   - (c) Exaggerated vertical lift on the hop.
   - (d) Flat-footed landing.
3. Mature stage.
   - (a) Rhythmical weight transfer throughout.
   - (b) Rhythmical use of arms but reduced during time of weight transfer.
   - (c) Low vertical lift on the hop.
   - (d) Toe landing.

**Visual Description**

1. Initial stage.

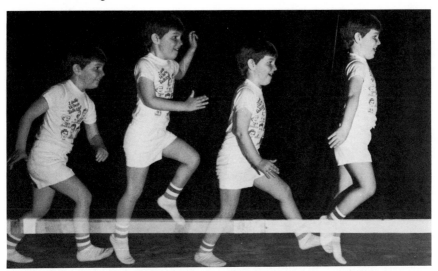

2. Elementary stage.

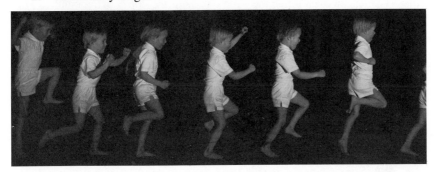

3. Mature stage.

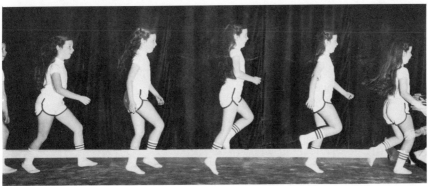

**Common Problems**

1. Segmented stepping and hopping action.
2. Poor rhythmical alteration.
3. Inability to use both sides of the body.
4. Exaggerated movements.
5. Landing flat-footed.
6. Exaggerated, inhibited, or unilateral arm movements.
7. Inability to move in a straight line.
8. Inability to skip backward and to the side.

## Climbing

Climbing is a fundamental movement similar to creeping. The primary difference between the two is that climbing requires the body weight to be pulled by the limbs in opposition to the force of gravity while creeping requires the body weight to be pushed by the limbs at right angles to the gravitational pull. Climbing may be performed with the legs alone, the arms alone, or with the legs and arms working together. The terrain over which the child climbs or the object being climbed (e.g., rope, pole, ladder) dictates the exact form to be taken. The following is a description of a vertical climbing pattern in which both the arms and the legs are used, as in climbing a ladder. It is based on my observations of children and is subject to verification and refinement.

**Developmental Sequence**

1. Initial stage.
   (a) Leans body weight forward toward the climbing surface to ensure balance.
   (b) Begins action with the feet.
   (c) Uses a follow step and a follow grip.
2. Elementary stage.
   (a) Tends to lead with the same foot and same hand.
   (b) Supports body weight with good balance.
   (c) Begins action with preferred foot.
   (d) Uses homolateral arm and leg action; appears in control.
3. Mature stage.
   (a) Good balance and body control.
   (b) Can lead off with either hand or leg.
   (c) Smooth, fluid, rapid motion.
   (d) Uses a contralateral arm-leg action.

**Visual Sequence**

1. Initial stage.

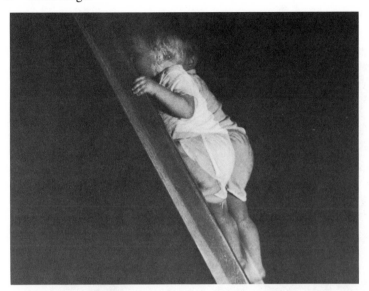

2. Elementary stage.

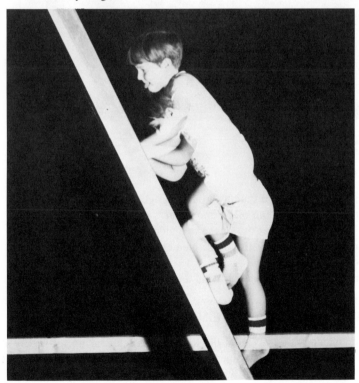

**3.** Mature stage.

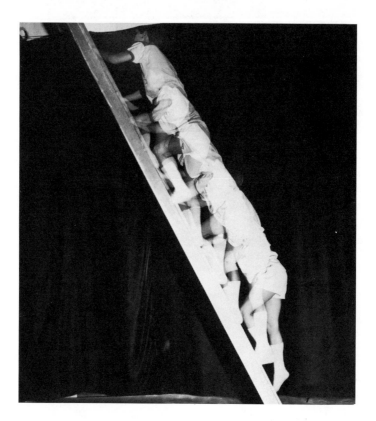

**Common Problems**

1. Failure to wrap the thumbs around the grasping object.
2. Improper sequencing of the movements of the limbs.
3. Uneven or irregular use of the two sides of the body.
4. Inability to transfer the basic elements to climbing other objects (e.g. rope, pole, ladder).
5. Inability to use alternating hand and/or foot placement.

## FUNDAMENTAL MANIPULATIVE MOVEMENTS

Gross motor manipulation involves the individual's relationship to objects and is characterized by giving force to objects and receiving force from them. Propulsive movements involve activities in which an object is moved away from the body.

Fundamental movements such as throwing, kicking, striking, and rolling a ball are involved. Absorptive movements involve activities that are concerned with positioning the body or a body part in the path of a moving object for the purpose of stopping or deflecting that object. Fundamental movements such as catching and trapping are involved. The essence of manipulative movements is that they combine two or more movements and are generally used in conjunction with other forms of movement. For example, propulsive movements are generally a composite of stepping, turning, swinging, and stretching. Absorptive movements generally consist of bending and stepping.

It is through the manipulation of objects that children are able to explore the relationship of moving objects in space. These movements involve making estimates of the path, distance, rate of travel, accuracy, and mass of the moving object. At the point of contact a check on previous estimates is possible. It is through such types of experimentation that children learn the nature and effect of the movement of objects. Because manipulative patterns commonly combine both locomotor and stabilizing movements, efficient use of them should not be expected at the same time that locomotor and stability abilities are developing. Only after these patterns have been fairly well established do we begin to see the emergence of efficient manipulative movements. The following is a description of several manipulative patterns of movement.

## Overhand Throwing

The overhand throw has been studied extensively over the past several years (Deach, 1951; Wild, 1938), with attention focused on form, accuracy, and distance. The components of the throw vary depending on which of these three factors the thrower is concentrating on and the starting position that is assumed. When viewing the overhand throw from the standpoint of the process or form, the following developmental sequence is apparent (McClenaghan, 1976; Roberton 1978a).

### Developmental Sequence

1. Initial stage.
   (a) The action is mainly from the elbow.
   (b) Elbow of the throwing arm remains in front of the body; action resembles a push.
   (c) Fingers spread at release.
   (d) Follow-through is forward and downward.
   (e) Trunk remains perpendicular to the target.
   (f) Little rotary action during the throw.
   (g) Body weight shifts slightly rearward to maintain balance.
   (h) Feet remain stationary.
   (i) There is often purposeless shifting of feet during preparation for the throw.

2. Elementary stage.
   (a) In preparation, the arm is swung upward, sideward, and backward to a position of elbow flexion.
   (b) Ball is held behind the head.
   (c) Arm is swung forward, high over the shoulder.
   (d) Trunk rotates toward the throwing side during the preparatory action.
   (e) Shoulders rotate toward throwing side.
   (f) Trunk flexes forward with forward motion of arm.
   (g) Definite forward shift of body weight.
   (h) Steps forward with leg on same side as throwing arm.
3. Mature stage.
   (a) Arm is swung backward in preparation.
   (b) Opposite elbow is raised for balance as a preparatory action in the throwing arm.
   (c) Throwing elbow moves forward horizontally as it extends.
   (d) Forearm rotates and thumb ends up pointing downward.
   (e) Trunk markedly rotates to throwing side during preparatory action.
   (f) Throwing shoulder drops slightly.
   (g) A definite rotation through hips, legs, spine, and shoulders during throw.
   (h) Weight during preparatory movement is on the rear foot.
   (i) As weight is shifted, there is a step with the opposite foot.

**Visual Description**

1. Initial stage.

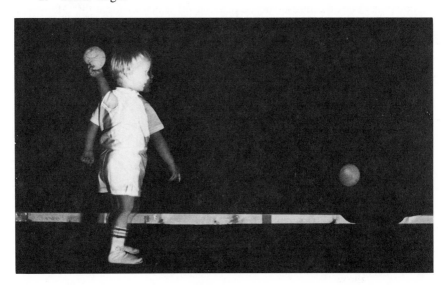

**2.** Elementary stage.

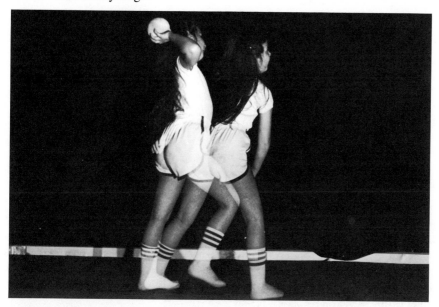

**3.** Mature stage.

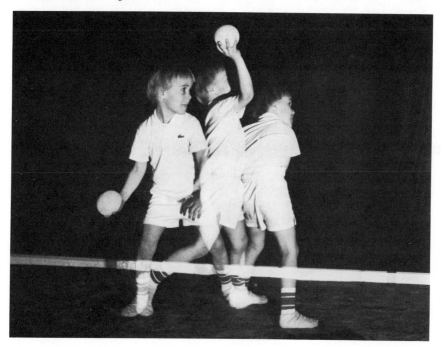

## Common Problems

1. Forward movement of the foot on the same side as the throwing arm.
2. Inhibited backswing.
3. Failure to rotate the hips as the throwing arm is brought forward.
4. Failure to step out on the leg opposite the throwing arm.
5. Poor rhythmical coordination of arm movement with body movement.
6. Inability to release the ball at the desired trajectory.
7. Loss of balance while throwing.
8. Upward rotation of the arm.

## Catching

The fundamental movement pattern of catching involves use of the hands to stop tossed objects. The elements of the underhand and overhand catch are essentially the same. The major difference is in the position of the hands upon impact with the object. The underhand catch is performed when the object to be caught is below the waist. The palms of the hands and the wrists are turned upward. When the object is above the waist, the palms face away from the individual in the direction of the flight of the object.

Several researchers have investigated the development of catching abilities in children (Guttridge, 1939; Pederson, 1973; Whiting, 1969). The following developmental sequence of catching is based on these and McClenaghan's (1976) study.

### Developmental Sequence

1. Initial stage.
   (a) There is often an avoidance reaction of turning the face away or protecting the face with arms (the avoidance reaction is learned and therefore may not be present).
   (b) Arms are extended and held in front of the body.
   (c) Body movement is limited until contact.
   (d) The catch resembles a scooping action.
   (e) Use of the body to trap ball.
   (f) Palms are held upward.
   (g) Fingers are extended and held tense.
   (h) Hands are not utilized in the catching action.
2. Elementary stage.
   (a) Avoidance reaction is limited to the eyes closing at contact with ball.
   (b) Elbows are held at the sides with an approximately 90° bend.

(c)    Since initial attempt at contact with the child's hands is often unsuccessful, the arms trap the ball.

(d)    Hands are held in opposition to each other; thumbs are held upward.

(e)    At contact the hands attempt to squeeze the ball in a poorly timed and uneven motion.

3.   Mature stage.

(a)    No avoidance reaction.

(b)    Eyes follow the ball into the hands.

(c)    Arms are held relaxed at the sides, and the forearms are held in front of the body.

(d)    Arms give on contact to absorb the force of the ball.

(e)    Arms adjust to the flight of the ball.

(f)    Thumbs are held in opposition to each other.

(g)    Hands grasp the ball in a well-timed, simultaneous motion.

(h)    Fingers grasp more effectively.

## Visual Description

1.   Initial stage.

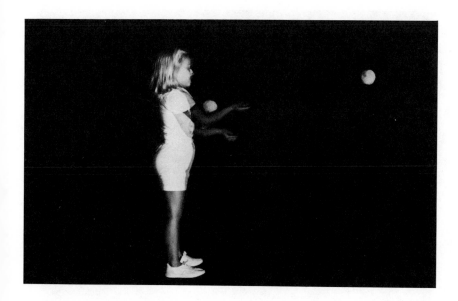

**2.** Elementary stage.

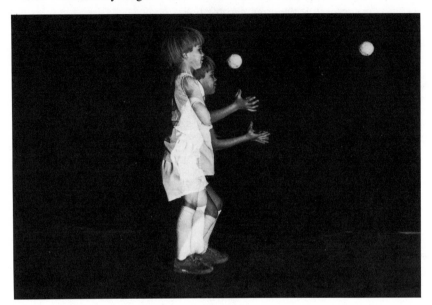

**3.** Mature stage.

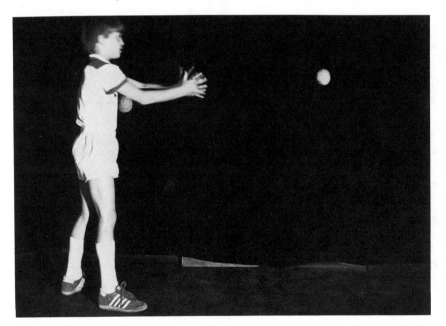

## Common Problems

1. Failure to maintain control of the object.
2. Failure to "give" with the catch.
3. Keeping the fingers rigid and straight in the direction of the object.
4. Failure to adjust the hand position to the height and trajectory of the object.
5. Inability to vary the catching pattern for objects of different weight and force.
6. Taking the eyes off the object.
7. Closing the eyes.
8. Inability to focus on, or track, the ball.
9. Improper stance, causing loss of balance when catching a fast-moving object.
10. Closing the hands either too early or too late.
11. Failure to keep the body in line with the ball.

## Kicking

Kicking is a form of striking in which the foot is used to impart force to an object directed toward a goal. Precise variations of the kicking action may be accomplished by making adjustments with the kicking leg and by bringing the arms and trunk into play. The primary factors that influence the type of kick used are: (1) the desired trajectory of the ball; and (2) the height of the ball when it is contacted. The fundamental kicking pattern for a stationary ground ball is the only common striking movement that does not use the arms and hands directly. The developmental aspects of kicking a stationary ball have been studied extensively by Deach (1951) and Seefeldt and Haubenstricker (1981). The developmental sequence that follows is based on these studies and the work of McClenaghan (1976).

### Developmental Sequence

1. Initial stage.
   (a) Movements are restricted during the kicking action.
   (b) Trunk remains erect.
   (c) Arms are used to maintain balance.
   (d) Movement of kicking leg is limited in the backswing.
   (e) Forward swing is short: there is little follow-through.
   (f) Child kicks "at" ball rather than kicking it squarely and following through.
   (g) A pushing rather than a striking action is predominant.
2. Elementary stage.
   (a) Preparatory backswing is centered at the knee.

    **(b)** Kicking leg tends to remain bent throughout the kick.

    **(c)** Follow-through is limited to the forward movement of the knee.

    **(d)** One or more deliberate steps are taken toward the ball.

**3.** Mature stage

    **(a)** Arms swing in opposition to each other during the kicking action.

    **(b)** Trunk bends at the waist during the follow-through.

    **(c)** Movement of the kicking leg is initiated at the hip.

    **(d)** Support leg bends slightly at contact.

    **(e)** Length of leg swing increases.

    **(f)** Follow-through is high; support foot rises to toes or leaves the surface entirely.

    **(g)** The approach to the ball is from a run or a leap.

### Visual Description

    **1.** Initial stage.

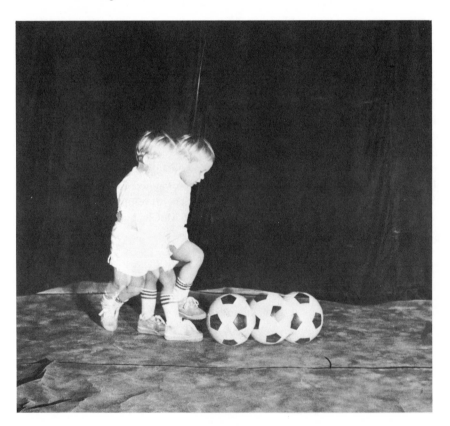

**2.**    Elementary stage.

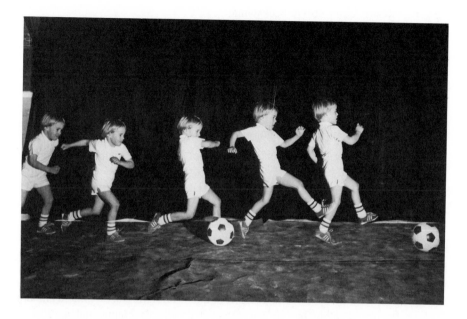

**3.**    Mature stage.

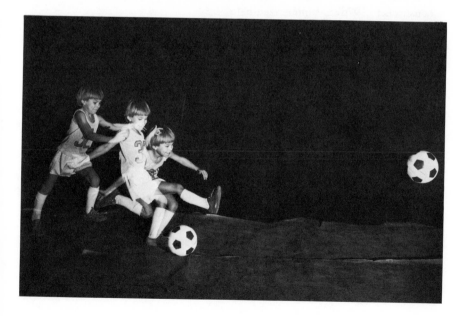

**Common Problems**

1.  Restricted or absent backswing.
2.  Failure to step forward with the nonkicking leg.
3.  Tendency to lose balance.
4.  Inability to kick with either foot.
5.  Inability to alter the speed of the kicked ball.
6.  Jabbing at the ball without any follow-through.
7.  Poor opposition of the arms and legs.
8.  Failure to use a summation of forces by the body to contribute to the force of the kick.
9.  Failure to contact the ball squarely, or missing it completely (eyes not focused on ball).
10. Failure to get adequate distance (lack of follow-through and force production).

## Striking

The first striking movements (other than kicking) appear in young children whenever they hit an object with an implement. Swinging at a ball in flight on a batting tee or on the ground is a familiar act to most children. Only a limited amount of scientific investigation has been conducted on the developmental aspects of striking in children (Deach, 1951; Halverson and Roberton, 1966, Seefeldt and Haubenstricker, 1976). The developmental sequence proposed by Seefeldt and Haubenstricker (1976) is summarized below.

**Developmental Sequence**

1.  Initial stage.
    (a) Motion is from back to front.
    (b) Feet are stationary.
    (c) Trunk faces direction of the tossed ball.
    (d) Elbow(s) fully flexed.
    (e) No trunk rotation.
    (f) Force comes from extension of flexed joints in a downward plane.
2.  Elementary stage.
    (a) Trunk turned to side in anticipation of the tossed ball.
    (b) Weight shifts to forward foot prior to ball contact.
    (c) Combined trunk and hip rotation.
    (d) Elbow(s) flexed at less acute angle.
    (e) Force comes from extension of flexed joints. Trunk rotation and forward movement are in an oblique plane.

**3.** Mature stage.
   **(a)** Trunk turned to side in anticipation of the tossed ball.
   **(b)** Weight shifts to back foot.
   **(c)** Hips rotate.
   **(d)** Transfer of weight is in a contralateral pattern.
   **(e)** Weight shift to the forward foot occurs while the object is still moving backward.
   **(f)** Striking occurs in a long, full arc in a horizontal pattern.
   **(g)** Weight shifts to forward foot at contact.

## Visual Description

**1.** Initial stage.

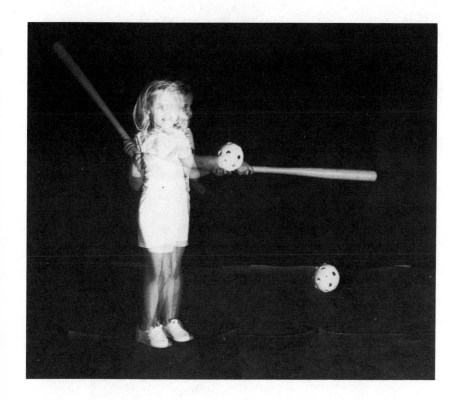

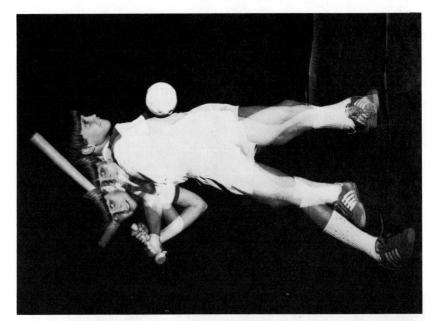

**3.** Mature stage.

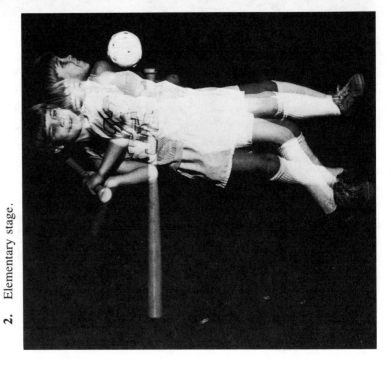

**2.** Elementary stage.

218

## Common Problems

1. Failure to focus on and track the ball.
2. Improper grip.
3. Failure to turn the side of the body in the direction of the intended flight.
4. Inability to sequence the movements in rapid succession in a coordinated manner.
5. Poor backswing.
6. "Chopping" swing.

## Dribbling

Dribbling a ball with one hand is a fundamental movement pattern that has received virtually no attention in the research literature on children. Dribbling is a complicated task requiring precise judgment of distance, force, and trajectory. Good figure-ground and depth perception are also required for efficient dribbling. The following proposed developmental sequence is based on my observational assessment of numerous children and is subject to verification and further refinement.

### Developmental Sequence

1. Initial stage.
   (a) Ball held with both hands.
   (b) Hands placed on sides of the ball, with palms facing each other.
   (c) Downward thrusting action with both arms.
   (d) Ball contacts surface close to body, may contact the foot.
   (e) Great variation in height of the bounce.
   (f) Repeated bounce and catch pattern.
2. Elementary stage.
   (a) Ball held with both hands, one on top and the other near the bottom.
   (b) Slight forward lean, with the ball brought to chest level to begin the action.
   (c) Downward thrust with top hand and arm.
   (d) Force of downward thrust inconsistent.
   (e) Hand slaps at ball for subsequent bounces.
   (f) Wrist flexes and extends and palm of hand contacts ball on each bounce.
   (g) Visually monitors ball.
   (h) Limited control of the ball while dribbling.
3. Mature stage.
   (a) Feet placed in narrow stride position, with foot opposite dribbling hand forward.
   (b) Slight forward trunk lean.
   (c) Ball held waist high.
   (d) Ball pushed toward ground, with follow-through of arm, wrist, and fingers.

(e) Controlled force of downward thrust.
(f) Repeated contact and pushing action initiated from the fingertips.
(g) Visual monitoring not necessary.
(h) Controlled directional dribbling.

## Visual Description

1. Initial stage.

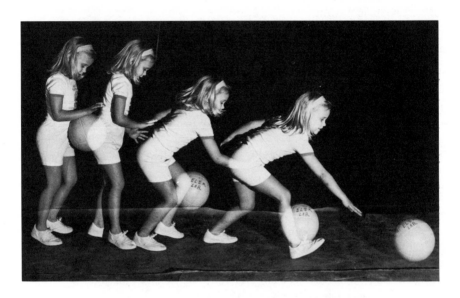

2. Elementary stage.

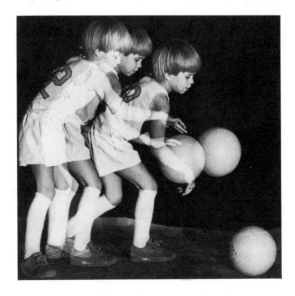

**3.** Mature stage.

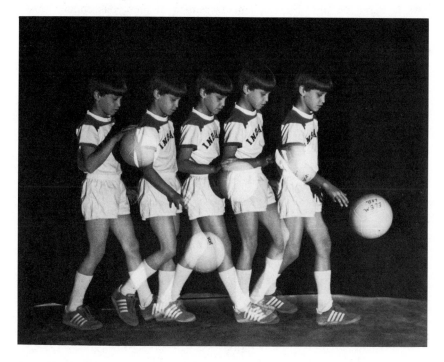

## Common Problems

**1.** Slapping at the ball instead of pushing it downward.

**2.** Inconsistent force applied to the downward thrust.

**3.** Failure to focus on and track the ball efficiently.

**4.** Inability to dribble with both hands.

**5.** Inability to dribble without visually monitoring the ball.

**6.** Insufficient follow-through.

**7.** Inability to move about under control while dribbling.

## Ball Rolling

Rolling an object is another fundamental movement pattern that has not been methodically studied. Ability in rolling a ball has most often been assessed by accuracy in knocking down bowling pins rather than from the standpoint of form. Numerous sport and recreational activities utilize the fundamental patterns found in rolling. Bowling, curling, shuffleboard, and the underhand pitch in softball utilize variations of the pattern found in mature rolling. The developmental sequence that follows is based on my observational assessment of numerous children and is subject to verification and further refinement.

### Developmental Sequence

1. Initial stage.
   (a) Straddle stance.
   (b) Ball is held with hands on the sides, with palms facing each other.
   (c) Acute bend at the waist, with backward pendulum motion of the arms.
   (d) Eyes monitor the ball.
   (e) Forward arm swing and trunk lift with the release of the ball.
2. Elementary stage.
   (a) Stride stance.
   (b) Ball held with one hand on bottom and the other on top.
   (c) Backward arm swing without weight transfer to the rear.
   (d) Limited knee bend.
   (e) Forward swing with limited follow-through.
   (f) Ball release between knee and waist level.
   (g) Eyes alternately monitor target and ball.
3. Mature stage.
   (a) Stride stance.
   (b) Ball held in hand corresponding to trailing leg.
   (c) Slight hip rotation and trunk lean forward.
   (d) Pronounced knee bend.
   (e) Forward swing with weight transference from rear to forward foot.
   (f) Release at knee level or below.
   (g) Eyes are on the target throughout.

### Visual Description

1. Initial stage.

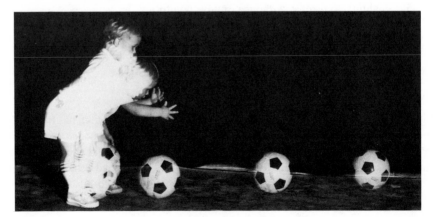

**2.**  Elementary stage.

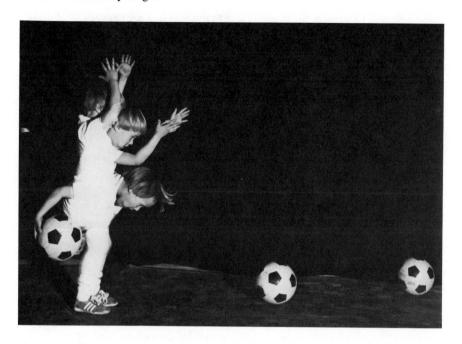

**3.**  Mature stage.

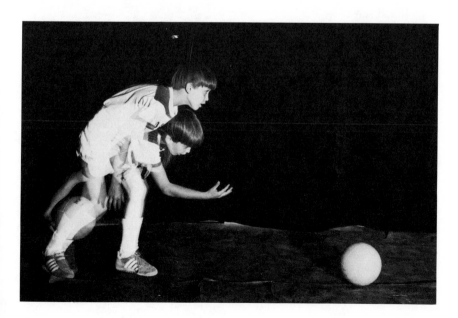

### Common Problems

1. Failure to transfer the body weight to the rear foot during the initial part of the action.
2. Failure to place the controlling hand directly under the ball.
3. Releasing the ball above waist level.
4. Failure to release the ball from a virtual pendular motion, causing it to veer to one side.
5. Lack of follow-through, resulting in a weak roll.
6. Swinging the arms too far backward or out to the side.
7. Failure to keep the eyes on the target.
8. Failure to step forward with the foot opposite the hand that holds the ball.
9. Inability to bring the ball to the side of the body.

## Trapping

Trapping an object is actually a form of catching in which the feet or body is used to absorb the force of the ball instead of the hands and arms. Trapping is a skill that must be highly refined in order to successfully play the game of soccer. With young children, however, trapping should be viewed very generally, that is, as the ability to stop a ball without use of the hands or arms. A developmental sequence for trapping in children follows. It is based on my observational assessment of numerous children and is subject to verification and further refinement.

### Developmental Sequence

1. Initial stage.
   (a) Trunk remains rigid.
   (b) No "give" with the ball as it makes contact.
   (c) Inability to absorb the force of the ball.
   (d) Difficulty getting in line with the object.
2. Elementary stage.
   (a) Poor visual tracking.
   (b) "Gives" with the ball, but movements are poorly timed and sequenced.
   (c) Can trap a rolled ball with relative ease but cannot trap a tossed ball.
   (d) Appears uncertain as to what body part to use.
   (e) Movements lack fluidity.
3. Mature stage.
   (a) Tracks ball throughout.
   (b) "Gives" with the body upon contact.
   (c) Can trap both rolled and tossed balls.
   (d) Can trap balls approaching at a moderate velocity.
   (f) Moves to intercept the ball with ease.

**Visual Sequence**

1. Initial stage.

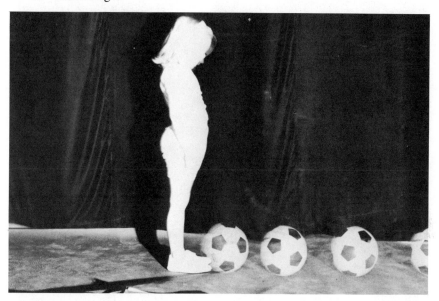

2. Elementary stage.

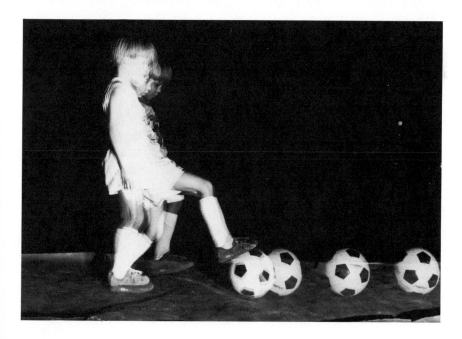

**3.** Mature stage.

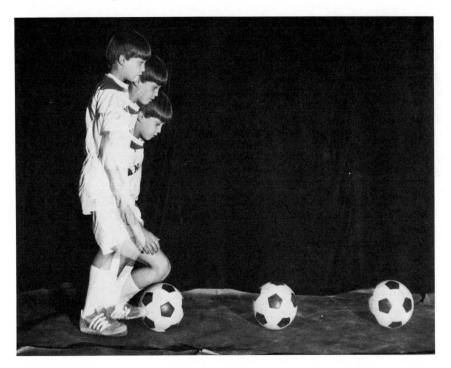

## Common Problems

1. Failure to position the body directly in the path of the ball.
2. Failure to keep the eyes fixed on the ball.
3. Failure to "give" as the ball contacts the body part.
4. Failure to angle an aerial ball downward toward the feet.
5. Causing the body to meet the ball instead of letting the ball meet the body.
6. Inability to maintain body balance when trapping in unusual or awkward positions.

## Volleying

Volleying is a form of striking in which an overhand pattern is used. It is a movement similar to the two-handed set shot that used to be popular in basketball and is similar to the overhead set shot used in power volleyball. The developmental sequence that follows is based on my observation of children and is subject to verification and refinement.

### Developmental Sequence

1. Initial stage.
   (a) Inability to accurately judge the path of the ball or balloon.
   (b) Inability to get under the ball.
   (c) Inability to contact the ball with both hands simultaneously.
2. Elementary stage.
   (a) Failure to visually track the ball.
   (b) Gets under the ball.
   (c) Slaps at the ball.
   (d) Action mainly from the hands and arms.
   (e) Little lift with the legs or follow-through.
   (f) Unable to control the direction or intended flight of the ball.
   (g) Wrists relax and ball often travels backward.
3. Mature stage.
   (a) Gets under the ball.
   (b) Good contact with fingertips.
   (c) Wrists remain stiff and arms follow-through.
   (d) Good summation of forces and utilization of the arms and legs.
   (e) Able to control the direction and intended flight of the ball.

### Visual Sequence

1. Initial stage.

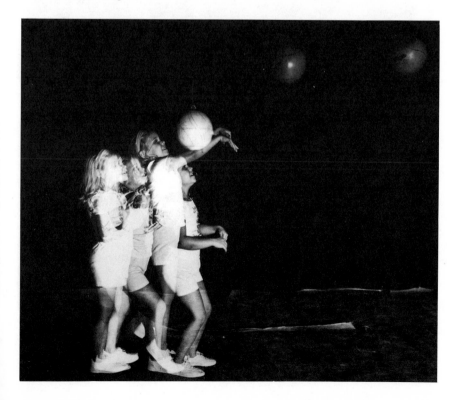

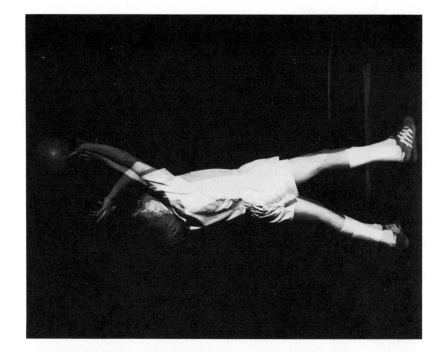

**3.** Mature stage.

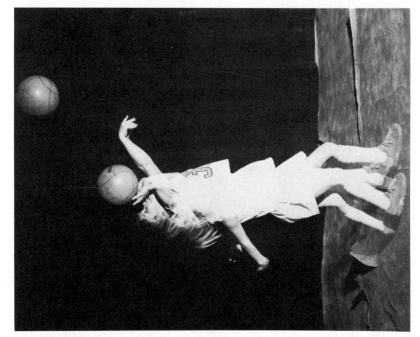

**2.** Elementary stage.

228

## Common Problems

1. Failure to keep the eyes on the ball.
2. Inability to accurately judge the flight of the ball and to properly time the movements of the body.
3. Failure to keep the fingers and wrists stiff.
4. Failure to extend all of the joints upon contacting the ball (lack of follow-through).
5. Inability to contact the ball with both hands simultaneously.
6. Slapping at the ball.
7. Poor positioning of the body under the ball.

## FUNDAMENTAL STABILITY MOVEMENTS

Stability is the most fundamental aspect of learning to move. It is through this dimension that children gain and maintain a point of origin for the explorations that they make in space. Stability involves the ability to maintain one's relationship to the force of gravity. This is true even though the nature of the application of the force may be altered as the requirements of the situation change, causing the general relationship of the body parts to the center of gravity to be altered. Movement experiences designed to enhance children's stability abilities enable them to develop flexibility in postural adjustments as they move in a variety of different and often unusual ways relative to their center of gravity, line of gravity, and base of support.

The ability to sense a shift in the relationship of the body parts that alter one's balance is required for efficient stability along with the ability to compensate rapidly and accurately for these changes with appropriate movements. These compensatory movements should ensure maintenance of balance, but they should not be overcompensating. They should be made only with those parts of the body required for compensation rather than readjusting the entire body to restore balance. Children's stability abilities should be flexible in order that they may make all kinds of movements under all sorts of conditions and still maintain their fundamental relationship to the force of gravity.

It should be noted here that the term stability as used in this text goes beyond the catch-all terms of *nonlocomotor* or *nonmanipulative* movements. The movement category of stability encompasses these terms but further implies maintenance of body control in movements that place a premium on maintaining balance. All movement involves an element of stability when viewed from the balance perspective. Therefore, strictly speaking, all locomotor and manipulative activities are, in part, stability movements. Certain fundamental movements may, however, be separated out from all others that place a premium on the controlled maintenance of equilibrium.

Axial movements and various static and dynamic balance postures are considered here as the major components of stability. Axial, or nonlocomotor, movements are orientation movements of the trunk or limbs while in a static position. Twisting, turning, bending, stretching, and swinging are all axial movements.

Postures are other body positions that place a premium on the maintenance of equilibrium while in a position of static or dynamic balance. Standing, sitting, inverted supports, rolling, stopping, dodging, and landing, as well as beam walking, stick balancing, and one-foot balances, are dynamic or static balance postures.

## Axial Movements

Axial movements are movements of the trunk or limbs that orient the body while it remains in a stationary position. Bending, stretching, twisting, turning, swinging, swaying, reaching, and lifting are axial movements. They are often combined with other movements to create more elaborate movement skills. Skilled performances in diving, gymnastics, figure skating, and modern dance typically incorporate a variety of axial movements along with various locomotor movements. Axial movements are included with a variety or manipulative skills in soccer, baseball, football, and track and field.

Little is known about the developmental sequence of axial movements. To date, no film analysis or observational studies have been conducted with children. The following represents a proposed developmental sequence for axial movements in general. It is based on observation of numerous children and is subject to further verification and refinement.

### Developmental Sequence

1. Initial stage.
   (a) Exaggerated base of support.
   (b) Momentary loss of balance.
   (c) Visual monitoring of the body and a model when possible.
   (d) Combined movements appear jerky and segmented.
   (e) Lack of fluid transition from one level or plane to another.
   (f) Only one action is possible at a time.
2. Elementary stage.
   (a) Good balance.
   (b) Appropriate base of support.
   (c) Requires visual model.
   (d) Does not have to monitor own body.
   (e) Good coordination of similar movements.
   (f) Poor transition in dissimilar movements.
   (g) Can combine two actions into one fluid movement.
3. Mature stage.
   (a) Smooth, rhythmical flow.

**(b)** Sequences several movements with ease.

**(c)** Vision not important.

**(d)** Appears totally in control.

**(e)** Can combine three or more movements into one fluid movement.

## Visual Description

**1.** Initial stage: twisting.

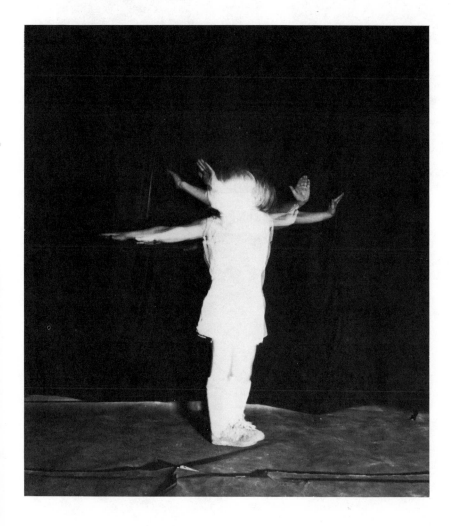

**2.** Elementary stage: stretching and bending.

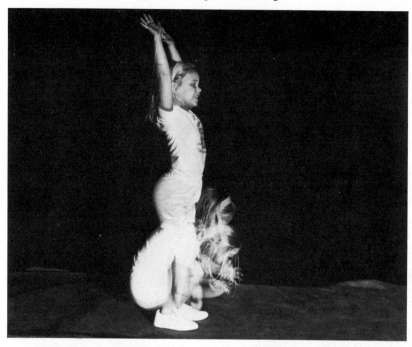

**3.** Mature stage: bending, stretching, and twisting.

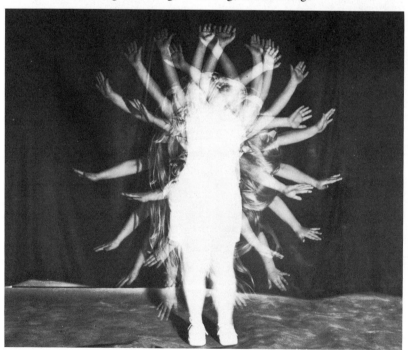

## Common Problems

1. Visually monitoring the body.
2. Visually mimicking a model.
3. Poor rhythmical coordination.
4. Segmented combination of movements.
5. Loss of balance.
6. Lack of smooth transition in the flow of movement.
7. Inability to perform at various tempos.
8. Inability to perform at different levels.

## Inverted Supports

Inverted supports involve postures in which the body assumes an upside-down position for a number of seconds before the movement is discontinued. Stabilization of the center of gravity and maintenance of the line of gravity within the base of support apply to the inverted posture as well as to the erect standing posture. An inverted supporting posture, however, utilizes either the head, hands, forearms, or upper arms (or a combination) as the base of support. The shoulders are above the point of support. The tip-up, tripod, headstand, and handstand are examples of skills that incorporate the fundamental pattern of the inverted support. To date, no developmental studies have been conducted with inverted supports. The following represents a developmental sequence based on my observation of numerous children, and is subject to verification and refinement.*

### Developmental Sequence

1. Initial stage.
   (a) Not able to maintain triangular three-point position.
   (b) Unable to assume any inverted three-point posture for one second or more.
   (c) Poor kinesthetic feel for unseen body parts.
   (d) Little coordinated control of movements.
2. Elementary stage.
   (a) Can maintain triangular three-point contact with surface.
   (b) Able to hold balance for two or three seconds, with frequent brief addition of fourth balance point.
   (c) Gradual improvement in monitoring of unseen body parts.
3. Mature stage.
   (a) Good surface contact position.
   (b) Good control of head and neck.
   (c) Good kinesthetic feel for body part location.

---

*Inverted postures requiring the head to serve as a balance point are not recommended for children prior to attainment of adequate muscle development in the neck (generally 4 years of age and older).

**(d)** Appears to be in good control of the body.

**(e)** Maintains an inverted three-point balance position for three or more seconds.

**(f)** Comes out of the static posture under control.

## Visual Description

1. Initial stage.

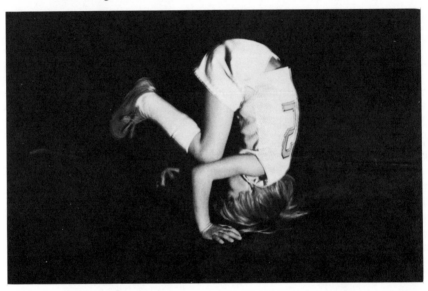

2. Elementary stage.

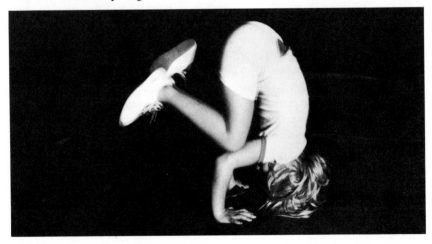

**3.** Mature stage.

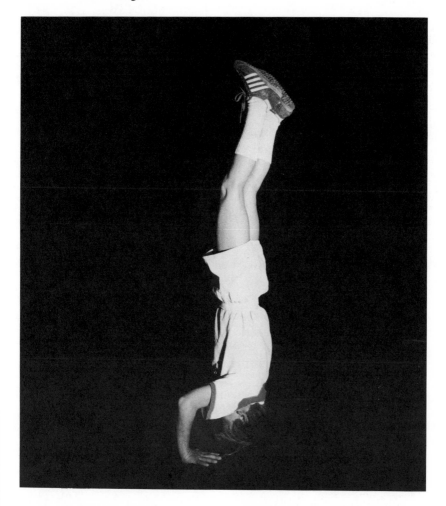

## Common Problems

1. Inability to accurately sense the location and position of body parts that are not visually monitored.
2. Inability to keep the line of gravity within the base of support.
3. Inadequate or exaggerated base of support.
4. Overbalancing by shifting the body's weight too far forward.

## Body Rolling

Body rolling postures, although actually locomotor in nature, require inordinate amounts of control of one's balance. Considerable disturbance of the fluid in the semicircular canals results from rolling actions. Therefore, they are regarded as fundamental stability movements. Body rolling movements may involve rolling forward, sideways, or backward. In each, the body is momentarily inverted and must maintain positional control as it travels through space. The sport skills of the forward and backward somersault are elaborations of the fundamental forward and backward rolling patterns. Walkovers and handsprings are sophisticated combinations of rolling patterns combined with transitional inverted supports.

Developmental studies of body rolling are not available. The following proposed sequence is based on my observation of children, and will require further verification and refinement.

### Developmental Sequence

1. Initial stage.
   (a) Head contacts surface.
   (b) Body curled in loose C position.
   (c) Inability to coordinate use of the arms.
   (d) Cannot get over backward or sideways.
   (e) Uncurls to L position after rolling forward.
2. Elementary stage.
   (a) After rolling forward, actions appear segmented.
   (b) Head leads action instead of inhibiting it.
   (c) Top of the head still touches the surface.
   (d) Body curled in tight C position at onset of roll.
   (e) Uncurls at completion of roll to a L position.
   (f) Hands and arms aid rolling action somewhat but supply little push-off.
   (g) Can perform only one roll at a time.
   (h) Back of head lightly touches surface.
3. Mature stage.
   (a) Head leads the action.
   (b) The head touches the surface very lightly.
   (c) Body remains in tight C throughout.
   (d) Arms aid in force production.
   (e) Momentum returns child to starting position.
   (f) Can perform consecutive rolls in control.

## Visual Description

**1.** Initial stage.

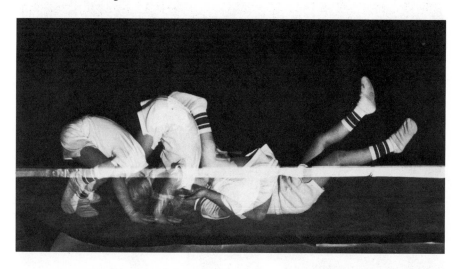

**2.** Elementary stage.

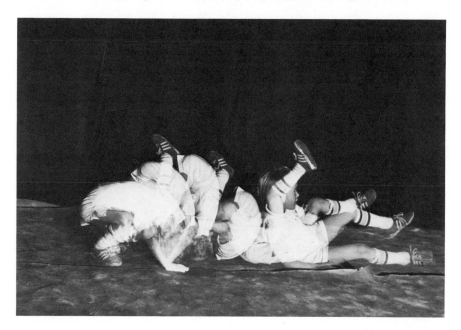

3. Mature stage.

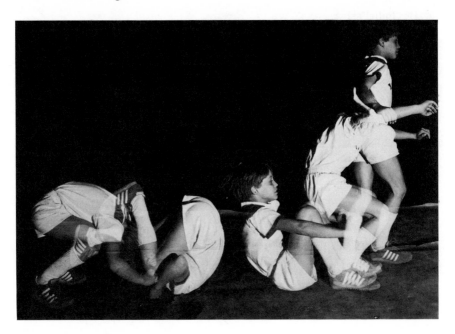

## Common Problems

1. Head forcefully touching surface.
2. Failure to curl body tightly.
3. Inability to push off with the arms.
4. Pushing off with one arm.
5. Failure to remain in tucked position.
6. Inability to perform consecutive rolls.
7. Feeling dizzy.
8. Failure to roll in a straight line.
9. Lack of sufficient momentum to complete one revolution.

## Dodging

Dodging is a fundamental stability pattern of movement that combines the locomotor movements of sliding with rapid changes in direction. Dodging involves rapid shifts in direction from side to side and requires good reaction time and speed of movement. Extensive developmental studies of dodging have not been conducted with children. Observational assessment of children does, however, provide the basis for the following sequence.

**Developmental Sequence**

1. Initial stage.
   (a) Segmented movements.
   (b) Body appears stiff.
   (c) Little knee bend.
   (d) Weight is on one foot.
   (e) Feet generally cross.
   (f) No deception.
2. Elementary stage.
   (a) Movements coordinated but little deception.
   (b) Performs better to one side than to the other.
   (c) Too much vertical lift.
   (d) Feet occasionally cross.
   (e) Little spring in movement.
   (f) Sometimes "outsmarts" self and becomes confused.
3. Mature stage.
   (a) Knees bent, slight trunk lean forward (ready position).
   (b) Fluid directional changes.
   (c) Performs equally well in all directions.
   (d) Head and shoulder fake.
   (e) Good lateral movement.

**Visual Description**

1. Initial stage.

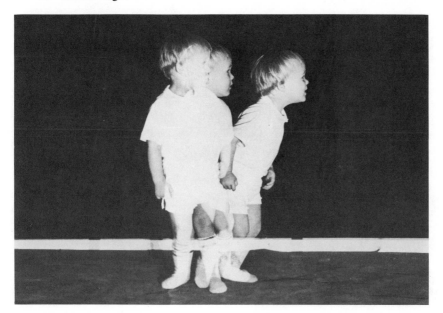

**2.** Elementary stage.

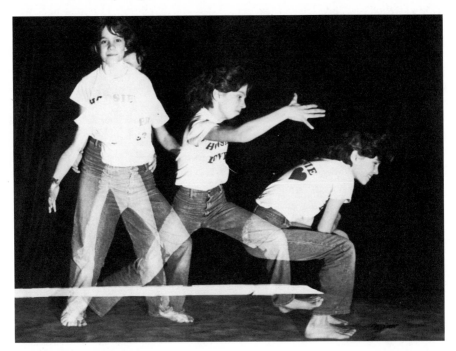

**3.** Mature stage.

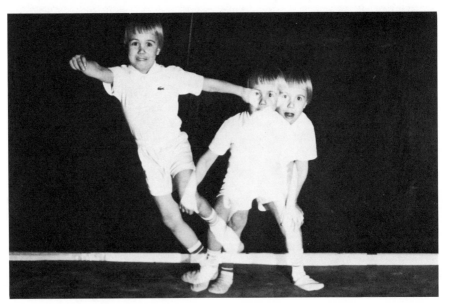

## Common Problems

1. Inability to shift the body weight in a fluid manner in the direction of the dodge.
2. Slow change of direction.
3. Crossing feet.
4. Hesitation.
5. Too much vertical lift.
6. Total body lead.
7. Inability to perform several dodging actions in rapid succession.
8. Monitoring body.
9. Rigid posture.

## One-Foot Balance

The one-foot balance is probably the most common measure of static balance ability. Several investigators have studied the one-foot balance with the eyes open or closed and the arms at the sides, folded, or on the hips (Cratty, 1979; De Oreo, 1971, 1980; Eckert and Rarick, 1975). Performance trends for balancing on one foot are reported in Chapter 13. The following appears to be the developmental sequence gleaned from these performance investigations, but it is subject to verification and refinement.

### Developmental Sequence

1. Initial stage.
    (a) Raises nonsupporting leg several inches so that thigh is nearly parallel with contact surface.
    (b) Either in or out of balance (no in between).
    (c) Overcompensates ("windmill" arms).
    (d) Inconsistent leg preference.
    (e) Balances with outside support.
    (f) Only momentary balance without support.
    (g) Eyes directed at feet.
2. Elementary stage.
    (a) May lift nonsupporting leg to a "tied-in" position on support leg.
    (b) Cannot balance with eyes closed.
    (c) Uses arms for balance but may "tie" one arm to the side of the body.
    (d) Performs better on dominant leg to a free position, by bending at the knee.
3. Mature stage.
    (a) Can balance with the eyes closed.
    (b) Uses arms and trunk as needed to maintain balance.
    (c) Lifts nonsupporting leg.

**(d)** Focuses on external object while balancing.

**(e)** Changes to nondominant leg without loss of balance.

**Visual Description**

1. Initial stage.

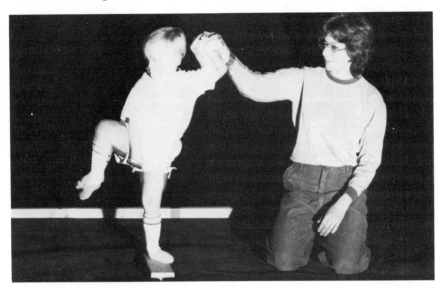

2. Elementary stage.

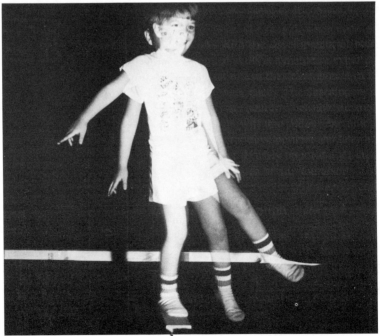

**3.** Mature stage.

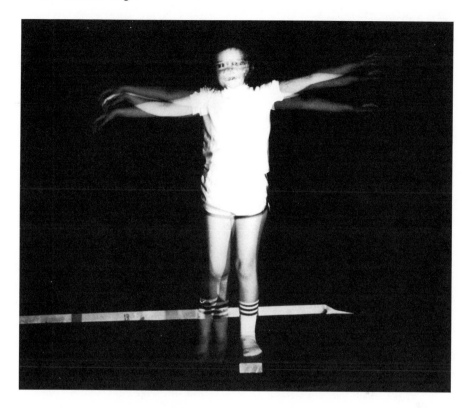

## Common Problems

1. "Tying" one arm to the side.
2. No compensating movements.
3. Inappropriate compensation of the arms.
4. Inability to use one or the other leg.
5. Inability to vary body position with control.
6. Inability to balance while holding objects.
7. Visually monitoring the support leg.
8. Overdependence on outside support.

## Beam Walk

The beam walk is the most frequently measured fundamental dynamic balance ability. A variety of investigations have been conducted, using walking boards that vary in length, width, and height from the supporting surface (De Oreo, 1971, 1980; Goetzinger, 1961; Seashore, 1949). Considerable information concerning the performance abilities of children from year to year is available (see Chapter 13), but little is known about the developmental sequence of the beam walking process itself. The following developmental sequence is based on my observational assessment of numerous children and is subject to refinement and verification.

### Developmental Sequence

1.  Initial stage.
    (a)  Balances with support.
    (b)  Walks forward while holding on to a spotter for support.
    (c)  Uses follow-step with dominant foot lead.
    (d)  Eyes focus on feet.
    (e)  Body rigid.
    (f)  No compensating movements.
2.  Elementary stage.
    (a)  Can walk a 2-in. beam but not a 1-in. beam.
    (b)  Uses a follow-step with dominant foot leading.
    (c)  Eyes focus on beam.
    (d)  May press one arm to the trunk while trying to balance with the other.
    (e)  Loses balance easily.
    (f)  Limited compensating movements.
    (g)  Can move forward, backward, and sideways but requires considerable concentration and effort.
3.  Mature stage.
    (a)  Can walk a 1-in. beam.
    (b)  Uses alternate stepping action.
    (c)  Eyes focus beyond the beam.
    (d)  Both arms used at will to aid balance.
    (e)  Can move forward, backward, and sideways with assurance and ease.
    (f)  Movements are fluid, relaxed, and in control.
    (g)  May lose balance occasionally.

**Visual Description**

1. Initial stage.

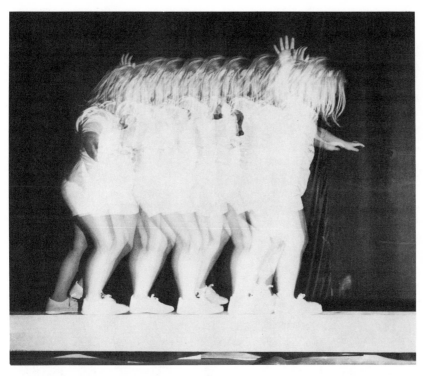

2. Elementary stage.

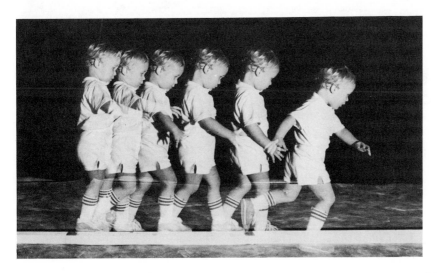

**3.** Mature stage.

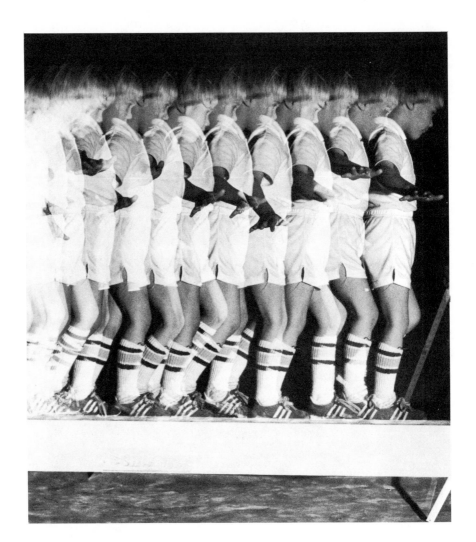

## Common Problems

1. Overdependence on spotter.
2. Visually monitors stepping leg.
3. "Tying" one arm in.
4. Rigid, hesitant movement.
5. Failure to actually negotiate the problem of balance.

**6.** Inability to perform without holding on to a spotter.

**7.** Poor rhythmical coordination of both sides of the body.

**8.** Overcompensating for loss of balance.

## DEVELOPMENTAL DIFFERENCES

When observing and analyzing the fundamental movement abilities of young children, it soon becomes apparent that there are various stages of development for each pattern of movement. It should also be obvious that differences in abilities exist between children, between patterns, and within patterns (McClenaghan and Gallahue, 1978a).

*Between children differences* should remind us of the principle of individuality in all learning. The sequence of progression through the initial, elementary, and mature stages is the same for most children. The rate, however, will vary, depending on both environmental and hereditary factors. Whether or not a child reaches the mature stage depends primarily on instruction, encouragement, and opportunities for practice. When these are absent, normal differences between children will be magnified.

*Differences between patterns* are seen in all children. A child may be at the initial stage in some, the elementary in other, and the mature in still others. Children do not progress at an even rate in the development of their fundamental movement abilities. Play and instructional experiences will greatly influence the rate of development of locomotor, manipulative, and stability abilities.

*Differences within patterns* are an interesting and often curious phenomenon. Within a given pattern, a child may exhibit a combination of initial, elementary, and mature elements. For example, in the throw, the arm action may be at the elementary stage, while the leg action is at the mature stage and the trunk action at the initial stage. Developmental differences within patterns are common and usually the result of: (1) incomplete modeling of the movements of others; (2) initial success with the inappropriate action; (3) failure to require an all-out effort; (4) inappropriate or restricted learning opportunities; or (5) incomplete sensorimotor integration.

Creative, diagnostic teaching can do much to aid the child in the balanced development of his or her fundamental movement abilities. Observational assessment of the child's movement abilities will enable the teacher to plan experiences and instructional strategies that will help the child develop mature patterns of movement. Once movement control has been established, these mature patterns may be further refined in terms of force production and accuracy in the sport-related movement phase. Failure to achieve proficiency in a wide variety of fundamental movement abilities will act as a barrier to the development of efficient and effective movement skills that may be applied to game, sport, and dance activities that are characteristic of the child's culture.

**Summary**

The fundamental movement pattern phase of development follows a sequential progression. The normal child, under optimal circumstances, will progress through the initial, elementary, and mature stages in a sequential manner. Developmental sequences for several fundamental movements have been identified through biomechanical assessment of children at different age levels. Developmental sequences have also been proposed, based on film, video tape, and observational assessment of numerous children. The question that should come to mind is: what effect does instruction have on attaining increasingly mature patterns of movement? In other words, is the increase in fundamental movement abilities due solely to maturation or do other factors play an important role? Miller (1978) investigated the facilitation of fundamental motor skill learning in children 3 to 5 years of age. She found that programs of instruction can increase fundamental movement pattern development beyond the level attained solely through maturation. She also found that an instructional program in skill development was more effective than a free-play program and that parents working under the direction of a physical education specialist can be as effective as physical education teachers alone in developing fundamental movement abilities in young children. Luedke (1980) found similar results, utilizing two different methods of instruction for the mature stage of throwing with fourth-grade boys and girls. Both instructional groups were more proficient in terms of form and performance, than a noninstructed control group. The results of these and other investigations indicate that the fundamental movement phase of development is greatly influenced by environmental factors. Success at higher skill levels will be directly influenced by the degree to which the child develops his or her fundamental movement abilities.

## CHAPTER HIGHLIGHTS

1. Classification of fundamental movements into initial, elementary, and mature stages is only one way of classifying basic movement.
2. Provided that there is ample opportunity, instruction, and encouragement, children are capable of achieving the mature stage of most fundamental motor skills by age 6.
3. Fundamental movements should be sufficiently flexible so that they can be altered as the requirements of the environment demand without deflecting attention from the purpose of the movement.
4. Fundamental movements may be dealt with in isolation or in combination with a variety of other movements.
5. Locomotor movements involve activities in which the body is projected in a vertical, horizontal, or diagonal plane relative to a fixed point on the ground.
6. Manipulative movements involve activities in which force is given to objects, or force is received from objects.

7. Manipulative movements may be classified as either propulsive or absorptive.
8. The ability to impart force to objects and receive force from objects enables the individual to come into meaningful physical contact with the environment.
9. Effective manipulation of objects requires considerable coordination of both sensory and motor systems of the body.
10. Attention to form, accuracy, or distance in the performance of movements will alter the parts of the particular action.
11. Stability is the most fundamental aspect of learning to move, because all movement involves an element of stability.
12. Axial movements involve movement of the limbs or trunk while the body remains in a static position.
13. Efficient performance of a variety of axial movements is basic to efficient performance of a number of games, sports, and rhythmic activities.
14. Stability movements place a premium on the maintenance of equilibrium while the body is in either a static or dynamic position.
15. Static balance refers to positions in which the body is required to maintain stability while the center of gravity remains fixed.
16. Static balance involves both upright and inverted body positions.
17. Dynamic balance refers to positions of the body in which the individual is required to maintain stability while the center of gravity is constantly shifting.
18. Numerous differences can be observed between children, between patterns, and within patterns in the performance of fundamental movement abilities.

## CRITICAL READINGS

Cooper J.M., M. Adrian, and R.B. Glassow: *Kinesiology,* St. Louis; Mosby, 1982, Chapters 8, 9, 17.

McClenaghan, B.A., and D.L. Gallahue: *Fundamental Movement: A Developmental and Remedial Approach,* Philadelphia: W.B. Saunders, 1978, Chapter 6.

Roberton, M.A.: "Stages in Motor Development," in M.V. Ridenour (ed.), *Motor Development, Issues and Applications,* Princeton, N.J.: Princeton, 1978.

Wickstrom, R.L.: *Fundamental Motor Patterns,* Philadelphia: Lea and Febiger, 1977, Chapters 3−8.

# CHAPTER 12

# Sport-Related Movement

Sport-related movement skills are merely mature fundamental movement patterns that have been further refined and combined with one another to form sport skills. Sport-related movement skills are task specific; but fundamental movements are not.

Most children should be *developmentally ready* to perform at the mature stage in virtually all fundamental movement patterns by age 6 and to begin the transition to the sport phase of motor development. However, many lag behind in their movement capabilities simply because of poor or absent instruction, little or no encouragement, and a general lack of opportunity for regular practice. We are all familiar with adults who throw a ball at the elementary stage or jump for distance using the pattern of movement characteristic of the 2- or 3-year-old child. We can logically expect the young child to perform at less than the mature level. It is not logical, however, for the older child, the adolescent, or the adult to perform fundamental movements at less than the mature level. Failure to develop mature forms of fundamental movement will have direct consequences on the individual's ability to perform task-specific skills at the sport-related movement phase. Progress through the general, specific, and specialized sport skill stages in a particular movement task is dependent on mature levels of performance at the fundamental movement pattern phase (Figure 12.1). For example, one could hardly expect to be successful in the game of softball if one's fundamental striking, throwing, catching, or running abilities were not at the mature level. There is a definite "proficiency

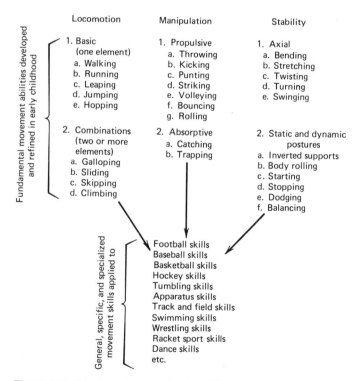

**Figure 12.1.** Fundamental movement abilities must be developed and refined prior to the introduction of sport and dance skills.

barrier'' (Seefeldt, 1980) between the fundamental movement pattern phase and the sport-related movement phase of development. The transition from one phase to another depends on mature patterns of movement being applied to a wide variety of general movement skills. If the patterns are less than mature, ability will, by necessity, be adversely affected.

This chapter focuses on the sport-related movement skill phase of development. Two important points should be kept in mind. First, even though the child may be cognitively and affectively ready to advance to this phase, advancement depends on successful completion specific aspects of the previous phase. Second, from one phase to another is not an all-or-none proposition. One is not required to be at the mature stage in all fundamental movements prior to advancing to subsequent stages. The 12-year-old, for example, who specialized early in gymnastics may be performing at a highly sophisticated level in several locomotor and stability movements and at the same time not be able to throw, catch, or kick a ball with the proficiency expected for his or her age and developmental level.

## DEVELOPMENTAL SEQUENCE OF SPORT-RELATED MOVEMENTS

After the child has achieved the mature stage in a particular fundamental movement pattern, little change occurs in the *form* of that movement ability during the sport-related movement phase. Refinement of the pattern and stylistic variations in form occur as greater skill (precision, accuracy, and control) is achieved, but the basic pattern remains unchanged (Wickstrom, 1977). However, dramatic changes in the performance level based primarily on increased physical abilities may be seen from year to year. As the child improves in strength, endurance, reaction time, speed of movement, coordination, and so forth, we can expect to see improved performance scores. Chapter 13 provides detailed discussion and comparison of physical abilities and the performance scores of children during childhood.

Within the sport skill phase, there are three separate but often overlapping stages. The onset of stages (general, specific, and specialized) during this phase of development depends on cognitive and affective factors within the child as well as neuromuscular factors. Factors *within* the individual and conditions within the environment stimulate the child to move from one stage to another.

One's fundamental movement patterns are little changed after reaching the mature stage, and physical abilities influence only the extent to which one's sport-related movement abilities are acted out in recreational or competitive situations. Therefore, *sport-related movement skills are mature fundamental movements that have been adapted to the specific requirements of a sport, game, or dance activity.* The extent to which these abilities are developed depends on a combination of factors. The three stages within the sport-related movement phase are outlined here.

*General stage.* This stage is characterized by the individual's first attempt to refine and combine mature movement patterns. There is heightened interest in sport, in pitting one's developing abilities against others', and in standards of performance and the skills of others. The child is interested in all sports and does not feel limited by physiological, anatomical, or environmental factors. Stress *begins* to be placed on accuracy and skill in the performance of games, lead-up activities, and a wide variety of sport-related movements. During this stage the individual works at "getting the idea" of how to perform the sport skill. Skill and proficiency are limited.

*Specific Stage.* During this stage the individual becomes aware of physical assets and limitations The individual begins to narrow his or her focus from all sports to certain types of sports. Stress is now placed on developing higher levels of proficiency. During this stage *practice* is the key to developing higher degrees of skill. The movement patterns characteristic of the beginner during the previous stage smooth out. More complex skills are refined and begin to be utilized in official sports for recreation and competition.

*Specialized Stage.* This stage is characterized by the individual's further limiting the scope of participation to a few activities that are engaged in frequently over a period of years. Further specialization and skill refinement occur here. Lifetime activities are chosen on the basis of abilities, ambitions, availability, and past experiences. Activity limitation is brought about by increased responsibilities and time demands. This is the "fine-tuning" stage. During this period the individual's performance is highly refined. Performance appears to be automatic, is highly reliable, and approaches the limits of the individual's capabilities.

It should be recognized that many individuals do not go through the development and refinement of sport-related movement skills in the sequence presented above. Children are often encouraged to refine the specialized skills involved in a particular sport at an early age. Early participation in sports is not detrimental, but too often this quest for specialization is done at the expense of the development of mature fundamental movement patterns and general movement skills in many forms of movement. Specialized skill development can be of value *if* it is not done at the expense of, or in the place of, a quality physical education program. It should only supplement the regular program in the form of after-school instruction or youth sport competition. If we as educators are aware of the importance of learning to move, and understand the developmental characteristics of children, we must reject the notion that *specialized* skill development is one of the purposes of the elementary school physical education program.

## GENERAL AND SPECIFIC MOVEMENT SKILLS

Under ideal conditions the general movement skill stage (i.e., the application of a wide variety of mature fundamental movement abilities) begins around age 7 or 8. The child's growing interest in his or her performance capabilities and sport, coupled with increasing cognitive sophistication and improved group interaction, tends to cause a surge of interest in being involved in organized competition. The growth in youth sport participation over the past fifteen years has been phenomenal. A 1975 survey estimated the number of participants in nonschool-sponsored youth sports at about 20 million (Athletic Institute, 1975). A recent study in Michigan revealed that every community in the sample group provided some form of competitive activity for children (Seefeldt and Gould, 1980). In fact, one would be hard pressed to find any sizable community in North America today that does not provide competitive sport experiences for its children through some form of nonschool-sponsored program. Youth sport is big, it is popular, and it is here to stay.

Youth sport can have detrimental as well as beneficial effects on children, all of which have been fully discussed in recent years. Youth sport provides an avenue for the child at the general or specific movement skill stage to further develop his or her abilities, get plenty of vigorous physical activity, and test developing skills against others in competitive situations. Competitive youth sport, however, should not be thought of as the only skill outlet for children. Participation in noncompetitive and leisure-time activity forms of cooperative recreation and dance also provides activity avenues for the child. Activities such as hiking, canoeing, fishing, jogging, new games, and the like, are alternative activities that can be enjoyed by children.

Tables 12.1 through 12.9 provide an overview of several sport-related skills and the various fundamental locomotor, manipulative, and stability movements that are involved in the performance of these activities.

## FOSTERING IMPROVEMENT*

By the third grade most children are beginning to develop *general* and *specific* movement skills. The emphasis on general and specific movement skills at this time results from the increase in the child's performance level potential. Both the children and the teacher are becoming more concerned with the degree of skill, accuracy, and form that is used in performing a movement. Student needs are the general concepts upon which teachers formulate their purposes for teaching. Probably the foremost concept is that the teacher's purpose is to help children *improve*. If teachers are concerned with children's improvement, they are aware of children's developmental needs and developmental potentials. By condensing the factual knowledge of developmental needs and developmental potentials into the operational goal of improvement, teachers do not get bogged down with where the children should be theoretically. The danger with these theoretical concerns is that

*A special thank you is extended to George Luedke, Southern Illinois University, Edwardsville, for his insightful contributions to this section.

**Table 12.1   Basketball Skills**

| Fundamental Movements | Related Sport Skill Movements | |
|---|---|---|
| **Manipulation** | | |
| Passing | Chest pass | Shovel pass |
| | Overhead pass | Push pass |
| | Baseball pass | |
| Shooting | Lay-up shot | Jump shot |
| | Two-hand set shot | |
| Bouncing | Stationary dribbling | Bounce pass |
| | Moving dribbling | |
| Catching | Pass above the waist | Rebounding |
| | Pass below the waist | Pass to the side |
| | | Jump ball reception |
| Volleying | Tipping | |
| | Center jump | |
| **Locomotion** | | |
| Running | In different directions while dribbling | |
| | In different directions without ball | |
| Sliding | Guarding while dribbling | |
| Leaping | Lay-up shot | |
| | Pass interception | |
| Jumping | Center jump | Rebounding |
| | Tip-in | Catching a high ball |
| **Stability** | | |
| Axial movements | Pivoting | |
| | Bending | |
| Dynamic balance | Compensation for rapid changes in direction, speed, and level of movement | |
| Dodging | Feinting with the ball | |

teachers will teach "theoretical" children rather than "real" children. The operational goal of improvement helps teachers to see children realistically at whatever level they are performing. The teachers' function then becomes one of evaluating and directing the learning experiences in order to bring about new successes for children.

The operational goal of improvement encompasses three other concepts that guide teachers in reaching this goal. The first of these concepts is *movement*

**Table 12.2  Contemporary Dance Skills**

| Fundamental Movements | Related Sport Skill Movements |
| --- | --- |
| **Locomotion** | |
| Walking | "Contemporary dance is an art form which utilizes a |
| Running | movement vocabulary specific to the particular |
| Leaping | creative effort being expressed. The choreographer |
| Jumping | utilizes movement as a vehicle of expression. |
| Hopping | Therefore, fundamental locomotor and stability |
| Galloping | movements serve as the means for conveying |
| Sliding | concepts and ideas."[a] |
| Skipping | |
| | |
| **Stability** | |
| Axial movements | bending, stretching, twisting, turning, reaching, lifting, falling, curling, pushing, pulling |
| Static and dynamic balance | Numerous balance skills requiring synchronizing rhythm and proper sequencing of movement |

[a]Personal communication from Fran Snygg, Associate Professor of Dance, Indiana University, December 16, 1980.

*control.* Here teachers are cognizant of the three categories of movement (stability, locomotion, and manipulation) and the Phases of Motor Development. Teachers are also aware of the need for variation and that learning moves from the general to the specific. By condensing this information into the concept of movement control, teachers again have a basis for analyzing their teaching effectiveness in this area of the child's growth and improvement.

The second concept under the goal of improvement is *emotional control.* Here teachers are concerned with children's understanding of themselves and others. Teachers rely heavily on their abilities to communicate with children and to teach them communication skills. These communication skills include discipline as well as experiences through which children can develop responsibility and self-control. The concept of emotional control gives teachers a guide for evaluating past experiences and designing new experiences.

The third and final concept is *learning enjoyment.* This concept also gives teachers a guide for evaluating and implementing their programs with children's improvement in mind. The objective here is for teachers to develop an eagerness to learn within each child. Success-oriented experiences and opportunities to receive praise and recognition reinforce the child's view of learning. By making the development of learning skills enjoyable, teachers hope to foster intrinsic motivation within the child.

The overall goal of improvement, with its three emphases of (1) movement control, (2) emotional control, and (3) learning enjoyment, gives teachers a compact philosophical construct that can serve as an operational guide to teaching action.

**Table 12.3 Football Skills**

| Fundamental Movements | Related Sport Skill Movements | |
|---|---|---|
| **Manipulation** | | |
| Throwing | Forward pass | Lateral |
| | Centering | |
| Kicking | Place kick | Field-goal kicking |
| | Punting | |
| Catching | Pass above the waist | Over the shoulder |
| | Pass below the waist | Across the midline |
| | Pass at waist level | Hand-off |
| Carrying | Fullback carry | |
| | One-arm carry | |
| **Locomotion** | | |
| Running | Ball carrying | |
| | Pursuit of ball carrier | |
| Sliding | Tackling | Blocking |
| Leaping and | Pass defense | |
| jumping | Pass reception | |
| **Stability** | | |
| Axial movements | Blocking | |
| | Tackling | |
| Static and dynamic | Blocking | Rolling |
| balance | Stances | Pushing |
| | Dodging a tackle | |

This construct can and should be modified by the teachers. Its purpose is not to limit teachers, but to provide operational guidelines to assure that their teaching is meaningful to children. Every teacher must rely on some sort of philosophical construct in the teaching situation. Teachers, for example, who have been teaching a number of years in a particular school system have no doubt developed a program designed to meet the students' needs. Because they understand *their* students' needs and potentialities, they have certain performance expectations for them. If these teachers were to take new teaching positions in other schools, they might temporarily lose their perspective of what they could expect of their new students. If they did not rely on a philosophical construct, there would be a good chance that they would impose performance expectations on their new students that were based on their knowledge of their former students. The purpose of the suggested

**Table 12.4   Softball/Baseball Skills**

| Fundamental Movements | Related Sport Skill Movements | |
|---|---|---|
| **Manipulation** | | |
| Throwing | Overhand throw for accuracy | |
| | Overhand throw for distance | |
| | Underhand toss | |
| | Overhand pitching | |
| | Underhand pitching | |
| Catching | Above-waist ball | Grounder |
| | Below-waist ball | Across midline |
| | Fly ball | Line drive |
| Striking | Batting | |
| | Bunting | |
| **Locomotion** | | |
| Running | Base running | |
| | Fielding | |
| Sliding | Fielding | |
| | Base sliding | |
| Leaping | Base running | Fielding |
| Jumping | Fielding | |
| **Stability** | | |
| Axial movements | Batting | |
| | Fielding | |
| | Pitching | |
| Dynamic balance | Compensation for rapid changes in direction, speed, and level of movement | |

philosophical construct is to give teachers a basis for keeping their teaching realistic, practical, and meaningful to the children.

**Summary**

The refinement of sport skill abilities may be viewed as occurring in three stages. In the general, or transitional, sport skill stage, it is crucial that a smooth transition be made from the mature fundamental movement pattern to corresponding sport skills. This transition will be hampered if the individual has not developed the mature pattern of movement necessary for performance of the sport skill. The teacher/coach must be alert to the proficiency with which the individual executes a

**Table 12.5   Soccer Skills**

| Fundamental Movements | Related Sport Skill Movements | |
|---|---|---|
| **Manipulation** | | |
| Kicking | Instep kick | Inside of foot kick |
| | Toe kick | Outside of foot kick |
| | Heel kick | Dribbling |
| | Corner kick | Passing |
| | Goal kick | Goalie punt |
| Striking | Heading | |
| | Juggling | |
| Catching | Goalie skills | |
| Throwing | Throw-in | |
| | Goalie throw | |
| Trapping | Sole trap | |
| | Double-knee trap | |
| | Stomach trap | |
| | Single-knee trap | |
| | Chest trap | |
| **Locomotion** | | |
| Running | With ball | |
| | Without ball | |
| Jumping and leaping | Heading | |
| Sliding | Marking | |
| **Stability** | | |
| Axial movements | Goalie skills | |
| | Field play skills | |
| Dynamic balance | Tackling | |
| | Dodging opponent | |
| | Feinting with ball | |

sport skill and not give in to the temptation of ignoring immature form as long as the outcome is satisfactory. All too often the teacher/coach focuses on the product rather than on the process, as evidenced by whether the ball goes through the hoop, or the batter gets on base, even if immature patterns of basket shooting or batting are used. There is no legitimate reason for not using the mature, mechanically correct, pattern in the performance of a sport skill. Use of a mature pattern of movement will, in the long run, enhance motor skill performance. However, once the mature level has been achieved, has become relatively automatic, and has been applied to

**Table 12.6   Track and Field Skills**

| *Fundamental Movements* | *Related Sport Skill Movements* | |
|---|---|---|
| **Manipulation** | | |
| Throwing | Shotput | Hammer |
| | Discus | |
| | Javelin | |
| | | |
| **Locomotion** | | |
| Running | Dashes | Pole-vault approach |
| | Middle distances | High-jump approach |
| | Long distances | Long-jump approach |
| | | |
| Leaping | Low hurdles | Running long-jump takeoff |
| | High hurdles | Pole-vault takeoff |
| | | |
| Jumping | High jump | |
| | Long jump | |
| | | |
| Vertical jump | High jump | |
| **Stability** | | |
| Axial movements | Pivoting and twisting (shotput, discus, javelin, and hammer) | |
| | | |
| Dynamic balance | Compensation for rapid changes in speed, direction, and level of movement | |

numerous sport-related situations, it is entirely appropriate to encourage unique individual variations in execution of the skill. The individual who does so is now at the specific movement skill stage.

At the specific movement skill stage, attention is focused on greater degrees of precision, accuracy, and control. Performance scores generally improve at a rapid rate, and the individual is cognitively more completely aware of the specific advantages and limitations of his or her body. The individual at this level is also influenced by a variety of social, cultural, and psychological factors in the selection and continued involvement in specific sport, dance, and recreational activities. The specialized movement skill stage is a continuation and further refinement of the previous stage. It is the pinnacle of the phases and stages of motor development. Specialized movement skills are closely aligned to the lifetime sport and recreational activities in which we all choose to actively take part. Failure to develop and refine the fundamental and sport skill abilities of the previous stages will have a negative effect on one's reaching this stage.

**Table 12.7   Racket Sport Skills**

| Fundamental Movements | Related Sport Skill Movements | |
|---|---|---|
| **Manipulation** | | |
| Striking | Forehand shot | Lob shot |
| | Backhand shot | Smash |
| | Overhead shot | Corner shot |
| | Sweep | Drop shot |
| **Locomotion** | | |
| Running | Net rush | |
| | Ball retrieval | |
| Sliding | Lateral movement to ball | |
| **Stability** | | |
| Axial movements | An aspect of all strokes (twisting, stretching, pivoting) | |
| Dynamic balance | Compensation for rapid changes in direction, level, and speed of movement | |

The goal of the teacher concerned with the motor development of children is to foster improvement in such a way that there is an orderly and developmentally sound progression through the fundamental and sport skill phases of development. Improvement in the movement control, emotional control, and learning enjoyment of the child serves as a practical philosophical construct around which to plan and implement the daily physical education lesson.

## CHAPTER HIGHLIGHTS

1. The child's performance level potential increases during later childhood and the preadolescent period and results in greater emphasis on general and specific movement skill development.
2. Specialized skill development in a specific sport often occurs prior to developing a sound base of fundamental movement abilities.
3. A sound base of fundamental movement abilities is essential to balanced motor development at higher skill levels.
4. Specialized skill development should not be a part of the developmentally based elementary school physical education curriculum.
5. The child's developmental potential in the general and specific movement skill phases is based on the foundation of movement patterns previously established.

**Table 12.8    Volleyball Skills**

| *Fundamental Movements* | *Related Sport Skill Movements* | |
|---|---|---|
| **Manipulation** | | |
| Striking | Overhand serve | Spike |
| | Underhand serve | Dink |
| Volleying | Set-up | |
| | Dig | |
| | | |
| **Locomotion** | | |
| Sliding | Lateral movement | |
| Running | Forward | |
| | Backward | |
| | | |
| Vertical jump | Diagonal | |
| | Spike | |
| **Stability** | | |
| Axial movements | | |
| | Found in general play (stretching, twisting, turning, falling, reaching) | |
| Dynamic balance | Rapid changes in speed, level, and direction of movement | |

6. Both structured and unstructured movement experiences are necessary in developing general and specific movement skills.

7. As the child's performance comes closer to the expected performance model, more specific tasks and information become important. Selection of the best ways to perform a skill becomes imperative.

8. Regardless of the skill level, movement variation can often be appropriate in furthering skill development or in motivating the child.

9. A return to or emphasis on mature fundamental movement patterns is essential prior to learning general and specific sport skills.

10. Activity selection and modification should be based on the teacher's knowledge of student capabilities and developmental needs.

11. Game-related general and specific sport skills take the form of lead-up activities. Lead-up activities emphasize various skill elements while approximating the official sport.

12. Competition may be used to motivate children to put forth greater effort and concentration in practicing correct or best ways to execute skills.

13. Youth sport competition is an important element in the lives of millions of children and requires competent leadership and developmentally appropriate experiences.

14. Basketball, football, soccer, softball, volleyball, dance, and other sport-related activities all require the use of specific movement skills that are based

**Table 12.9 Gymnastic Skills**

| Fundamental Movements | Related Sport Skill Movements | |
|---|---|---|
| **Locomotion** | | |
| Running | Approach | |
| Vertical jumping | Back flip | |
| | Front flip | |
| Skipping | Skip step | |
| Leaping | Various stunts | |
| **Stability** | | |
| Axial movements | One or more found in numerous stunts and apparatus skills (bending, stretching, twisting, turning, falling, reaching, pivoting) | |
| Static balance | Integral part of all stationary tricks and landing on dismounts | |
| Inverted supports | | Tip-up headstand |
| | | Tripod handstand |
| Body rolling | Forward roll | Back walkover |
| | Backward roll | Front walkover |
| Dynamic balance | Compensation for changes in direction, level, and speed of movement | |

on the three categories of movement (stabilization, locomotion, and manipulation).

## CRITICAL READINGS

Cooper, J.M., M. Adrian, and R.B. Glassow: *Kinesology*, St. Louis: Mosby, 1982, Chapters 10—21.

De Oreo, K.: "Refining Locomotor Skills" and "Refining Nonlocomotor Skills," in C. Corbin (ed.), *A Textbook of Motor Development*, Dubuque, Iowa: W.C. Brown, 1980, pp. 59—74.

Lawther, J.D.: *The Learning and Performance of Physical Skills*, Englewood Cliffs, N.J.: Prentice-Hall, 1977, Chapter 5.

Martens, R., and V. Seefeldt: *Guidelines for Youth Sports*, Washington, D.C.: AAHPERD, 1979.

Martens, R., et al.: *Coaching Young Athletes*, Champaign, Illinois: Human Kinetics, 1981.

# ABILITIES OF CHILDREN

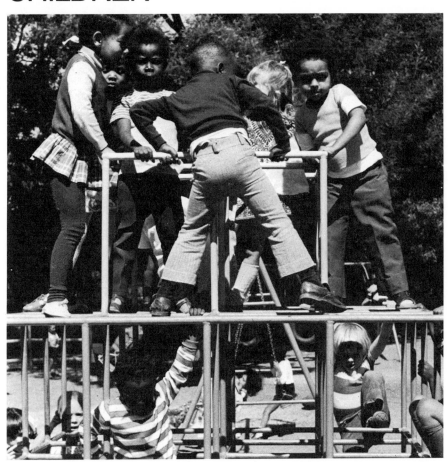

# Physical Abilities
# of Children

The physical fitness and motor fitness of children should be of great concern to all and not just the physical educator and physician. In the last several years the fitness level of boys and girls in North America has become of great concern to many. This concern was highlighted by the results of a test of minimum muscular efficiency (Kraus-Weber Test) that was administered to several thousand American and European children. The results of this historic study indicated that the performance of American children was significantly poorer than that of their European counterparts. In fact, over 55 percent of the Americans failed the test, as compared to less than 10 percent of the European youths. Although the comparison has been criticized for several reasons, it pointed out the important fact that American children are often in poor physical condition.

As a result of the Kraus-Hirschland study (1954), the President, Dwight D. Eisenhower, established the President's Council on Youth Fitness in an effort to promote the upgrading of the physical fitness of our nation's children. Since that time the President's Council and others concerned with the fitness level of our youth have made many important contributions toward that goal. The American Alliance for Health, Physical Education, Recreation, and Dance (AAHPERD) has developed a Youth Fitness Test that is probably the most widely used standardized physical fitness test throughout the United States. This test was developed for boys and girls in the fourth grade and above. The importance of gaining and maintaining a higher level of fitness has been promoted by the Fitness Council through publications, newspaper articles, and television spots. The importance of movement, motor development, and good physical education programs as a means of enhancing the fitness level of children has also been promoted.

The fact remains, however, that a great many of our children are still unfit. Two factors seem to have contributed greatly to this state of affairs. First, the impact of the importance and need for enhancing physical fitness has been centered on children in middle childhood through adolescence and on into adulthood. Until recently, little attention has been focused on the fitness needs of children during the preschool and elementary school years. As a result, our knowledge of the fitness of children and their capacity for work is limited. This has given rise to the second factor, namely, the child's "heart myth" and other basically false assumptions concerning the fitness of children.

According to the child's heart myth, there is a discrepancy in the development of the heart and blood vessels in children, and as a result, vigorous exercise should be avoided at the risk of straining the heart. This widely believed myth has been disproven by Karpovich (1937), Astrand (1952), and others, and is reflected in Corbin's (1980) statement that "a healthy child can not physiologically injure the heart permanently through exercise unless the heart is already weakened" (p. 20). Another erroneous assumption is that young children play all day and get plenty of vigorous physical activity. The crowded conditions of apartment living and city dwelling for many, along with the ever-present television set and its fascination, has created a sedentary society of children. Children need regular, vigorous physical activity every day, and the only way they will get it is through a drastic reorganization of their daily routines. Vigorous exercise and physical activity have been shown to be important factors in normal healthy growth.

## PHYSICAL FITNESS ABILITIES

Although there has been extensive study in the area of physical fitness over the past several years, comparatively little is known about the physical fitness of children. A review of the literature on fitness reveals a marked lack of information, particularly on children under 8 years of age. Most tests of physical fitness require the individual to go ''all out'' and perform at his or her maximum. Anyone familiar with young children will recognize the difficulty of this situation. The problems lie in: (1) being able to sufficiently motivate the youngster for maximal performance, (2) accurately determining whether a maximum effort has been achieved, and (3) overcoming the fears of anxious parents. Experts working with young children have an almost untouched area for the study of physical fitness. The problems of conducting investigations of this nature are many, but carefully controlled, patient research will yield much valuable information. Cardiovascular endurance, muscular strength, muscular endurance, and flexibility are generally considered to be the components of physical fitness. Each of these components is discussed briefly in the following paragraphs and illustrated in Figure 13.1.

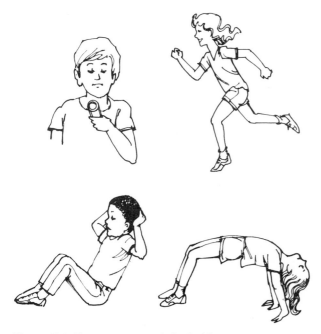

**Figure 13.1.** The components of physical fitness.

## Cardiovascular Endurance

Cardiovascular endurance is an aspect of muscular endurance, specific to the heart, lungs, and vascular system. It refers to the ability to perform numerous repetitions of a stressful activity requiring considerable use of the circulatory and respiratory systems.

Maximal aerobic power as measured by maximal oxygen uptake (Max $Vo_2$) is a universally accepted means of measuring status and change in cardiovascular fitness. It is not, however, universally accepted or understood how to express maximal aerobic ability in relation to body size. The literature concerning the aerobic capacity of children, particularly children under 8 years of age, is sparse. Young children make difficult subjects, and the testing environment is limited to the extent of the interest in putting forth a maximal effort. Bailey et al. (1978) indicated that knowing how maximal aerobic power relates to body mass and body size is very important when dealing with children. "In fitness training studies on children there is a problem in determining if changes and maximal aerobic power are a result of training, growth or both, since increasing size may result in changes similar to the training effect" (p. 140−141). Bailey and his colleagues studied 200 Canadian boys for ten years beginning when the boys were 7 years old. The subjects received no special instruction or activity other than the performance of a yearly treadmill test of their aerobic capacity. The results of this study revealed yearly increases in their oxygen utilization. However, when the data were expressed in terms of the amount of oxygen utilized in proportion to body weight (liters per minute per kilogram of body weight) no consistent pattern with increasing age emerged. This finding indicates that the aerobic capacity of an individual is related in part to body weight and in part to age.

Andersen et al. (1978) conductd a nine-year longitudinal study of aerobic capacity with Norwegian boys and girls ranging in age from 8 to 12 years. The results of their investigation indicated that gains in aerobic power were greater than could be expected from growth in body size alone. Fitness expressed on the basis of body weight and on lean body mass increased as the children became older. The authors attributed this linear trend toward improved aerobic capacity over time and without special training to informal environmental stimulation and not simply changes in body size.

Sometimes heart rate responses to exercise are used as a crude measure of cardiovascular endurance in young children because of the difficulty in gathering Max $Vo_2$ data. Mrzena and Macuek (1978) tested children 3 to 5 years old on the treadmill. Each subject was required to walk or run for five minutes at a level grade with the treadmill set at three different speeds (3, 4, and 5 km/h). The highest heart rates were recorded at 142 beats per minute. Another group performed the treadmill task at 4 km/h while the grade was increased from 5 to 10 to 15°. This group produced heart rates averaging 162 beats per minute. It was noted by the investigators that when the treadmill speed was increased to 6 km/h and the inclination to 20°, "the children were not able to increase the step frequency and lost their balance" (p. 31). The maximum aerobic capacity of preschool children is certainly greater than the scores obtained in this experiment, but the maturity of movement as well as the psychological and emotional state of the young child will determine the degree of cooperation and effort put forth.

In an investigation by Parizkova (1977), heart rates of 160 beats per minute were recorded in a bench stepping task with 3-year-old children. The children had considerable difficulty maintaining the cadence of thirty steps per minute on the low bench without the investigator holding one hand and stepping with the children. The children in this investigation also had difficulty maintaining the task even though normal play heart rates of young children often exceed 200 beats per minute. Cumming and Hnatiuk (1980) reported that normal maximal heart rates for children range from 180 to 234 beats per minute. This investigation again reminds us of the extreme difficulty in achieving a maximal effort for a sustained period of time with young children. A study by Montoye (1970) used a three-minute step test to evaluate an entire community. The results of Montoye's investigation indicate that resting, exercise, and recovery heart rates decrease with age between ages 10 and 20 and to a lesser degree between ages 20 and 35. Children are capable of working at much higher heart rates than previously expected.

Although it is now clear that children are capable of achieving maximal heart rates at or above their adult counterparts, it is doubtful that such levels are obtained during the daily routines of the vast majority of children. Gilliam and his colleagues (1981) confirmed this hypothesis in an experiment in which they monitored the heart rate patterns of 6- and 7-year-olds during a two-month summer period. The results of this investigation in which twenty-two boys and eighteen girls wore a small heart monitoring device for twelve hours daily during their normal daily routine revealed:

> The voluntary activity patterns of the children studied may not be adequate in terms of duration and intensity, to promote cardiovascular health. . . . our data and others' show children . . . very seldom experience physical activity of high enough intensity to promote cardiovascular health. Furthermore, our data show that boys are more active than girls. (p. 67)

Although the data on young children are inconclusive with regard to maximum aerobic capacity as measured by maximal oxygen consumption and exercise heart rates, we do know that their abilities are similar to those of adults when corrected for body size. We know also that the aerobic working capacity of an individual develops early in life and is dependent, in part, on the life style of the individual child. Sedentary children will not develop the same degree of cardiovascular endurance as their active counterparts. Activities such as running, peddling a tricycle or bicycle, and swimming should be a part of daily life experiences of all children.

## Muscular Strength

Muscular strength is the ability of the body to exert force. In its purest sense, it is the ability to exert *one* maximum effort. Children engaged in daily active play are doing much to enhance their leg strength by running and bicycling. Their arm strength is developed through such activities as lifting, carrying objects, handling tools, and swinging on the monkey bars. Strength may be classified as isotonic or isometric. *Isometric strength* involves exerting force on an immovable object. The muscle contracts, but there is little change in its length. *Isotonic strength,* on the other hand, refers to the ability of a muscle to go through its full range of motion. The muscles involved contract, but they also shorten and lengthen during the activity. A barbell curl and a bench press are examples of isotonic strength activities.

Strength is commonly measured by using a dynamometer or tensiometer. These devices are highly reliable when utilized by trained personnel. The dynamometer is calibrated and designed to measure grip strength, leg strength, and back strength. The cable tensiometer is more versatile than the dynamometer in that it permits measurement of many different muscle groups. The classic longitudinal studies conducted by Clarke (1971) utilized eighteen different cable tensiometer tests and revealed yearly strength increments in boys between 7 and 17 years. After age 12 or 13, girls tend to differ markedly from boys in their strength. According to Corbin (1980), girls without training tend to level off at this age, but boys continue to gain in strength. It seems probable that the strength levels of preschool and primary grade boys and girls are similar, with the edge being given to boys based on their tendency to be slightly taller and heavier than girls. Unfortunately, virtually nothing is known about the muscular strength of the young child.

Relatively few longitudinal investigations have been conducted into the development of strength in children at all ages. The information that is available, however, indicates consistency in the development of strength in children over time. In fact, strength has been shown to increase more rapidly than muscle size during childhood (Armussen, 1973). This is probably due to the increasing skill and coordination with which a maximal contraction may be performed and indicates the interrelationship between strength, coordination, and motor performance in children.

Although strength is a relatively stable quality throughout childhood, the prediction of strength at later years from measures taken in childhood has met with little success. The "strong" child at age 8, for example, will not necessarily make the greatest gains in strength from childhood through adolescence. Neither will the "weak" child necessarily make the least gains in strength from childhood through adolescence. The rapid change in body size, which is positively correlated with strength, and the individual variability of growth patterns make prediction a precarious venture.

Boys tend to be stronger than girls, particularly in the upper extremities, at all ages, and the differences are magnified with age (Armussen, 1973). The extra gain in strength by boys during puberty is due to the increase in the production of male sex hormones that influence the increase in muscularity. Female adolescents do not markedly increase in their muscularity. Therefore, boys may be thought of as stronger than girls because of the sheer quantity of muscle mass rather than any qualitative differences. Mean strength values for girls do not increase after puberty, while those for boys continue to make dramatic changes. The average adult female is only about 80 percent as strong as her male counterpart, even when corrections are made for differences in size (Rarick and Dobbins, 1975).

Early-maturing boys and girls are stronger than their chronological-age peers. They also show an earlier surge in strength development (Jones, 1949). This early surge in strength often proves extremely beneficial in youth sport activities that require strength and endurance. With systematic training, it is possible to accelerate the development of strength in children (Armussen, 1973). The opitmal age, frequency, duration, and intensity of strength training for children are not known. The possible negative effects of *intense* training may contraindicate special strength training programs for children. Considerably more research needs to be conducted in this area before the final answer may be given.

## Muscular Endurance

Muscular endurance is the ability of a muscle or a group of muscles to perform work repeatedly against moderate resistance. Muscular endurance is similar to muscular strength in terms of the activities performed but it differs in emphasis. Strength-building activities require overloading the muscles to a greater extent than endurance activities. Endurance-building activities require less of an overload on the muscle but more repetitions. Therefore, endurance may be thought of as the ability to continue in strength performance. Children performing sit-ups, push-ups, and pull-ups are actually engaged in endurance activities even though strength is required for any movement to begin. These three activities are among the most often used measures of muscular endurance, and according to Montoye (1970), they are among the best tests available.

The daily uninhibited play routines of most young children, when viewed in toto are excellent examples of endurance that most adults would find difficult to duplicate in terms of relative endurance. Relative endurance refers to the child's endurance level adjusted to body weight. It stands to reason that the adult's gross level of endurance and fitness is generally greater than that of the child, but when one's body weight is divided into the total fitness score, differences are less pronounced.

The results of the bent knee sit-up test and the flexed arm hang test administered as a part of both the AAHPERD Youth Fitness Test (1980) and the CAHPER Manitoba Physical Fitness Performance Test* (1980) reveal developmental changes in muscular endurance. On both of these measures, boys and girls showed a tendency toward considerable improvement during childhood, followed by a gradual leveling-off of performance.

The bent knee sit-up test is a measure of isotonic abdominal endurance. Boys and girls perform at nearly the same level until age 8, when boys begin to show superiority until the prepubescent years of 11 and 12. At his point girls slightly out perform the boys. From about age 13 onward, boys continue to improve in average performance but at a less rapid pace after age 15. Girls tend to level off at ages 13 and 14 and decline slightly thereafter. In both the Canadian and the American children, the upsurge in performancae by boys during adolescence can be explained by their increased muscularity; girls did not continue to improve perhaps because of the greater amounts of fatty tissue in proportion to lean muscle mass. The tendency to level off in performance during later adolescence could also be a matter of motivation and lack of all-out test-taking cooperation instead of purely physiological factors. These are important points to consider. One must be careful *not* to imply that no matter how hard girls try to improve their performance, they will not be able to do so.

The isometric endurance flexed arm hang administered to both boys and girls on the Manitoba Physical Fitness Performance Test (CAHPER, 1980) also revealed developmental differences between the sexes. Boys tend to improve their score slightly from age 5 onward, with a preadolescent lull followed by rapid improvement through age 18. Girls, on the other hand, improve somewhat until age 11 or 12, whereupon they achieved a plateau until age 15, and showed a slight decline thereafter. Hunsicker and Reiff (1977) reported similar findings with American girls on the flexed arm hang. The performance of both boys and girls was quite similar from age 5 to age 8, but began to diverge radically after that in favor of the boys. The results of the pull-up measure on the Youth Fitness Test for boys indicate steady increments with age in this endurance measure (Hunsicker and Reiff, 1977). There is little difference in boys between ages 7 and 12, but after the onset of puberty, there is a dramatic increase in pull-up scores for boys.

The results of both the AAHPERD Youth Fitness Test and the Manitoba Physical Fitness Performance Test serve as vivid examples of the developmental aspects of muscular endurance. Namely:

1. The performance levels of both boys and girls are similar during early and middle childhood.

---

*The Monitoba Physical Fitness Performance Test is reported here because it is one of the very few tests available with norms for children from age 5 to age 18. It has been administered to over 10,000 Canadian children living in the province of Manitoba and yields information similar to the AAHPERD Youth Fitness Test.

**2.** Girls tend to outperform boys on some measures of muscular endurance during the preadolescent period.

**3.** Girls tend to level off and even decline in their muscular endurance performance after age 12.

**4.** Boys make rapid gains in muscular endurance throughout adolescence.

The differences exhibited between boys and girls and the span of years in which improved performances can be expected on measures of muscular endurance should be examined carefully. Although boys can be expected to outperform girls in measures of endurance and strength due to anatomical and physiological advantages, there is no adequate biological explanation of differences in the span of years over which relative improvement may be seen. A reasonable explanation may be encountered in social and cultural differences and child-rearing differences between males and females. Although our North American culture has undergone radical changes in the last several years in its view of girls and women being involved in physical activity, it is apparent that there are often discrepancies in the opportunities, encouragement, and instruction that girls receive in vigorous physical activity.

## Flexibility

Flexibility is the ability of the various joints of the body to move through their full range of motion. There are two types of flexibility: static and dynamic. *Static,* or *extent flexibility* is the ability to flex the trunk of the body in different directions. *Dynamic flexibility* is the ability to perform stretching muscular contractions of various limbs of the body. Flexibility is joint specific and can be improved with practice. Hupperich and Sigerseth (1950) indicated, however, that dynamic flexibility in the shoulder, knee, and thigh joints decreases with age in children as evidenced by their investigation of girls 6, 9, and 12 years of age. Their investigation revealed also that static flexibility increased with age. Clarke (1975) reviewed the research on flexibility in 1975 and concluded that flexibility begins to decline in boys around age 10 and in girls around age 12. This confirms Leighton's (1956) study of the flexibility of boys ages 10 to 18. His investigation revealed that the frequent assumption that boys have a high level of flexibility during childhood and adolescence is questionable. Boys showed no consistent pattern of increasing or maintaining flexibility with age, but did show a definite tendency toward decreased flexibility with age. DiNucci (1976) reported that girls performed better than boys on five different measures of flexibility at all ages.

The sit and reach test utilized in the Manitoba Physical Fitness Performance Test yielded interesting results but they were somewhat in contradiction with the results of the studies just mentioned. The average distance reached when attempting to touch one's toes as measured by a modified Wells and Dillon flexometer decreased for girls until age 12, at which time they, too, began to make steady increases through age 18.

The apparently contradictory results of these investigations may be puzzling until one recalls that flexibility is joint specific. Increases in one joint area do not imply a general trait of increased flexibility in all other joints. Cultural differences may also be evident between the American and the Canadian children. We often assume that all of today's preschool and elementary school children are involved in plenty of vigorous physical activity that would promote the progressive development and maintenance of flexibility. However, this assumption is not based in fact, as evidenced by the sedentary life style of millions of youngsters. Based on the available information on felxibility, we can assume that:

1. Flexibility is joint specific.
2. Cultural differences may influence flexibility scores.
3. Girls tend to be more flexible than boys during childhood and adolescence.
4. Strength development need not hinder flexibility development.
5. Activity levels are a better indicator of flexibility than age.

## PHYSICAL FITNESS AND MOVEMENT ABILITIES

The interaction between the components of physical fitness and physical activity is obvious. Performance of any movement task whether it be at the rudimentary, fundamental, or sport skill level requires varying degrees of cardiovascular fitness, muscular strength, muscular endurance, and joint flexibility. All movement involves overcoming inertia, and in order to overcome inertia, a force must be exerted. In order to exert that force, one must possess some degree of strength. If a movement task is to be performed repeatedly, as with dribbling a ball, endurance is also required. If the action is to be repeated over an extended period of time at a rapid pace, as in dribbling a ball up and down a basketball court, both cardiovascular endurance and flexibility are required. The reciprocal nature of the components of physical fitness may also be viewed from the standpoint that performance of movement activities maintains and develops higher levels of physical fitness. The components of physical fitness are inseparable from movement activity. Rarely, if ever, is a movement activity performed that does not involve some aspect of strength, endurance, or flexibility.

It is not possible under normal conditions to isolate the basic components of skill performance. However, tests have been devised that, by their very nature, require more of one component of fitness than another. It is through this indirect means of measuring physical fitness that we are able to determine *estimates* of one's functional health (Table 13.1).

**Table 13.1  Common Measures of the Components of Physical Fitness and a Synthesis of Findings**

| Physical Fitness Component | Common Tests | Specific Aspect Measured | Synthesis of Findings |
|---|---|---|---|
| Cardiovascular endurance | Step test | Physical work capacity | Maximum $O_2$ estimates are tenuous with young children. Children can achieve maximum $O_2$ values similar to adults when corrected for body weight. Maximal heart rates decrease with age. Trend for improved Max $Vo_2$ values in both boys and girls with age. Girls level off after age 12 or so. Both continue to improve. |
| | 12-minute run, treadmill test | Aerobic endurance, Max $Vo_2$ | |
| Muscular strength | Hand dynamometer | Grip strength | Annual increase for boys from age 7 on. Girls tend to level off after age 12. Boys slow prior to puberty, then gain rapidly throughout adolescence. Boys superior to girls at all ages. |
| | Back and leg dynamometer | Back and leg strength | |
| | Cable tensiometer | Joint strength | |
| Muscular endurance | Push-ups | Upper body endurance | Similar abilities throughout childhood slightly in favor of boys on most items. Lull in performance prior to age 12. Large increases in boys from 12 to 16, then a leveling off. Girls show no significant increases without special training after age 12. |
| | Sit-ups | Abdominal endurance | |
| | Flexed arm hang | Upper body endurance | |
| | Pull-ups | Upper body endurance | |
| Flexibility | Bend and reach | Hip joint flexibility | Flexibility is joint specific. Girls tend to be more flexible than boys at all ages. Flexibility decreases with reduced activity levels. |
| | Sit and reach | Hip joint flexibility | |

## MOTOR FITNESS ABILITIES

Considerable research has been conducted on the motor performance of the adolescent, adult, and skilled performer. The literature is replete with information dealing with their performance levels, biomechanics, and neurophysiological capabilities, but relatively little has been done with preschool and elementary school children. The situation is much the same as with physical fitness. Only recently have investigators begun to more closely analyze the motor abilities of children. Recent studies on the specific factors that make up the child's motor fitness abilities indicate that a well-defined structure is present during early childhood but that these factors may differ somewhat from those of older age groups (Peterson et al., 1974; Seefeldt, 1980a). There is a factor structure of motor abilities in children generally consisting of four or five items depending on the age level investigated (Bergel, 1978; Peterson et al., 1974; Rarick and Dobbins, 1975). *Movement control factors* of balance (both static and dynamic balance) and coordination (both gross motor and eye-hand coordination), coupled with the *movement force factors* of speed, agility, and power, tend to emerge as the components that most influence motor performance. The movement control factors (balance and coordination) are of particular importance during early childhood when the child is gaining control of his or her fundamental movement abilities. The force production factors (speed, agility, and power) begin to assume greater importance after the child has gained control of his or her fundamental movements and passes into the sport-related movement phase of later childhood.

It should be remembered that as with the components of physical fitness, ones motor abilities are intricately interrelated with movement skill acquisition (Figure 13.2). One depends in large part on the other. Without adequate motor abilities, the child's level of skill acquisition will be limited. And without adequate skill acquisition, the level of attainment of motor fitness components will be impeded. The components of motor fitness are discussed here, illustrated in Figure 13.3, and synthesized in Table 13.2.

### Coordination

Coordination is the ability to integrate separate motor systems with varying sensory modalities into efficient patterns of movement. The more complicated the movement tasks, the greater the level of coordination necessary for efficient performance. Coordination is interrelated with the motor abilities of balance, speed, and agility, but not closely aligned with strength and endurance (Barrow and McGee, 1978). Coordinated behavior requires the child to perform specific movements in a series both quickly and accurately. Movement must be synchronous, rhythmical, and properly sequenced in order to be coordinated.

Eye-hand and eye-foot coordination are characterized by integrating visual information with limb action. Movements must be visually controlled and precise in

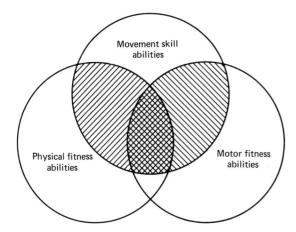

**Figure 13.2** The interrelated nature of the child's movement, physical fitness, and motor fitness abilities.

order to project, make contact with, or receive an external object. Bouncing, catching, throwing, kicking, and trapping a ball all require considerable amounts of visual input integrated with motor output in order to result in efficient coordinated movement.

Gross body coordination in children involves moving the body rapidly while performing various fundamental movement skills. Peterson et al. (1974) have indicated that measures such as the shuttle run, 30-yd dash, various hopping and skipping tests, and the standing long jump load high with the factor of gross body coordination. Gross body coordination and eye-hand and eye-foot coordination appear to improve with age in a roughly linear fashion. Also, the performance of boys tends to be superior to that of girls throughout childhood (Frederick, 1977; Van Slooten, 1973).

## Balance

Balance is the ability to maintain the equilibrium of one's body when it is placed in various positions. Balance is basic to all movement and is influenced by a variety of factors. Maintenance of balance is influenced by visual, tactile-kinesthetic, and vestibular stimulation.

Vision plays an important role in balance with young children. Cratty and Martin (1969) found that boys and girls age 6 and under could not balance on one foot with their eyes closed. But by age 7, they were able to maintain balance with their eyes closed, and balancing ability continued to improve with age. Use of the eyes enables the child to focus on a reference point in order to maintain balance.

The eyes also enable the young child to visually monitor the body during a static or dynamic balance task.

Tactile and kinesthetic abilities play an important role in balance. The famous rod-and-frame experiments conducted by Wapner and Werner (1957) emphasize the importance of the tactile and kinethetic senses. Verticality of a luminous rod in a frame was predicted by subjects seated in a darkened room and tilted to one side. The hypothesis was that children do not have control of their kinesthetic abilities to the point of being able to compensate for changes in body tilt and therefore must rely on visual information for accurate prediction of verticality. The experiment by Comalli et al. (1959) confirmed this hypothesis and revealed that in subjects from 6 to 16 years of age the rod appeared to be vertical when it was actually tilted in the same direction as the individual. Older subjects (age 16 to age 50) were able to more accurately locate the apparent vertical plane but often overcompensated and predicted verticality of the rod in the opposite direction from their own tilt. In other words, tactile and kinesthetic abilities tend to improve with age and contribute to balance more in adults than in children (Parker, 1980).

Balance is profoundly influenced by the vestibular apparatus. The fluid contained in the semicircular canals and the otolith plays a key role in maintaining equilibrium. The receptors in the semicircular canal respond to changes in angular acceleration (dynamic and rotational balance). While the otolith receptors respond to linear accelerations (static balance), the movement of hairs (macula) in either the otolith or the semicircular canals triggers nerve impulses by changing the electrical potential of adjoining nerve cells (Parker, 1980). Movement of the body and gravity are sensed by these vestibular receptors and aid the individual in being aware of both static and dynamic postural changes as well as of changes in acceleration. The vestibular apparatus coordinates with the visual, tactile, and kinesthetic systems in governing balance. It appears that vestibular development in terms of balance occurs very early in life and that the vestibular apparatus is structurally complete at birth. However, the body musculature and the other sensory modalities involved in maintaining balance must further mature and be integrated with vestibular clues in order to be of real use to the child in maintaining either static or dynamic balance.

Balance is often defined as static or dynamic. *Static balance* refers to the ability of the body to maintain equilibrium in a stationary position. Balancing on one foot, standing on a balance board, and performing a stick balance are common means of assessing static balance abilities. Research on the static balance abilities of children shows a linear trend toward improved performance with age from ages 2 through 12 (De Oreo, 1971, Keogh, 1965; Van Slooten, 1973). Prior to age 2 children generally are not able to perform a one-foot static balance task, probably because of their still-developing abilities to maintain a controlled upright posture. De Oreo (1980) indicated that clear-cut boy-girl differences are *not* seen in static balance performance as with other motor performance tasks. In fact, girls tend to be more proficient than boys until about age 7 or 8, whereupon the boys catch up. Both sexes level off in performance around age 8, prior to a surge in abilities from age 9 to age 12.

**Table 13.2   Common Measures and the Components of Motor Fitness and a Synthesis of Findings**

| Motor Fitness Component | Common Tests | Specific Aspect Measured | Synthesis of Findings |
|---|---|---|---|
| Coordination | Cable jump | Gross body coordination | Year by year improvement with age in gross body coordination. Boys superior from age 6 on in eye-hand and eye-foot coordination. |
| | Hopping for accuracy | Gross body coordination | |
| | Skipping | Gross body coordination | |
| | Ball dribble | Eye-hand coordination | |
| | Foot dribble | Eye-hand coordination | |
| Balance | Beam walk | Dynamic balance | Year by year improvement with age. Girls often outperform boys, especially in dynamic balance activities until about age 8. Abilities similar thereafter. |
| | Stick balance | Static balance | |
| | One-foot stand | Static balance | |
| Speed | 20-yd dash | Running speed | Year by year improvement with age. Boys and girls similar until age 6 or 7, at which time boys make more rapid improvements. Boys superior to girls at all ages. |
| | 30-yd dash | Running speed | |
| Agility | Shuttle run | Running agility | Year by year improvement with age. Girls begin to level off after age 13. Boys continue to make improvements. |
| Power | Vertical jump | Leg strength and speed | Year by year improvement with age. Boys outperform girls at all age levels. |
| | Standing long jump | Leg strength and speed | |
| | Distance throw | Upper arm strength and speed | |
| | Velocity throw | Upper arm strength and speed | |

*Dynamic balance* refers to the ability to maintain equilibrium when moving from point to point. Balance beam walking tests are used most often as measures of dynamic balance in children. The available literature on dynamic balance indicates a trend similar to static balance. Girls are often more proficient than boys until age 8 or 9, whereupon they perform at similar levels (De Oreo, 1971; Frederick, 1977). Both slow in their progress around age 9, prior to making rapid gains to age 12 (Goetzinger, 1961; Heath, 1949).

## Speed

Speed is the ability to cover a short distance in as short a period of time as possible. Speed is influenced by reaction time (the amount of elapsed time from the signal "go" to the first movements of the body) as well as movement time (the time elapsed from the initial movement to completion of the activity). Reaction time depends on the speed with which the initial stimulus is processed through the efferent and afferent neural pathways and is integrated with the initial response pattern. Reaction time has been shown to decrease in children as they get older.

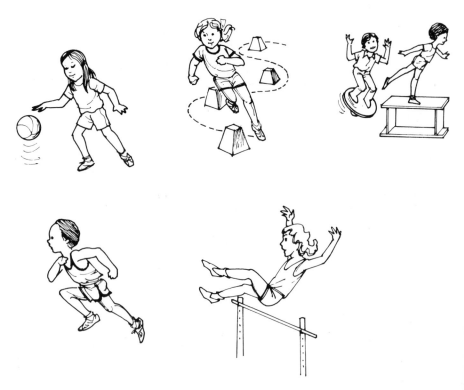

**Figure 13.3.** The components of motor fitness.

Cratty (1979) reported that the information available concerning simple reaction time indicates that it is about twice as long in 5-year-olds as it is in adults for an identical task and that there is rapid improvement from age 3 to age 5. These developmental differences are probably due to neurological maturation and differences in the information processing capabilities of children and adults.

Speed of movement in children is most generally measured through various tests of running speed. Frederick (1977), in testing the running speed of five groups of children 3 to 5 years of age on the 20-yd dash found linear improvement with age but no sex differences. In a study of the running speed of elementary school children, Keogh (1965) found that boys and girls are similar in running speed at ages 6 and 7, but boys were superior from age 8 to 12. Both boys and girls improve with age at about 1 ft per second per year from ages 6 to 11 (Cratty, 1979). Keogh also found similar improvement and boy-girl differences in the 50-ft hop for speed, although girls tended to perform better than boys on hopping and jumping tasks that require greater precision and accuracy of movement.

Speed of movement generally improves until about age 12 in both boys and girls. After this, however, girls tend to level off in their performance and boys tend to continue improving throughout the teenage years (AAHPER, 1976). The movement speed of both boys and girls may be fostered during childhood and beyond through opportunities for vigorous physical activity that incorporate short bursts of speed.

## Agility

Agility is the ability to change the direction of the body rapidly and accurately as it moves from one point to another as fast as possible. It is the ability to make quick and accurate shifts in body position during movement. A variety of agility runs have been used as indirect measures of agility. Unfortunately, the wide variety of ways in which these scores have been obtained makes it impossible to compare studies. Scores from the 30-ft shuttle run used as a measure of running agility in both the AAHPER Youth Fitness Test and the Manitoba Physical Fitness Performance Test yield some complementary results. The Manitoba Test results indicate that from ages 5 to 13 both boys and girls improve their average shuttle run times annually, with boys having a slight edge in speed of about half a second (CAHPER, 1980). The AAHPER Test (1976) indicates that boys improve at a faster rate than girls from age 12 onward. Girls on both tests clearly level off in their agility scores after age 13, while boys continue to make annual improvements.

## Power

Power is the ability to perform a maximum effort in as short a period as possible. Power is sometimes referred to as "explosive strength" and represents the product of strength times speed. This combination of strength and speed is exhibited in children's activities that require jumping, striking, throwing for distance, and other explosive, "all-out" efforts. The speed of contraction of the muscles involved, as well as the strength and coordinated use of these muscles, determines the degree of power of the individual.

Because power involves a combination of motor abilities, it is difficult, if not impossible, to obtain a pure measure of this component. The often-used throwing and jumping measures can only give us an indirect indication of power because of the obvious requirements for skill involved in both of these tasks. Frederick (1977) did, however, find significant yearly increments in vertical jump, standing long jump, and distance throwing tasks for children ages 3 through 5. Also, the boys outperformed the girls on all measures at all age levels. The same results were found by Keogh (1965) for boys and girls from 6 to 12 years of age and by Van Slooten (1973) for children 6 to 9 years of age on the throw for distance, but with sex differences magnified beyond age 7. Luedke's (1980) excellent review of the literature on throwing supports these studies.

Similar linear improvements and differences between boys and girls may be seen in the standing long jump from age 3 through age 5 (Frederick, 1977), 6 through 12 (Keogh, 1965), and 10 through 17 (AAHPER, 1976). Differences in throwing velocity based on age and sex have also been shown in samples of children from 6 to 14 years old (Glassow and Kruse, 1960; Luedke, 1980). However, differences from age to age and between sexes are closely related to yearly strength and speed of movement increments as well as to the varying sociocultural influences on boys and girls.

## CHILDHOOD OBESITY

We are living today in a world far different from that of our ancestors. Vigorous physical exertion is not a necessary part of the daily life pattern of most people. Today, most exercise, if it occurs, is planned and is not an integral part of one's existence. In addition to a reduction in the exercise required in our daily lives, we also enjoy, for the present, an abundance of available food. Thus it is possible for an individual to consume a large amount of food while using up little of the energy contained in that food. The maintenance of body weight is relatively simple. It requires maintaining a balance between the number of calories taken into the body in the form of food and the number of calories burned through exercise and other daily activities. If more calories are consumed than are burned over a period of time, obesity is the eventual result.

Fat has a number of constructive functions. It is a reserve source of energy; it is a vehicle for fat-soluble vitamins; it provides protection and support to the body parts, insulating the body from the cold; and in proper proportion, it enhances the appearance of the body. However, to serve these functions, the proportion of fat desired in individuals is about 15 percent for males and 22.5 percent for females

(Wilmore, 1974). The full-term infant has about 16 percent fat, much of which develops during the last two months of the gestation period (Documenta, 1970). Ideally, there is very little change in the percentage of body fat in proportion to total body weight from birth to adulthood. However, the percentage of body fat may range from a low of about 8 percent (typical of the long-distance, ectomorphic-built, runner) to as high as 50 percent (characteristic of the very obese). It is estimated that there are over 70 million overweight Americans (Wilmore, 1974). In North America the percentage of lean body mass decreases with age and the percentage of body fat is the most important determiner of obesity. A person's weight is less crucial than how much fat compared to lean body mass constitutes his or her body. In fact, Kaufmann (1975) stated that "body composition is the *only* valid criterion for determining what obesity is" (p. 77).

Obesity places additional stress on the circulatory, respiratory, and metabolic systems and may cause, or intensify, disorders in these systems. Armstrong et al. (1951) found that the mortality rate for obese men was 79 percent higher than for a normal risk group in setting standards for life insurance policies. Investigations by Joslin et al. (1952) have shown a strong correlation between obesity and the onset of diabetes. In addition, obese individuals, particularly children and young adults, often suffer ridicule from their peers and discrimination by adults (Mayer, 1968).

The primary causes of obesity in young children with normal hormonal balances are excessive eating and lack of exercise, or a combination of both, which often results in a vicious cycle in which poor eating and exercise habits are formed and carried on into adult life. The child who is urged to clean the plate at every meal, yet who is not encouraged to exercise regularly, has the potential for a serious weight problem.

An area of interest to many who study obesity is the activity levels of obese children. A study by Bruch (1940) examined 160 obese children. It was found that 76 percent of the boys and 88 percent of the girls were rated as inactive when compared to normal youngsters. Further studies by M. L. Johnson and his colleagues (1956) compared the caloric intake and activity of normal and obese girls. It was found that the obese girls spend less than half as much time at physical activity as the nonobese group. These studies indicate that dieting is not the complete, nor even the best, solution to obesity in children. In fact, since their food intake may be normal, dieting may cause serious deficiencies in the nutrients required for proper growth and health. Since a major cause of obesity in children is lack of activity, increases in this area may be the best and most healthful solution to the problem.

Many studies show that obesity runs in families, due either to heredity or environmental factors. Mayer (1968) found that the chances of obesity are 10 percent for children with parents of normal weight, 40 percent if one parent is obese, and 70 percent if both parents are obese. Again, the cause seems to be lack of regular vigorous activity, rather than dietary excesses or hormonal imbalances.

Studies indicate that poor dietary and exercise patterns established early in life may increase the chances of obesity as an adult due to an increase in the number of fat cells. Oscai (1973) has indicated that exercise in early life may reduce the number of fat cells formed by the body. The exercise habits developed during childhood may have a pronounced influence on the possible development of obesity in later life. Although hereditary, environmental, and nutritional factors play a role, regular, *vigorous* physical activity may be the most important variable in preventing obesity.

Figure 13.4 depicts the evolution of the typical fat cell. The primitive fat cell has an irregular shape, a central nucleus, and large amounts of cytoplasm surrounding the nucleus. In the first stage, droplets of fat appear mixed with the cytoplasm. In the second stage, these droplets grow. In the third stage, the fat droplets enlarge and finally merge into one large droplet, with the nucleus pushed to the top of the cell. The fat cell has become bloated with fat substances. It has

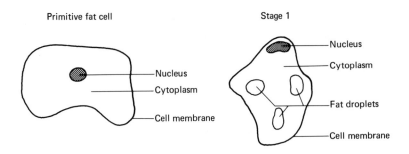

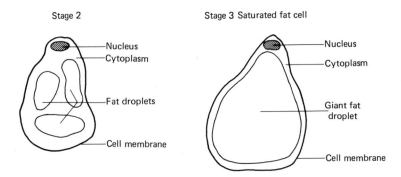

**Figure 13.4.** Evolution of the typical fat cell.

become *fat*. As a person becomes obese, the percentage of body fat increases by storing more and more fat substance in the fat cells (Kaufman, 1975). It is now believed that fat cells are difficult to destroy. When a person loses weight, the amount of fat decreases but the number of fat cells remains constant. The fat cells become thin, but they remain in the body. This along with differences in metabolic rates may help to explain why some people have great difficulty losing and keeping excess fat off while others have equal difficulty gaining weight. Kaufman (1975) states that "there is strong evidence that if an individual is obese as a child, he has a 90 percent chance of being obese as an adult" (p.78). A growing body of evidence (Stein et al., 1981) implicates obesity as a factor in the development of atherosclerosis and coronary heart disease.

Enos et al. (1955) and McNamera et al. (1971) autopsied teenage soldiers killed in Korea and Vietnam, respectively. The results of their post-mortem investigations revealed that coronary and aortic atherosclerosis were present in no less than one third of the soldiers autopsied. One of the major suspected risk factors in the development of atherosclerosis and subsequent chronic heart disease is the early development of obesity (Stein et al., 1981). It is, however, not yet known whether limiting weight gain during childhood will have any long-term influence on adult weight gain and on reduction of the risk of chronic heart disease (Fisch et al., 1975).

## ANOREXIA NERVOSA

A problem as perplexing and potentially as dangerous as obesity is anorexia nervosa, which is characterized by an aversion to the consumption of food and an obsession with being "too fat" even when clearly underweight. These self-starvers can lose 25 to 50 percent of their normal body weight in the pursuit of thinness. They start dieting and, although emaciated, continue to refuse food because they see themselves as fat.

The incidence of anorexia nervosa is on the rise. It is particularly prevalent among adolescent girls. Bruch (1979) contends that anorexia nervosa is increasing so much that probably every family doctor will sooner or later be confronted with an anorectic patient. About 10 percent of all cases of anorexia nervosa are fatal, and many others become chronic invalids (Rothenberg, 1976).

Characteristically, there is no true loss of appetite or awareness of hunger pains corresponding to the body's need for food. Some actually brainwash themselves into believing that the pain actually feels good. In about 25 percent of the cases, food refusal alternates with eating binges. Anorectics become obsessed with the whole idea of food. They think about it, talk about it, collect recipes, and often force their family members to overeat (Bruch, 1979).

In an effort to remove unwanted food from the body, many anorectics resort to self-induced vomiting, or excessive use of enemas, laxatives and diuretics. All this may result in a serious disturbance of the body's electrolyte balance, which may play a role in cases that end in death (Minuchin et al., 1978).

Anorectics pursue their goal of thinness not only through food restriction but through exhausting exercise. Many were interested in sports before the illness. Exercise then becomes a solitary activity, a way to burn off calories or show endurance. In spite of their weakness due to extreme loss of weight, many display incredible energy and are hyperactive. Anorectics drive themselves to unbelievable feats to demonstrate that they can live up to the ideal of mind over body (Bruch, 1979).

Many anorectics do not want the curves and roundness associated with the developing adolescent body, and they are often terrified of dealing with sexual matters. By starving themselves, they can remain children forever with no menstrual periods or development of secondary sex characteristics (Bruch, 1979).

Anorectics are usually described as having been outstandingly good children. They were the pride and joy of their parents and teachers. Psychiatrists have come to recognize the overwhelming sense of ineffectiveness under which the victims operate. They camouflage their self-doubt with perfect, conforming behavior. The extreme control they exercise over their bodies provides them with a sense of accomplishment. Even a slight weight gain may result in depression and self-hatred (Bruch, 1979).

The anorectic child often grows up in a family with highly enmeshed patterns, and close, interpersonal contact becomes important to her or him. Loyalty and protection are more valuable to the anorectic than autonomy and self-realization. The individual learns to subordinate the self. The expectation from learning a skill, for example, is not competence, but approval. The reward is love and not knowledge. The family of anorectic children is typically child-oriented. The child grows up protected by parents who over focus on the child's well-being. Because the child sees family members focusing on her or his actions and commenting on them, an obsessive concern for perfection often develops. The anorectic is both extremely self-conscious and alert to other people's signals. Overinvolvement with the family often creates a developmental lag in dealing with the outside world (Minuchin et al., 1978).

Some early warning signals of anorexia nervosa are:

1.  Overidentification with a doctor-prescribed weight-control program.
2.  Obsession with dieting and talk of food.
3.  Social isolation accompanying slimness.
4.  No participation in the courting behavior of classmates.
5.  Sudden increased involvement in athletics, usually of a solitary nature.
6.  Exaggerated concern with achieving high academic grades.
7.  Overconcern with being overweight.
8.  Failure to consume food, followed by food binges.
9.  Aversion to most foods.

Society is partly to blame for the increase in anorexia nervosa. The lean, slender form is glorified by the society we live in. It propagates the idea that being thin symbolizes beauty, desirability, and self-control and is a magic key to a happier life. Educators may be among the first to recognize a case of anorexia nervosa. They should be able to recognize the early stages of the illness while it is still reversible. Once it has lasted any length of time, it becomes exceedingly difficult to treat.

## Summary

Maximal oxygen consumption (Max $Vo_2$) refers to the largest quantity of oxygen an individual can consume during physical work while breathing air at sea level. It is a measure of one's maximum ability to transmit oxygen to the tissues of the body. An increase in one's aerobic capacity is an excellent indicator of a higher energy output. Astrand (1952) indicates that improvement in Max $Vo_2$ is possible but by only about 20 percent. Genetic inheritance plays a crucial role in the ability to consume oxygen. Maximal oxygen consumption tends to improve as a function of age until about age 18 to 20. Improvement thereafter is primarily a function of training. Women possess about 75 percent of the capacity of men to consume oxygen. The differences between males and females prior to puberty are largely unexplored. The entire area of oxygen consumption in children has been investigated by relatively few researchers, and the results have often been conflicting. This is due largely to the questionable reliability and reproducibility of Max $Vo_2$ measures with children.

Numerous studies have reported increases in Max $Vo_2$ with training in children (C.H. Brown, et al., 1972; Massicotte and MacNab, 1974; Vrijens, 1978). However, several studies have failed to show a training effect with children (Cumming and Friesen, 1967; Cumming et al., 1969; Daniels and Oldridge, 1971; Ekbolm, 1969). This discrepancy in results is probably due to the fact that young children are not predisposed to all-out physical exertion. The use of scientific gadgets, the enduring of pain, and the length of time involved in data collection all make the results of any training study with children subject to further verification.

Cardiovascular endurance is probably improvable in children much the same as it is in adults. Children simply need to be *motivated* to perform, become familiar with *pacing* themselves, and engage in *intensive* physical work over time.

The primary concern of the parent and teacher should not be how to improve maximum oxygen utilization but how to develop movement abilities and sufficiently motivate the child to the point that he or she improves as a function of a daily self-programmed regimen of vigorous physical activity. The teacher of preschool and primary grade children needs to focus on developing and refining fundamental movement abilities. The intermediate and upper grade teacher needs to apply these movement abilities to a variety of game, sport, and dance activities that provide an avenue for enhancing maximum oxygen utilization and other fitness abilities.

Although specific questions remain unanswered, there is agreement among researchers regarding the advisability of vigorous physical activity in children. The growth patterns of almost all the internal organs are in proportion to the remainder of the body. Hence the lungs, heart, and so forth, *are* able to cope with the demands placed on them. Physical trials indicate that the muscular system will flag and result in body collapse long before any damage is done to the heart. (Cunningham et al., 1977). Proportional to their mass, young children can transport and utilize oxygen volumes comparable to adults (Cumming and Hnatiuk, 1980). There seems to be no appreciable difference in the fatigability patterns between children and high school youth and adults.

The general consensus among researchers is that a sound heart cannot be injured by vigorous physical activity. Precautionary measures need, of course, be taken in the case of a child with a suspected or known cardiac and/or pulmonary dysfunction.

Muscular strength, muscular endurance, and flexibility are also components of physical fitness. They are related to one's positive state of health in much the same way as is cardiovascular endurance. Good levels of physical fitness tend to reduce the likelihood of suffering from numerous physical ailments. The components of physical fitness improve with age but not in a linear fashion. There is a strong tendency to make small gains during early and later childhood, followed by a lull during the preadolescent period. During adolescence boys often make rapid gains in all measures of physical fitness, while girls tend to level off and sometimes to decline in their performance scores after age 15.

The motor fitness components of coordination and balance are closely aligned with the development of movement control during early childhood. Once good control has been established, the child is able to focus on improvement in the force components of motor fitness. Speed, agility, and power improve dramatically during later childhood much the same way as balance and coordination improve during early childhood. There is a linear trend for improvement in all measures of motor fitness. The motor abilities of both boys and girls improve with age and effort, with boys outperforming girls at all levels except during the prepubescent period.

Physical fitness has been measured in children and youth in a number of ways. The AAHPER Youth Fitness Test was one of the first fitness tests devised based on specifically developed norms, and has been the most widely used fitness test in America. Recently, however, a new fitness test has been devised that is based on a different rationale of what it takes to be fit. The AAHPERD Lifetime Health Related Physical Fitness Test (1980) is composed of four items: (1) the nine-minute run for distance, or 1 mile run for time, (2) the sum of the triceps and subscapular skinfold measurements, (3) the one-minute bent-knee sit-up test, and (4) the sit and reach test. These items measure cardiorespiratory endurance, body composition, and the musculoskeletal function of the lower back and abdomen. This new test emphasizes that one does not have to be an athlete to be fit and views fitness as a continuum, with no single level of achievement mandated for all. Instead, minimum fitness levels compatible with optimal health are established.

## CHAPTER HIGHLIGHTS

1. There has been a growing realization of the importance of and necessity for vigorous physical activity for children and youth as well as adolescents and adults.
2. The normal daily routine of millions of North American children tends to exclude opportunities for regular vigorous physical activity.
3. Accurately determining the fitness levels of young children is difficult and time-consuming. Therefore, information concerning children under 8 years of age is limited.
4. The components of physical fitness are generally considered to be: cardiovascular endurance, muscular strength, muscular endurance, and flexibility.
5. Cardiovascular endurance is measured by determining the volume of oxygen consumed per kilogram of body weight.
6. Numerous indirect measures of Max $Vo_2$ have been devised and yield an indirect measure of aerobic capacity.
7. Children can achieve Max $Vo_2$ values similar to adult values, when corrected for body weight.
8. The sedentary child will not develop the same degree of aerobic fitness as his or her active counterpart.
9. Muscular strength may be classified as isotonic or isometric and involves one maximum exertion.
10. Strength improves in a linear fashion over age throughout childhood.
11. Predicting strength scores in later years on the basis of strength scores achieved during childhood is imprecise.
12. Boys tend to be stronger than girls at all ages even when body weight corrections are made.
13. Early maturers are stronger than later maturers. This condition often offers advantages in youth sport activities.
14. Endurance levels of children approach and often exceed those of adults when adjusted for body weight.
15. Endurance levels are similar for boys and girls prior to puberty, at which time boys improve at a more rapid pace and to higher levels.
16. Differences in endurance levels between sexes and among sexes may be partially accounted for by differences in achievement motivation levels when being tested.
17. Flexibility is joint specific and as such has often revealed conflicting results in research measures of this fitness component.
18. Age is a poor predictor of flexibility. Activity levels offer a better guide.
19. Physical fitness abilities, motor fitness abilities, and movement abilities are

interrelated. One affects the other and none operates in isolation of the others except in some controlled research settings.

20. Factor analytic studies with young children tend to indicate that the components of motor fitness (motor ability) may be grouped into a movement control factor and a movement force factor.

21. Balance and coordination are considered to be movement control factors, while speed, agility, and power are regarded as movement force factors.

22. The components of motor fitness, although generally subject to improvement over age, do not reveal a linear trend to do so.

23. Coordinated movement requires integration of sensory and motor systems into a congruent and harmonious action pattern.

24. Balance is critical to all movement behavior and is influenced by a variety of sensory mechanisms. Disturbance of any of these systems will have negative results on both static and dynamic balance behavior.

25. Speed, agility, and power are all influenced by both reaction time and movement time and improve up to about age 12 in most boys and girls. Improvement beyond this time requires special training.

26. Obesity is a national health problem that may be counteracted during childhood.

27. Poor diet and exercise patterns greatly increase the possibility of obesity. The obese child is likely to be an obese adult.

28. Anorexia nervosa is an emotional problem characterized by an aversion to food and fear of being too fat.

29. Anorexia nervosa is much more prevalent in our society today than it was just ten or fifteen years ago and may be traced in part to society's overconcern for a slim, trim figure or physique.

30. Anorexia nervosa is especially prevalent in adolescent girls, is easy to spot, but is very difficult to counteract.

## CRITICAL READINGS

AAHPERD: "Health Related Fitness," in *Journal of Physical Education and Recreation* (S. Plowman, Feature coordinator), 52, 1, 26–39, 1981.

Cratty, B.J.: *Perceptual and Motor Development in Infants and Children,* Englewood Cliffs, N.J.: Prentice-Hall, 1979, pp. 196–222.

Gilliam, T.B., et al.: "Physical Activity Patterns Determined by Heart Rate Monitoring in 6–7-Year-Old Children," *Medicine and Science In Sports and Exercise,* 13, 1, 65–77, 1981.

Hunsicker, P., and G. Reiff: "Youth Fitness Report 1958–1965–1975," in *Journal of Physical Education and Recreation,* 48, 32, 1977.

Stein, E.A., et al.: "Coronary Risk Factors in the Young," *Annual Reviews of Medicine,* 32, 601–613, 1981.

## CHAPTER 14

# Perceptual-Motor Abilities of Children

Perceptual development plays an important role in cognitive functioning, and as a result one is complexly intertwined with the other. The greatest development of perceptual abilities occurs during the preschool and primary years. Movement activities have been shown to be an important facilitator of perceptual development in young children. As a result, the term *perceptual-motor* has come into wide usage in recent years. Perceptual-motor abilities and readiness for learning are closely interrelated in young children. Perceptual-motor (movement) activities serve as an important mode through which fundamental readiness and academic concepts can be developed and reinforced. Based on this, the perceptual-motor development of children and its influence on academic concept readiness is the primary focus of this chapter.

The development of perceptual-motor abilities involves the complex interaction of perceptual, motor, and cognitive processes. Depending on the orientation of the reader, perceptual-motor experiences may be considered primarily as psychomotor *or* cognitive in nature. The variation in perspective stems from the purpose for which perceptual-motor activities are being performed. It has been documented that practice in perceptual-motor activities will enhance perceptual motor abilities (psychomotor perspective) (H. Smith, 1970). It has, however, been correspondingly demonstrated that practice in perceptual-motor activities will reinforce and aid in the development of academic concept development (cognitive perspective) (Cratty, 1972). Piaget lends support to this position with his stress on the sensorimotor phase of development in cognitive functioning. Perceptual-motor development is an important aspect of the cognitive domain that may be linked to academic concept readiness.

## PERCEPTUAL DEVELOPMENT IN INFANCY

From the moment of birth, the infant begins the process of learning how to interact with the environment. This interaction is a perceptual as well as a motor process. The term *perception* refers to "any process by which we gain immediate awareness of what is happening outside ourselves" (Bower, 1977, p. 1). In order to gain immediate information about the outside world, we must rely on our various senses. For our purposes we will discuss perceptual development separately, but caution must be taken not to separate the two in your thinking. The hyphen in the term perceptual-motor signifies the dependency of voluntary motor activity on perception and the dependency, in part, of the development of perceptual capacities on motor activity. This does not mean, however, that both perceptual and motor abilities will develop at the same time and at the same rate. Some perceptual abilities develop earlier and are independent of movement although they will eventually be paired during childhood.

Newborns receive all sorts of sensory stimulation (visual, auditory, olfactory, gustatory, tactual, and kinesthetic) through the various sense modalities. They make responses to these stimuli, but these responses have limited utility and are more or less automatic. Newborns are unable to integrate these sensory impressions that impinge on the cortex with stored information in order for meaning to be attached to these sensations. Only when sensory stimuli can be integrated with stored data do these sensations take on meaning for the infant and warrant being called *percep-tions*.

Newborns attach little or no meaning to sensory stimuli. The ability to integrate stored data with incoming data has not developed sufficiently. For example, light rays impinging on the eyes register on the retinas and are transmitted to appropriate nerve centers in the sensory areas of the cortex. The newborn's reaction is simple (sensation); if the light is dim the pupils dilate, and if the light is bright the pupils constrict and some of the stimulation is shut off (consensual pupillary reflex). Soon the infant blinks as the stimulus approaches. These simple reflex actions persist throughout life, but after a while the infant begins to attach meaning to the visual stimuli received. Soon a certain face becomes "mother." A blob is identified as having either three or four sides. Later it is identified as a triangle or as a square. The youngster now attends to certain stimuli and begins to apply basic meaning to them. The powers of visual perception are now developing.

The development of perceptual abilities is of considerable importance. McCandless (1967) has stated that:

> An adult functions well or poorly, succeeds or fails, depending on the way he manages his behavior in terms of his perception of himself and the world around him, and on how his perceptions fit with those of the people among whom he lives. His sense organs, the meaning he gives to the sensations he receives and his responses to the stimuli determine this consonance or disconance. (p. 22)

As with the development of motor abilities in the infant, the development of perceptual skills is a matter of experience as well as maturation. Maturation plays an important role in the development of increased acuity of perception, but most of it is due to experience. The learning opportunities that the child and the adult have primarily account for the sophistication of their perceptual modalities. Only through experience will the infant be able to acquire these capabilities. The infant's sensorimotor development and later perceptual-motor development are basic to later functioning. If early opportunities are severely inhibited or retarded, we may expect later abilities to be limited also.

## Visual Perception

At birth, the infant's eyes have all of the parts necessary for sight and are completely formed with the exception of the fovea, which is incompletely developed. There is also an immaturity of the ocular muscles. These two factors result in poor fixation, focusing, and coordination of eye movements. The blinking and lacrimal apparatuses are poorly developed at birth, and the neonate is unable to shed tears until one to seven weeks after birth. It is debatable whether the newborn possesses color vision because of the amount of rhodopsin (visual purple) present in the rods and cones of the eye. Fixation, tracking, acuity, color preference, and visual discrimination develop rapidly during the early weeks and months of life. Table 14.1 presents a list of the major developmental aspects of infant visual perception, along with the approximate age at which they begin to emerge.

In order to obtain information about the infant's perceptual abilities, a variety of measures may be obtained. Changes in general motor activity, physiological changes, reflexive movements, and voluntary motor responses are the primary means by which the researcher is able to determine whether the infant is responding to the experimental conditions. A change in one or more of these processes provides cues to the infant's developmental level and response to the experimentally produced situation. Recent research (Bower, 1974) has devised new means of evaluating infant perception. As more information becomes available, it becomes obvious that the infant is capable of far more sophisticated abilities than previously thought possible.

**Table 14.1    Developmental Aspects of Selected Infant Visual Perceptual Abilities**

| Visual Quality | Selected Abilities | Approximate Age of Onset |
|---|---|---|
| Sensitivity to light (McCandless, 1967) The visual apparatus is complete in the newborn and is first put to use by adjusting to varying intensities of the light source. | Consensual pupillary reflex (contraction and dilation of the pupils) | Birth 2 to 3 hours |
| | Strabismus | Birth to 14 days |
| | Turns head toward light source | Birth |
| | Closes eyes if light is bright | Birth |
| | Tightens eyelids when asleep | Birth |
| | More active in dim light than bright light | 0 to 1 year |
| Fixation (Bower, 1966; Jeffrey, 1966; Zubek, 1954) Fixation is probably monocular and essentially reflexive during the first six weeks of life. | Fixates one eye on bright objects | Birth |
| | Fixates both eyes on bright objects | 2 to 3 days |
| | Turns head from one stationary bright surface to another | 11 days |
| | Follows an object in motion, keeping the head stationary | 23 days |
| | Directs eyes toward an object | 10 weeks |

**Table 14.1** (Continued)

| Visual Quality | Selected Abilities | Approximate Age of Onset |
|---|---|---|
| Tracking (Field, 1976; Haith, 1966; Pratt, 1954)<br>Tracking forms the basis for later crucial avoidance and approach reactions, and develops far sooner than the motor component. | Horizontal<br>Vertical<br>Diagonal<br>Circular | Begins at birth. Time of onset is inconsistent, but the sequence is fixed. |
| Color discrimination and preference (Spears, 1964)<br>Inconsistent evidence. Color vision may or may not be present at birth depending on the amount of rhodopsin present. | Color vision<br>Color preference<br>Prefers shape to color<br>Reacts to color | Birth?<br>4 months<br>15 days<br>4 months |
| Form, shape, and pattern discrimination (Bower, 1977; Fantz, 1963; Hershenson, 1964; Lewis et al., 1966)<br>Discrimination begins early and develops rapidly in complexity. The human face is the favorite of all objects. | Prefers patterned objects to plain<br>Imitates facial gestures<br>Prefers human face to all other objects<br>Size and shape constancy<br>Discriminates between two- and three-dimensional figures<br>Geometric shape discrimination | Neonate<br><br>Neonate<br>Neonate<br><br>2 months<br>3 months<br><br>6 months |
| Visual acuity (McCandless, 1967)<br>the length of focus increases daily as the eye matures. | Organically complete visual apparatus<br>Length of focus 4 to 10 in.<br>Length of focus about 36 in.<br>Length of focus about 100 ft | Birth<br><br>Birth to 1 week<br>3 months<br>1 year |
| Depth perception (Bower, 1966; Cruikshank, 1941; Gibson, 1960)<br>Monocular vision at birth soon gives way to binocular vision and perception of depth | Monocular vision<br>Binocular vision<br>Depth perception | Birth<br>1 month<br>6 months |

## Auditory, Olfactory, and Gustatory Perception

Available research data concerning the development of auditory, olfactory, and gustatory perceptions in the human infant are much less complete than for the visual modality. In the area of auditory perception we find that as with vision the development of auditory abilities does not unfold naturally without the influence of the environment. Environmental conditions influence the extent of development of audition. The *ear* is structurally complete at birth, and the infant is capable of hearing just as soon as the amniotic fluid drains (usually within a day or two after birth). The fetus responds to sound before birth, and the neonate reacts primarily to the loudness and duration of sound. (Bernard & Sontag, 1947)

**Table 14.2  Developmental Aspect of Selected Infant Auditory, Olfactory, and Gustatory Abilities**

| Perceptual Quality | Selected Abilities | Approximate Age of Onset |
|---|---|---|
| Auditory perception (hearing) (Bower, 1977; Levanthal and Lipsett, 1964; Wertheimer, 1961) The ear is structurally complete at birth, and the newborn can respond to sound. | Responds to loud, sharp sounds | Prenatal |
| | Ability to localize sounds | Birth |
| | Reacts primarily to loudness and duration | Birth |
| | Crude pitch discrimination | 1 to 4 days |
| | Responds to tonal differences | 3 to 6 months |
| | Reacts with pleasure to parent's voice | 5 to 6 months |
| Olfactory perception (smell) (Bower, 1977; Engen et al., 1963) The olfactory mechanism is structurally complete at birth, and the newborn responds crudely to various odors. | Responds to odors | Neonate |
| | Reduced sensitivity upon repeated application of the simuli ("habituation") | Neonate |
| | Does not distinguish between pleasant and unpleasant odors | Neonate |
| | Discrimination abilities improve with practice | Infancy |
| | Shows preference for certain odors | Infancy |
| Gustatory perception (taste) (Pratt, 1954; Bower, 1977) The newborn reacts to variation in sweet, sour, and bitter tastes. Little research data are available on this modality. | Shows preference in tastes (prefers sweet to sour, and sour to bitter) | Neonate |

The research on olfactory and gustatory perception is much more sparse than on hearing. It is difficult to separate the developmental sequence of smell and taste simply because the nose and mouth are closely connected, and stimuli applied to one are likely to affect the other. The newborn does, however, appear to react to certain odors, although this may be due more to the pain caused by the pungent odors used than to smell. Newborns react to taste, preferring sweet tastes to sour ones and sour tastes to bitter ones. Table 14.2 presents a list of the major developmental aspects of infant auditory, gustatory, and olfactory perception.

## PERCEPTUAL DEVELOPMENT IN CHILDHOOD

By the time the child reaches 2 years of age, the ocular apparatus is mature. The eyeball is nearly adult size and weight. All anatomical and physiological aspects of the eye are complete, but the perceptual abilities of the young child are still incomplete. Although the child is able to fixate on objects, track them, and make accurate judgments of size and shape, numerous refinements still need to be made. The young child is unable to intercept a tossed ball with any degree of control (Payne, 1981). Difficulty with letter and number reversals is commonly experienced (Davidson, 1934; Rudel and Teuber, 1963). Children's perception of moving objects is poorly developed (Wapner, and Werner, 1957) as are figure-ground perceptual abilities (Gallahue, 1968), and perception of distance (Smith and Smith, 1966).

The extent to which movement plays a role in visual perceptual development is not known. Held and his colleagues (1961, 1963, 1964, 1965), O.W. Smith and P.C. Smith (1966), and Riesen and Aarons (1959) all speculated on the importance of movement in the development and refinement of visual perceptual abilities. They have conducted investigations based on the hypothesis that self-produced movement is both a necessary and a sufficient condition for visual-motor adjustment to occur within a visually altered environment. They contend that without movement, visual perceptual adjustments will not occur, and that the muscles and the motor aspect of the nervous system are intimately involved with perception, with one being dependent on the other. The concept of a relationship between movement activity and perceptual development has also been indirectly supported by the decline in performance on perceptual and motor deprivation experiments (Hebb, 1949; Riesen and Aarons, 1959), and experiments testing visual perceptual adjustment to an optically rearranged environment (Held and Blossom, 1961; Held and Mikaelian, 1964; Hoepner, 1967; Gallahue, 1982).

The fact remains, however, that the results of each of these experiments are only speculative at best when applied to the development of perceptual abilities in children. At this juncture we still do not know the extent of the role that movement plays in perceptual development. It is probably safe to say, however, that movement is a sufficient condition for encouraging the development of perceptual abilities.

Whether it is in fact a *necessary* condition is doubtful, but this conclusion must await further experimentation.

## PERCEPTUAL-MOTOR DEVELOPMENT IN CHILDREN

The visual perceptual abilities of young children are not the same as in adults. Children's visual world is in the developmental stages and is therefore restricted. The development of perceptual abilities significantly inhibits or enhances children's movement performance. From the previous section we have seen that the converse of this may be true; that is, movement performance may significantly inhibit or enhance the development of the children's perceptual abilities. The child restricted in perceptual development often encounters difficulties in performing perceptual-motor tasks.

The realization that the process of perception is not entirely innate enables one to hypothesize that the quality and quantity of movement experiences afforded young children are related to some extent to the development of their perceptual abilities. The initial responses of young children are motor responses, and all future perceptual and conceptual data are based, in part, on these initial responses. Young children must establish a broad base of motor experience in order for these higher learnings to develop properly. Meaningfulness is imposed on perceptual stimulation through movement. The matching of percetual and motor data is thought by many to be necessary for the child to establish a stable spatial world (Barsch, 1965; Kephart, 1971). The more motor and perceptual learning experiences that children have, the greater the opportunity to make this ''perceptual-motor match'' and to develop a plasticity of response to various movement situations.

Unfortunately, the complexity of our modern society often deters the development of many perceptual-motor abilities. The environment in which today's children are raised is so complicated and dangerous that they are constantly being warned not to touch or to stay away from situations that potentially offer great amounts of motor and perceptual information. Children often grow up in a large city, or in an apartment building, and seldom are given the opportunity to climb a tree, walk a fence, jump a stream, or ride a horse. They often miss out on many of the experiences that children ought to have as a part of their daily life experiences, in order to develop their movement abilities. The lack of these movement experiences and the adaptability of response that comes with practice and repetition often deter perceptual development.

Artificial means must be devised to provide additional experiences and practice in the perceptual-motor activities that modern society is unable to provide naturally. Providing children with substitute experiences that they are unable to get or fully explore on their own may have a positive effect on the development of their visual perceptual abilities. This would seem to support the position that the motor development specialist should be an essential person in the child's educational curriculum. A sound physical education program will contribute to the development of children's perceptual-motor skills and help develop many of the basic readiness skills prerequisite to success in school.

Physical education literature is replete with developmental skills and activities. For several years, many physical education and classroom teachers have been promoting learning readiness through physical activities. The majority have not been fully aware of the magnitude of the contribution that they have been making to children's development.

The development and refinement of children's *spatial world* and their *temporal world* are two of the primary contributions of perceptual-motor training programs. The jargon used in programs across North America varies greatly. There does seem, however, to be general agreement that the following perceptual-motor qualities are among the most important to be developed and reinforced in children by the motor development specialist.

## Body Awareness

The term *body awareness* is often used in conjunction with the terms *body image* and *body schema*. Each term refers to the developing capacity of young children to

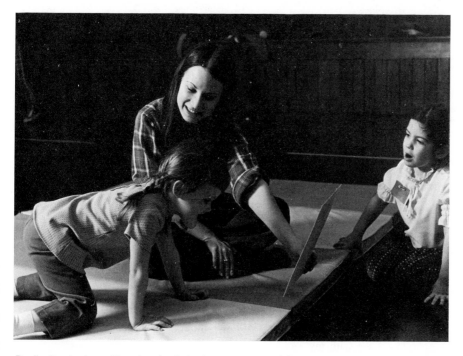

Duplicating body positions is a basic body awareness activity.

accurately discriminate among their body parts. The ability to differentiate among one's body parts and to gain a greater understanding of the nature of the body occurs in three areas. The first of these is *knowledge of the body parts*. This means being able to accurately locate the numerous parts of the body on oneself and on others. Second is *knowledge of what the body parts can do*. This refers to the child's developing abilities to recognize the parts of a given act and the body's actual potential for performing it. *Knowledge of how to make the body parts move efficiently* is the third component of body awareness. This refers to the ability to reorganize the body parts for a particular motor act and the actual performance of a movement task. The following are examples of movement activities that may be used to enhance the various components of body awareness.

**I.** Knowledge of the body parts.
　　　Touch your_____.
　　　**A.** head.

| | |
|---|---|
| **1.** Hair. | **9.** Lips. |
| **2.** Forehead. | **10.** Tongue. |
| **3.** Eyebrows. | **11.** Teeth. |
| **4.** Eyelashes. | **12.** Chin. |
| **5.** Eyes. | **13.** Ears. |
| **6.** Nose. | **14.** Earlobes. |
| **7.** Nostrils. | **15.** Neck. |
| **8.** Cheeks. | |

　　　**B.** Trunk.

| | |
|---|---|
| **1.** Chest. | **4.** Waist. |
| **2.** Stomach. | **5.** Side. |
| **3.** Hips. | |

　　　**C.** Arms.

| | |
|---|---|
| **1.** Shoulders. | **6.** Thumb. |
| **2.** Elbows. | **7.** Palm. |
| **3.** Forearms. | **8.** Wrist. |
| **4.** Hands. | **9.** Knuckles. |
| **5.** Fingers. | **10.** Fingernails. |

　　　**D.** Legs.

| | |
|---|---|
| **1.** Thighs. | **5.** Instep. |
| **2.** Knees. | **6.** Toes. |
| **3.** Calves. | **7.** Heels. |
| **4.** Ankles. | |

**II.** Knowledge of what the body parts can do.
　　　**A.** Head.
　　　　　**1.** I see with my_____.
　　　　　**2.** I hear with my_____.

    **3.** I smell with my_____.
    **4.** I taste with my_____.
    **5.** I lick with my_____.
    **6.** I blink with my_____.
    **7.** I talk with my_____.
    **8.** I kiss with my_____.
    **9.** I wrinkle my_____.
    **10.** I wear earrings on my_____.
**B.** Trunk.
    **1.** I carry a knapsack on my_____.
    **2.** Food goes to my_____.
    **3.** I wear a belt around my_____.
    **4.** I fold my arms across my_____.
    **5.** I bend at the_____.
**C.** Arms.
    **1.** I shrug my_____.
    **2.** I bend at the_____.
    **3.** I clap with my_____.
    **4.** I snap my_____.
    **5.** I wave with my_____.
    **6.** I point with my_____.
    **7.** I grasp with my_____.
    **8.** I carry heavy things on my_____.
    **9.** I color with my_____.
    **10.** I throw with my_____.
**D.** Legs.
    **1.** I kick with my_____.
    **2.** I bend at the_____.
    **3.** I squat on my_____.
    **4.** I kneel on my_____.
    **5.** I stand on my_____.
**III.** Knowledge of how to make the parts move efficiently.
    **A.** Coupling movements.
        **1.** Touch your nose to your shoulder.
        **2.** Touch your ear to your knee.
        **3.** Touch your knee to your toes.
        **4.** Touch your elbow to your knee.
        **5.** Touch your forehead to your thigh.
        **6.** Touch your elbow to your waist.
        **7.** Touch your head to your thigh.
        **8.** Touch your back to your heels.
        **9.** Touch your forearms to your calves.
        **10.** Touch your toes to your ear.

**B.** Specific body part movements.

| | |
|---|---|
| **1.** Click your heels. | **6.** Arch your back. |
| **2.** Pike at the hips. | **7.** Jut your chin out. |
| **3.** Tuck your trunk. | **8.** Pop your lips. |
| **4.** Shrug your shoulders. | **9.** Snap your fingers. |
| **5.** Stick out your chest. | **10.** Wiggle your nose. |

## Spatial Awareness

Spatial awareness is a basic component of perceptual-motor development that may be divided into two subcategories: (1) *knowledge of how much space the body occupies* and (2) *the ability to project the body effectively into external space.* Knowledge of how much space the body occupies and its relationship to external objects may be developed through a variety of movement activities. With practice and experience, children progress from their egocentric world of locating everything in external space relative to themselves (*egocentric localization*) to the development of an objective frame of reference (*objective localization*). For example, preschoolers determine the location of an object relative to where they are standing. Older children are, however, able to locate an object relative to its proximity to other nearby objects without regard to the location of their body.

As adults, our spatial awareness is generally adequate, but we may still encounter difficulties in locating the relative position of various objects. For example, when reading a road map while traveling through unfamiliar territory, many people become confused as to whether they are traveling north, south, east, or west. Difficulty is often encountered in deciding to turn right or left while looking at the map, without almost literally placing oneself on the map in order to project a mental image of which direction to turn. The absence of familiar landmarks and the impersonality of the road map make it difficult for many to objectively localize themselves in space relative to this particular task. Young children encounter much the same difficulty but on a broader scale. They must first learn to orient themselves subjectively in space and then proceed ever so carefully to venture out into unfamiliar surroundings in which subjective clues are useless. Providing children with opportunities to develop spatial awareness is an important attribute of a good movement education program that recognizes the importance of perceptual-motor development. The following is a list of examples of how spatial awareness may be enhanced in children.

**I.** How much space does the body occupy?
   **A.** Walk between two chairs.
   **B.** Step over objects at various heights.

    **C.** Walk or crawl under an object.

    **D.** Crawl through a tunnel (inner tubes will do).

    **E.** Estimate the size of various body parts.

    **F.** Compare body part size to other objects.

    **G.** Estimate your height on a chalkboard and then compare with actual height.

    **H.** Trace your body on a sheet of newsprint.

    **I.** Estimate how many steps it will take to get to the other end of the gymnasium and then see how close you came.

    **J.** Make yourself as small, tall, fat, or skinny as you can.

**II.** Projecting the body into external space.

    **A.** Follow one-step directions from point A to point B, using familiar objects in the room (desk, table, window, etc.).

    **B.** Follow two- and three-step directions from point A to point B and then C and D, using familiar objects in the room.

    **C.** Follow one-step directions outdoors from point A to point B without the use of familiar landmarks.

    **D.** Follow two- and three-step directions outdoors from point A to point B and then C and D without the use of familiar landmarks.

    **E.** Place a long rope on the floor in a certain configuration. Have the children walk on the rope with their eyes open. Repeat with the eyes closed.

    **F.** Draw a pattern on the floor. Have the children walk the pattern with their eyes open and then repeat the walk with their eyes closed.

    **G.** Draw a simple pattern (circle, square, or triangle) on the board. Have the children walk the same pattern on the floor.

    **H.** Give the children a task card indicating the location of a hidden object through a series of clues that require objective localization.

    **I.** Teach the children how to use a compass and locate various objects.

    **J.** Using a compass, determine the location of certain areas on a map of your school, community, city, or state.

## Directional Awareness

An area of great concern to many teachers is that of directional awareness. It is through directional awareness that children are able to give dimension to objects in external space. The concepts of left–right, up–down, top–bottom, in–out, and front–back are enhanced through movement activities that place emphasis on direction. Directional awareness is commonly divided into two subcategories: *laterality* and *directionality*.

    Laterality refers to an *internal* awareness or feel for the various dimensions of the body with regard to their location and direction. Children who have adequately developed the concept of laterality do not need to rely on external cues for determining direction. They do not need, for example, to have a ribbon tied to their wrist to remind them which is their left and which is their right hand. They do not need to rely on cues such as the location of their watch or ring to provide information about direction. The concept of laterality seems so basic to most adults that it is difficult to conceive how anyone could possibly not develop laterality. However, we need only to look into the rear-view mirror of our car to have directions reversed and sometimes confused. Backing up a trailer hitched to a car or truck is an experience that most of us prefer to avoid because of the difficulty we encounter in deciding whether to turn the wheel to the left or right. The pilot, astronaut, and deep-sea diver must possess a high degree of laterality or "feel" for determining up from down and left from right.

Directionality is the *external* projection of laterality. It gives dimension to objects in space. True directionality depends on adequately established laterality. Directionality is important to parents and teachers because it is a basic component in learning how to read. Children who do not have fully established directionality will often encounter difficulties in discriminating between various letters of the alphabet. For example, the letters *b*, *d*, *p*, and *q* are all similar. The only difference lies in the direction of the "ball" and the "stick" that make up the letters. As a result, the child encounters considerable difficulty in discriminating between several letters of the alphabet. Entire words may even be reversed for the child with a directionality problem. The word *cat* may be read as *tac*, or *bad* may be read as *dab* because of the inability to project direction into external space. Some children encounter difficulty in the top−bottom dimension, which is more basic than the left−right dimension. They may write and see words upside down and are totally confused when it comes to reading.

It should be pointed out that establishing directional awareness is a developmental process and relies on both maturation and experience. It is perfectly normal for the 4- and 5-year-old to experience confusion in direction. We should, however, be concerned for the 6- and 7-year-old child who is consistently experiencing these confusions because this is the time when most schools traditionally begin instruction in reading. Adequately developed directional awareness is one important readiness skill necessary for success in reading, and movement is one way in which this important perceptual-motor concept may be developed. The following are examples of movement activities useful in helping children develop directional awareness. They have not been separated into laterality and directionality here because of the author's conviction that the two cannot be effectively dealt with independently of one another in movement.

**I.** Movement commands utilizing directional clues.
   **A.** Stand in front of (behind) Jennifer.
   **B.** Step out on your left (right) foot.

    **C.** Move clockwise (counterclockwise).

    **D.** Stand to the right (left) of_____.

    **E.** Run between (around) the chairs.

**II.** Moving in different directions.

    **A.** Forward.                      **E.** Left.

    **B.** Sideward.                  **F.** Right.

    **C.** Backward.                  **G.** Upward.

    **D.** Diagonally.                 **H.** Downward.

**III.** Moving with other people.

    **A.** Stand in front of (behind)_____.    **D.** Stand to the left (right) of_____.

    **B.** Step under (over)_____.          **E.** Stand between_____and_____.

    **C.** Stand near (far)_____.

**IV.** Moving with an object (hoop, wand, etc.).

    **A.** Left−right.                **D.** Front−back.

    **B.** Top−bottom.             **E.** On−in.

    **C.** Over−under.

**V.** Moving on an object.

    **A.** Carpet squares can be used as steppingstones to teach left−right concepts of footedness.

    **B.** With footprints or handprints on the floor or wall, match left and right.

    **C.** Balance beam activities performed unilaterally or bilaterally are beneficial.

    **D.** Moving through a mat maze made from folding mats placed in such a way that left−right decisions have to be made is beneficial.

    **E.** Obstacle course activities that require the use of left and right in a prescribed manner are beneficial.

## Temporal Awareness

The preceding discussion of the various aspects of perceptual-motor development dealt with the development of the child's spatial world. Body awareness, spatial awareness, and directional awareness are closely interrelated and combine to help children make sense out of their spatial world. Temporal awareness, on the other hand, is concerned with the development of an adequate time structure in children. It is developed and refined at the same time the child's spatial world is developing.

    Temporal awareness is intricately related to the coordinated interaction of various muscular systems and sensory modalities. The terms *eye-hand coordination* and *eye-foot coordination* have been used for years to reflect the interrelationship of these processes. The individual with a well-developed time dimension is the one that we refer to as coordinated. One who has not fully established this is often called clumsy or awkward.

    Everything that we do possesses an element of time. There is a beginning point and an end point, and no matter how minute, there is a measurable span of time between the two. It is important that children learn how to function efficiently in this time dimension as well as in the space dimension. Without one the other cannot develop to its fullest potential.

*Rhythm* is the basic and most important aspect of developing a stable temporal world. The term has many meanings but is described here as the synchronous recurrence of events related in such a manner that they form recognizable patterns. Rhythmic movement involves the synchronous sequencing of events in time. Rhythm is crucial in the performance of any act in a coordinated manner. Cooper (1982) tape-recorded the sounds of the movement pattern of selected sport skills in outstanding performers. The sounds made by these performers were transcribed into musical notation illustrating that a recordable rhythmical element was present. The recorded rhythms of these outstanding athletes were beaten out on a drum in several teaching situations with beginners. The results were startling in that the beginners learned the movements of the champions more rapidly when this technique was used than in a standard teaching situation. Cooper and Andrews (1975) concluded that "it appears that beginning performers can profit by listening to and emulating certain elements of the rhythmic pattern of the good performers. Teachers should take full advantage of this phenomenon" (p. 66). Surely this statement applies to children as well as athletes. We must recognize the rhythmic element in all efficient movement, and in so doing be sure that we emphasize the rhythmic component of all movement.

H. Smith (1970) indicated that children begin to make temporal discriminations through the auditory modality before the visual and that there is transfer from the auditory to the visual but not the reverse. Activities that require performing movement tasks to auditory rhythmic patterns should begin with young children and be a part of their daily lives. The activity possibilities are endless. Moving to various forms of musical accompaniment ranging from the beat of a drum to instrumental selections can be an important contributor to temporal awareness. The following is a partial list of activities that may be used with young children to help them develop a more efficient time structure.

I. Rhythmic activities (with accompaniment).
    A. Move to various tempos.
    B. Move to various accents.
    C. Move to various intensities.
    D. Move to various rhythmical patterns.
    E. Perform fundamental locomotor movements to music.
    F. Singing rhythms.
    G. Basic folk dances.
II. Movement and drama (with accompaniment).
    A. Mimetics.           C. Puppetry.
    B. Finger plays.     D. Creative dance.

**III.** Ball activities.
   **A.** Tracking a swinging ball.
   **B.** Striking a stationary suspended ball.
   **C.** Striking a swinging suspended ball.
   **D.** Kicking a stationary ball.
   **E.** Kicking a moving ball.
**IV.** Rhythmic ball activities.
   **A.** Bounce and catch to music.
   **B.** Toss to self and catch to music.
   **C.** Toss to partner and catch to music.
   **D.** Volley to music (use a balloon).
   **E.** Combine bouncing, tossing, and catching to music.

## Perceptual-Motor Training Programs

During the past several years perceptual-motor training programs have sprung up across North America. During the 1960s and early 1970s several of these programs were given considerable exposure in the popular press. Based on these articles and the claims of some, many people formed the impression that these programs were panaceas for the development of cognitive and motor abilities. Considerable confusion and speculation developed over the values and purposes of perceptual-motor training programs. Programs adhering to one technique or another emerged almost overnight. All too often, people were inadequately trained, ill informed, and frankly, not clear on just what they were trying to accomplish. The smoke has now cleared, and concerned educators have taken a closer, more objective look at perceptual-motor training programs and their role in the total educational spectrum. Instead of claiming they are panaceas or adhering to one training technique or another, many are viewing perceptual-motor programs as important facilitators of readiness development. Perceptual-motor activities are being recognized as important contributors to the *general* readiness of children for learning. The contribution of perceptual-motor activities to *specific* perceptual readiness skills is being closely reexamined.

Readiness programs may be classified as *concept developing,* and *concept reinforcing*. Concept developing programs are generally designed for children who for a variety of reasons have been limited or restricted in their experiential background (e.g., socioeconomic class, prolonged illness, ethnic background, television). Head Start programs and Frostig's (1969) developmental program are examples of concept developing programs, in which a variety of multisensory experiences including perceptual-motor activities are used as a means of developing fundamental readiness skills.

Concept reinforcing programs are those in which movement is used in *conjunction* with traditional classroom techniques to develop basic cognitive understandings. In this type of program, movement is used as an aid or vehicle for reinforcing cognitive concepts dealt with in the nursery school or primary grade classroom. Cratty (1973), Humphrey (1974), and others have outlined a variety of concept reinforcing activities for use by young children.

Remedial training programs are the third and most controversial type of perceptual-motor training program. They have been established as a means of alleviating perceptual inadequacies and increasing academic achievement. Programs have been developed by Delacato (1959), Getman (1952), Kephart (1971), and others in attempts to aid cognitive development through perceptual-motor remediation techniques. The avowed purpose of these programs is to enhance academic achievement. There is, however, little solid support for this claim although abundant testimony and opinions are available. Figure 14.1 presents an overview of the various types of perceptual-motor training programs.

## Readiness and Remediation

Research indicates that as children pass through the normal developmental stages, their perceptual abilities become more acute and refined. This is due partly to the increasing complexity of the neuromuscular apparatus and sensory receptors and partly to the increasing of children's ability to explore and move throughout their environment. Piaget's (1954) work has traced the gradual development of perception from crude, meaningless sensations to the perception of a stable spatial world. His stages of development rely heavily on motor information as a primary information gathering process. As the perceptual world of children develops, they try to construct it with as much stability as they can in order to reduce variability as far as possible. As a result, they learn to differentiate between those things that can

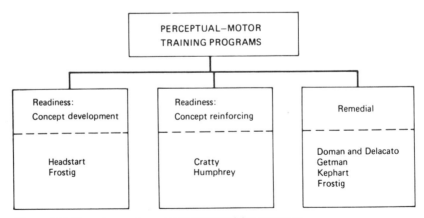

**Figure 14.1** Three types of perceptual-motor training programs.

be ignored, are easily predictable, or are wholly unforeseen and must be observed and examined in order to be understood, according to Piaget and others. Movement plays an important role in this process of developing perceptual readiness for cognitive tasks. Table 14.3 provides a comparison of Piaget's stages of development with those proposed by Kephart, and by this author.

The majority of our perceptions, and visual perceptions in particular, result from the elaboration and modificaiton of these basic reactions by experience and learning. When we speak of children being perceptually ready to learn, we are, in fact, referring to a point in time in which they have sufficiently developed their basic perceptual and conceptual learning tasks. Perceptual readiness for learning is a developmental process, and perceptual-motor activities play an important part in helping young children achieve a *general* stage of readiness. *Specific* perceptual readiness skills, such as visual perceptual readiness for reading, *may* be affected by the quality and quantity of the perceptual-motor experiences engaged in by children, but this has not been conclusively demonstrated in controlled research studies.

The process of being able to read (as well as other important tasks) involves a number of abilities of which visual perceptual ability is an important one. The reading process may be considered in terms of three basic areas, namely, language, skill, and perception. Considerable research has been conducted in the first two areas, but the third has only begun to be explored. The perceptual phase of reading involves the identification and recognition of words on a printed page. Form and shape perception may be enhanced through movement as well as directional awareness of up, down, left, and right. All are important factors associated with word identification and recognition.

The period of the greatest amount of perceptual-motor development is between age 3 and age 7. These are the crucial years preceding and during the time that children begin to learn to read. They are perceptually ready to read when they have developed a sufficient backlog of information that enables them to encode and decode sensory impressions at a given point in time with the benefit of previous learning experiences of high quality as well as quantity. A sufficient number of children enter the first grade with a lag in their perceptual abilities to warrant programs in readiness training that utilize perceptual-motor development activities as one of many avenues for intervention. The movement education portion of the school day can play an important role in helping many of these children catch up with their peers.

## Research Findings

Research efforts are continually being made in an attempt to document the virtues of perceptual-motor training programs on readiness and remedial aspects of perceptual and cognitive development. Each new research effort stimulates new questions and problems. The results that are available are not conclusive, but there is ample

**Table 14.3  Comparison of Piaget's, Kephart's, and Gallahue's Phases and Stages of Development**

| Approximate Chronological Age | Piaget's Intellectual Evolution | Kephart's Developmental Sequences | Gallahue's Phases of Motor Development |
|---|---|---|---|
| 0 to 6 months | Sensorimotor phase<br>Use of reflexes<br>Primary circular reactions<br>Coordination of prehension and vision, secondary circular reactions | Reflexive stage<br><br>Motor stage<br>Rudimentary motor pattern development | Reflexive phase<br>Encoding stage<br><br>Decoding stage |
| 6 to 12 months | Secondary schemata<br>Discovery of new means, tertiary circular reactions | Balance<br>Receipt and propulsion, Globular Form | Rudimentary phase<br>Reflex inhibition stage |
| 1 to 2 years | Beginnings of insight and cause/effect relationships<br>Egocentric organization<br>Perceptive movement | Motor-perceptual stage<br>Laterality<br>Hand-eye coordination<br>Gross motor pattern development<br>Syncretic form<br>Form recognition | Preinitial stage |
| 2 to 4 years | Preoperational thought phase<br>Perceptually oriented, period from self-satisfying behavior to rudimentary social behavior<br>Awareness of a conceptual hierarchy, beginnings of cognition | | Fundamental movement phase<br>Initial stage<br><br>Elementary stage |

| Age | | | |
|---|---|---|---|
| 4 to 6 years | Beginning abstractions | Perceptual-motor stage<br>Directionality<br>Eye-hand coordination<br>Perceptual stage<br>Form perception<br>Constructive form<br>Form reproduction | Mature stage |
| 7 to 10 years | Concrete operations phase<br>Additive composition,<br>reversibility, associativity,<br>identity, deductive reasoning<br>Relationships<br>Classification | Perceptual cognitive stage | Sport-related movement phase<br>General stage |
| 11 years and over | Formal operations phase<br>Intellectual maturity<br>Symbolic operations<br>Abstract thinking<br>Propositional thinking | Cognitive perceptual stage<br>Cognitive stage | Specific stage<br>Specialized stage |

evidence to suggest that perceptual-motor training programs are making a positive contribution to the motor, and perceptual development of children. In reviewing the literature, one may discover several generalizations that lend support to and have specific implications for the elementary education and physical education specialist concerned with the prevention and remediation of perceptual-motor learning disabilities. Some of the concepts that arise out of this research are:

1.  Not all learning disabilities are perceptual-motor in nature. Some may be due to problems in perceptual functioning. Others may be due to problems in concept formulation.

2.  Perceptual-motor deficits may or may not lead to learning disabilities in a given child. Despite this fact, diagnosis and remediation of problems is worthwhile if only for the expanded competencies, both physical and emotional (self-concept), that result from such remediation.

3.  Diagnostic tools for assessment are at this time in a rather primitive state. Distinct elements in the perceptual-motor spectrum have yet to be identified. Diagnostic tests cannot yet validly isolate separate factors.

4.  Low-level functional deficits (perceptual-motor tasks) seem to be associated with high-level functional deficits (perceptual-cognitive tasks). This is to say that children who perform poorly on tasks of high complexity (reading and arithmetic) also tend to perform poorly on low complexity tasks (laterality, directionality, midline).

5.  Intramodal abilities develop before intermodal abilities. This means that children learn to use each of the senses separately before they can interrelate them and use more than one mode at a time.

6.  The most efficient learning mode seems to be vision although learning is enhanced when information is presented to or processed by two or more modes at the same time. That is, the child is likely to learn more if presented information visually and auditorily at the same time than if presented information through only one mode at a time.

7.  Not all children are at the same perceptual level on entering the first grade. Perceptual development is a process of both maturation and experience, and children therefore develop at their own individual rates.

8.  Adequate perception (auditory, visual, tactile-kinesthetic) is prerequisite to success in school. Inaccurate perceptions lead to difficulties in academic concept formation. Perceptual readiness is an important aspect of total readiness for learning.

9.  Perceptual abilities can be improved through specialized training programs.

10. A program of perceptual-motor assessment can be useful at the preschool or kindergarten level to identify potential readiness lags in children and to adjust the curriculum to their strengths and weaknesses.

11.  Deprivation of perceptual-motor experiences at an early age may hinder the development of the child's perceptual abilities.

12.  Perceptual-motor training programs enhance the development of auditory, visual, and tactile-kinesthetic perceptual abilities in young children.

13.  Perceptual-motor activities should be included as part of readiness training programs.

14.  Some studies show a casual relationship between certain perceptual-motor abilities and reading achievement among selected groups of slow, normal, and above-average-intelligence children.

15.  A physical education program oriented toward the movement education concept provides many of the movement experiences that contribute to the development of the child's perceptual-motor abilities.

In conclusion, when we say that a child is "ready" to learn, we are, in fact, referring to a point in time when the child through maturation and learning has sufficiently developed the perceptual and motor abilities to be able to benefit measurably from higher-order perceptual and cognitive tasks. Movement experiences serve as a vehicle by which these capabilities are developed and refined. Children learn by doing. The physical educator plays an important role in the development of the young child's perceptual-motor abilities through a varied program of movement experiences that values the worth of each individual child.

## ASSESSING PERCEPTUAL-MOTOR DEVELOPMENT

During the past several years numerous measures of perceptual-motor development have been constructed. Generally, these tests were developed as measures for children who had been classified as "slow learners," "brain-damaged," or "neurologically impaired." They have been used with varying degrees of success. A list of selected tests of perceptual-motor functioning may be found at the conclusion of this chapter. The classroom teacher and physical education teacher are the first to pick up "subjective" cues of possible perceptual-motor difficulties in preschool and primary grade children. The validity of these subjective observations must not be discounted or minimized. On the contrary, the careful daily observation of children's behavior can be very valuable and reliable in detecting potential lags in development. It is suggested that the teacher refer students suspected of a developmental lag to the school psychologist for testing and specific delineation of the problem. The results of the testing should be shared with the parents and the teachers with whom the child comes in contact. In this way they can form an effective team to eliminate or diminish the difficulty. The checklist of cues that follow may aid the teacher in more accurately informal assessment of children with a potential perceptual-motor problem.

### Checklist of Possible Perceptual-Motor Dysfunctions

This checklist is designed to serve only as a subjective indicator of *possible* perceptual-motor difficulties. There is very little interrelationship among these variables and there is no predictable pattern for determining difficulties. Failure in several of these items *may*, however, lead the teacher to seek further information through more objective evaluative procedures.

1. Has trouble holding or maintaining balance.———
2. Appears clumsy.———
3. Cannot carry body well in motion.———
4. Appears to be generally awkward in activities requiring coordination.———
5. Does not readily distinguish left from right.———
6. In locomotor skills, performs movements with more efficiency on one side than the other.———
7. Reverses letters and numbers with regularity.———
8. Is not able to hop or skip properly.———
9. Has difficulty making changes in movement.———
10. Has difficulty performing combinations of simple movements.———
11. Has difficulty in gauging space with respect to the body, and bumps into and collides with objects and other children.———
12. Tends to be accident-prone.———
13. Has poor hand-eye coordination.———
14. Has difficulty handling the simple tools of physical education (beanbags, balls, and other objects that involve a visual-motor relationship).———
15. Has persistent poor general appearance.———
    (a) Shirt tail always out.———
    (b) Shoes constantly untied.———
    (c) Fly incessantly unzipped.———
    (d) Socks bagged around ankles.———
    (e) Hair uncombed.———
16. Is inattentive.———
17. Does not follow directions, or is able to follow verbal but not written directions, or vice versa.———
18. Has speech difficulties.———
    (a) Talks too loudly.———
    (b) Talks too softly.———
    (c) Slurs words.———
19. Poor body posture.———
20. Has hearing difficulties.———
    (a) Always turns head to one side.———
    (b) Holds or prefers one ear over the other.———
21. Has difficulty negotiating stairs.———

**22.** Daydreams excessively.———
**23.** Is excessively messy in work.———
    **(a)** Goes out of the lines.———
    **(b)** Inconsistency of letter size, etc.———
    **(c)** General sloppiness.———
**24.** Is unable to copy objects (words, numbers, letters, etc.).———

## Summary

Perceptual-motor training programs possess many of the same elements as any quality physical education program. Many of the movement skills taught in the perceptual-motor curriculum, whether it be a readiness or a remedial program, parallel those taught in regular preschool and elementary school physical education classes. The goals of each program are obviously different. Where as a primary goal of the physical education program is to develop movement control through practice and instruction in a variety of movement activities, the goal of the perceptual-motor program is to enhance perceptual-motor abilities through practice and instruction in a variety of movement activities.

Perceptual-motor training programs that purport to enhance academic achievement or to promote specific readiness for schoolwork do so amid considerable controversy and a lack of research support. Public testimony and opinion have served for years as the basis of support for perceptual-motor training programs. This is not adequate in today's world of accountability. However, the value of perceptual-motor experiences to a general state of readiness should not be dismissed. Enhancement of body, spatial, directional, and temporal awareness as a means of guiding the child toward improved movement control and efficiency in fundamental movement is worthwhile in itself. Practice in perceptual-motor activities will enhance perceptual-motor abilities. Whether these abilities have a *direct* effect on academic performance is questionable. One can be assured, however, that they do play an important role in developing and refining the child's movement abilities.

A comparison of the Phases of Motor Development with Kephart's developmental sequence and Piaget's cognitive phases of development was presented in Table 14.3. Careful review of these models reveals the interrelated nature of the perceptual, motor, and cognitive processes. The magnitude of this relationship and the conditions necessary for improved functioning in each area await further well-controlled scientific research.

## CHAPTER HIGHLIGHTS

1. The infant's perceptual abilities begin developing at birth and are generally refined by age 7.
2. Development of perceptual abilities depends, in part, on movement.

3. All voluntary movement involves an element of perception.
4. Perceptual and motor abilities do not necessarily develop at the same time and at the same rate.
5. Recent research indicates that the neonate and infant have more sophisticated perceptual abilities than expected.
6. Vision is the primary perceptual modality. The auditory, olfactory, and gustatory modalities are important but have not been studied as closely as visual perception.
7. Visual, tactile, and kinesthetic perception are of particular importance to the movement behavior of the child.
8. The extent of the role of movement in visual perceptual development is not known. Movement has been shown to be a sufficient condition for developing selected visual perceptual abilities, but it has not been shown to be a necessary condition.
9. The child restricted or behind in perceptual development often encounters problems developing perceptual-motor abilities.
10. Practice in perceptual-motor activities will enhance perceptual-motor abilities.
11. There is insufficient evidence to support the claim that practice in perceptual-motor activities will enhance academic achievement.
12. Bodily, spatial, directional, and temporal awareness are four perceptual-motor components that may be enhanced through a quality physical education program.
13. Perceptual-motor programs may be thought of as readiness and remedial in nature. Ample testimony is available to support both, but research evidence is lacking at the present time.
14. Both formal and informal assessment instruments have been devised to assess perceptual-motor abilities. These subjective instruments must be thought of only in terms of providing clues to possible developmental difficulties and not as a means of labeling children.

## CRITICAL READINGS

Bower, T.G.R.: *Development in Infancy*, San Francisco: W.H. Freeman, 1974, Chapters 2, 4, 5.

Bower, T.G.R.: *The Perceptual World of the Child*, Cambridge, Mass.: Harvard University Press, 1977.

De Oreo, K., and H. Williams: "Characteristics of Visual Perception," in C.B. Corbin (ed.), *A Textbook of Motor Development*, Dubuque, Iowa: W.C. Brown, 1980, pp. 148–173.

Seefeldt, V., "Perceptual-Motor Programs," in J. Wilmore (ed.), *Exercise and Sports Science Reviews*, New York: Academic Press, 1974, pp. 265–288.

## SELECTED MEASURES OF PERCEPTUAL-MOTOR FUNCTIONING IN CHILDREN

Berry, K.E.: *Developmental Test of Visual-Motor Integration,* Follett Educational Corporation, Chicago, Ill.

Bender, Laura: *Bender Visual Motor Gestalt Test,* The Psychological Corporation, New York, N.Y.

Cheves, R.: *Pupil Record of Educational Behavior,* Teaching Resources Corporation, Boston, Mass.

Doll, E.: *Oseretsky Motor Proficiency Tests,* American Guidance Service, Inc., Circle Pines, Minn.

Frostig, Marianne, and D. Horne: *The Marianne Frostig Developmental Test of Visual Perception,* Consulting Psychologists Press, Palo Alto, Calif.

Katz, J.: *Kindergarten Auditory Screening Test,* Follett Educational Corporation, Chicago, Ill.

Kirk, Samuel, et al.: *The Illinois Test of Psycholinguistic Abilities,* University of Illinois Press, Urbana, Ill.

*Perceptual Testing-Training Kit for First Grade Teachers,* Winter Haven Lions Research Foundation, Inc., Winter Haven, Fla.

*Perceptual Testing-Training Kit for Kindergarten Teachers,* Winter Haven Lions Research Foundation, Inc., Winter Haven, Fla.

Roach, Edward, and N. Kephart: *The Purdue Perceptual-Motor Survey,* Charles E. Merrill, Columbus, Ohio.

Valett, Robert: *Valett Developmental Survey of Basic Learning Abilities,* Fearon Publishers, Palo Alto, Calif.

Wepman, J.: *Auditory Discrimination Test,* Language Research Associates, Chicago, Ill.

# 15

# The Self-Concept of Children

Do you remember when you were a child with nothing to do but play for hours and hours each day? Do you remember the excitement of that first climb to the top of the monkey bars, your first successful ride on your two-wheeler, or your first swim all the way across the pool? We can all remember as children how good it felt to succeed and can probably even remember a time or two when we did not. Those successes and failures of childhood may seem quite remote and meaningless to us now, but as a child they were important events in our lives. Events that had an influence on what and who we are today. Many of these events centered around our early play experiences, because how children feel about themselves is greatly determined by play experiences, both successful and unsuccessful.

Children are active, energetic, and emerging beings. Much of their life is spent in play and active exploration of their ever-expanding world. The so-called play world of children occupies a large portion of their day and is of central importance to them. It is an important avenue by which children come to learn more about themselves, their bodies, and their potential for movement. The development of many basic affective concepts have their roots in the carefree, exhilarating world of play.

Self-concept is an important aspect of children's affective behavior that is influenced through the world of games, play, and vigorous movement. Because the establishment of a stable, positive self-concept is so crucial to effective functioning in our lives, its development is too crucial to be left to chance. The important contribution that movement and vigorous physical activity can make to forming a good self-concept should not be overlooked. As parents and teachers we should be genuinely interested in the development of a good self-concept in our children. In the past the important link between physical activity and self-concept has often been given only lip service. In this chapter we will examine self-concept development and the potential for movement to enhance self-concept.

## WHAT IS SELF-CONCEPT?

Self-image, self-esteem, self-respect, self-confidence, and ego are terms used to describe essentially the same thing, namely, one's estimate of personal worth or worthlessness. Although these terms have subtle differences in meaning, they are often used interchangeably and add up to the sum total of how we feel about ourselves and how we think others feel about us. It is that feeling of "I can" or "I can't," "I'm good," or "I'm bad," that we all possess.

Self-concept may be thought of as awareness of one's personal characteristics, attributes, and limitations and the way in which these characteristics are both like and unlike others. The notion of self-esteem is also included in this definition, because it refers to the value one places on oneself and one's behavior. Self-esteem and self-concept are closely related and referred to interchangeably because value judgments are frequently involved in what children learn about themselves from other people.

What makes people different from each other and makes them uniquely

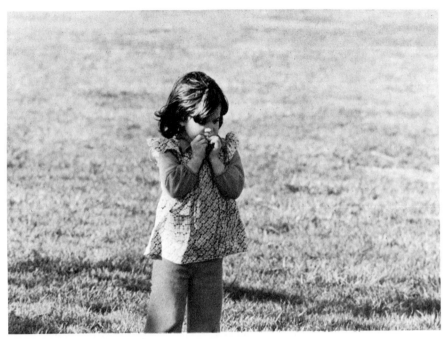

Self-concept is that feeling of "I can" or "I can't."

themselves and not someone else is their self-concept and view of the world as *they* know it. The sum of their experiences and their feelings about these experiences contribute to this mental model. We find out about ourselves in many ways. By choosing, trying things out, experimenting, and exploring, we discover who we are, what we can do, and what we cannot do. Not only do we *discover* who we are, but through our experiences we contribute to the making or formation of our unique identity. Each new choice adds something to our backlog of experience and hence to our world and to ourselves.

Self-concept is *learned,* and its development begins at least at birth. Some authorities argue that the emotional state of the expectant mother, ranging from a relaxed, happy pregnancy to a tension-filled, traumatic pregnancy, may have a dramatic affect on the unborn child. Yamamoto (1972) states that:

> some studies have suggested that stress experiences by a pregnant mother can alter the movements of the fetus from normal to hyperactive—the mother should know that a physically healthy child has a greater chance for adequate psychological development, since the concept of a child's physical self plays an important part in the entirety of the self-concept. (pp. 181–182)

The early months of life mark the first tangible beginnings of self-concept development. The tenderness, warmth, and love displayed between parent and child convey the first feeling of "I am loved" and "I am valued." The infant's sense of well-being is affected by the emotional state of the parent and attention to his or her physical needs. The fulfillment of psychological needs is just as important, for the infant needs to establish a sense of trust, security, recognition, and love. Trust is a basic issue to be resolved in the early mother-infant relationship. Mothers and fathers create a sense of trust in their children by combining sensitive care of their baby's needs with a firm sense of personal trustworthiness. Erikson was probably the first to recognize the establishment of a sense of trust during the early months of life. His stage of "trust versus mistrust" is rooted in the child's developing a sense of being loved and valued in a world that has constancy and permanence.

The toddler experiences the satisfaction of mastering the art of walking successfully or solving a problem with a new toy. This development of a sense of autonomy is an important facilitator of a positive self-concept, influenced greatly by parents, teachers, and other central adults in the life of the child. These individuals have a unique opportunity to selectively reinforce the child's learning about herself or himself. This is done through consistent acceptance, with both respect and concern and provision for freedom and independence within carefully defined limits. Much of what the young child learns is imitative, and this learning is not restricted to overt action. Feeling and attitudes can also be learned through imitation. As a result, the type of model that central adults project determines many of the attitudes and feelings that the child develops.

Gradually, the child develops a greater sense of independence. During the sixth or seventh year, the child begins to shift his or her frame of reference from the home and family to the school and the teacher. The sphere of "significant others" that have an impact on the developing self expands. Teachers as well as the peer group begin to exert greater influence. The teacher becomes a primary model for the child, and there is a great desire to please. Martinek and Zaichkowsky (1977) found that the teacher's expectations of the child's performance level had a definite impact on self-concept from the second through the sixth grades. A study by Zaichkowsky et al. (1975) revealed that the teacher's level of expectancy for children in a physical activity was positively correlated with self-concept scores. In other words, those expected to do well had higher self-concepts than those expected to do poorly. The implications of these findings are enormous when applied to the teacher/learner, or coach/athlete dyad.

The teenager feels good about the accomplishment of new and difficult tasks and the newly found sense of independence that accompanies performing meaning-ful work and earning money. The thoughtful parent recognizes the importance of the peer group at this level and the importance of assisting in the gradual establishment of a sense of mature independence. Self-concept can be enhanced continually throughout life through the pride of accomplishment and the sense of

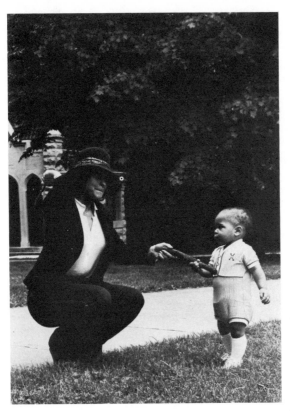

Playful interaction between parent and child is an important facilitator of self-concept development.

being needed, loved, and valued. When using the term *self,* we find that it includes more than one's personal physical self. It also includes and is affected by all of those persons and groups with whom we identify. Our family, friends, acquaintances, church, school, and place of business are all persons or institutions with which we identify.

Our conviction of personal worth and effectiveness develops chiefly through successful experiences in coping, according to Maynard (1973). For one to have confidence one must be able to cope. One must be willing to accept oneself as well as others who are different. Children who can cope are adaptable rather than rigid in their behavior. They are diligent, can concentrate on a task, and can work through difficulties. Confidence in oneself is developed through the joy of finding what one does well—of doing anything really well. Motor abilities and movement skills are only one avenue by which self-image may be enhanced. It is, however, a very important one for most children, because so much of their daily life experiences are centered around the need for efficient and effective movement.

In short, self-concept is the sum total of our life's experiences. It is our personal estimate of self-worth based on what we think of ourselves and what we think others think of us. Self-concept is developed through successful experiences in coping throughout our daily lives and doing something well. Movement plays an important role in enhancing or limiting self-concept development in children, because it is a central focus in their lives. High positive value is placed by both children and adults on successful performance in physical activities, as evidenced by the hero status of many college and professional athletes and the high positive peer group acceptance of the skilled performer.

## SOCIAL STATUS AND MOVEMENT SKILL

The relationship between children's social status and their performance in movement activities has been a subject of interest to researchers for many years. Numerous studies point out that there is indeed a link between high positive peer group acceptance and ability in games and sports, especially in boys. Tuddenham (1951) has pointed out that central in the boys' constellation of values is athletic skill, predicated upon motor coordination, strength, size, and physical maturity.

Skill level is often controlled by factors that are outside the child's influence. Such things as physical stature, health-related conditions, and lack of experience and quality instruction make it impossible for many children to meet the values of their peer group. As a result, they often suffer for it in terms of feelings of inferiority, rejection, and poor self-image. Tuddenham has stated that personal insecurity and social maladjustment often have their roots in this area.

When considering the effect of skill level on the social status of young girls, the available literature present a somewhat different picture. The results of Tuddenham's (1951) classic study indicated that girls are less dependent than boys on the possession of specific physical skills. Cratty (1967) does indicate, however, that it does seem important for girls to be moderately skillful in motor performance between the approximate ages of 5 and 14 years, but after that superior motor performance in other than a few "acceptable" sports (golf, tennis, horseback riding, etc.) can *detract* from a girl's popularity. It appears that the tremendous changes we are witnessing in the role of women in our society and the recent surge of interest in all forms of competitive athletics for girls and women may soon prove Tuddenham's and Cratty's researches to be generally outdated. The upsurge of interest in participation in traditionally male activities such as Little League baseball and the Soap-Box Derby, along with increased intramural and interscholastic competition for girls, has clearly indicated a change in the social status of physical activity for females. The vast majority of recent self-concept research has shown little in the way of sex differences between boys and girls (Felker, 1974; Erhartic, 1977; Martinek and Zaichowsky, 1977; Piers, 1969). Martinek and Zaichowsky have, however, documented a definite tendency for reduced self-concept during puberty for both sexes.

When applied to young children, it is safe to hypothesize that boys and girls from about age 4 or 5 years onward are either positively or negatively affected by their performance abilities in games, sports, and dance activities. Although this is not the only avenue of influence on the child's self-concept, we must recognize that it is an important one, one that we should be sure to properly guide and nurture through concerned guidance and developmentally appropriate experiences.

## POSSIBLE CONSEQUENCES OF A POOR SELF-CONCEPT

A poor self-concept is reflected in the feelings of "I can't," "I'm always wrong," or "I'm worthless." Children who feel bad about themselves and the world they know are not likely to feel better about the part of the world they do not know. As a result, they often reflect the attitude of caring little to explore that world. This is simply because it does not look inviting and appears hostile and full of possibilities for humiliation and defeat. Holt (1970) makes the point that this hostile and threatening new world becomes one that does not lure the child out but thrusts in on him or her, invading those few fairly safe places where even a small sense of who and where he or she is are threatened. Children with a negative self-concept come to view the world they do not know as even worse than the world they are familiar with.

Children who feel themselves to be of little worth due to repeated failures often fall back on the protective strategy of deliberate failure. Deliberate failure serving as a self-protecitve device can be explained by the principle that you cannot fall out of bed when you are sleeping on the floor. In other words, children who view themselves as complete failures will not even be tempted to try. They avoid the "agony of defeat" because they feel that the "thrill of victory" is a hopeless cause.

Children with a poor self-concept are also negatively affected by what they think others think of them (Yawkey, 1980). Children, as well as adults, tend to live up to the expectations of others, or at least to what these expectations are perceived to be. Teachers are of tremendous importance in shaping children's basic attitudes toward themselves in relation to school. During the elementary years a significant correlation exists between children's perception of their teachers' feelings toward them and their own self-image. Teachers who place a great deal of emphasis and value on self-concept tend to be associated with students who hold a positive view of themselves. The use of such terms as *stupid, dumb, always wrong, bad boy (girl), trouble-maker,* and *lousy* all have a tremendous impact on children. These spoken words, as well as our unspoken indications of disapproval, dismay, disgust, anger, and surprise, have an effect on what children think others think of them. Given enough negative information, the child soon learns the role that he or she feels is expected. Children with a negative self-image tend to live up to their perceived negative role. As a result, a cycle of failure and perceived expectation of failure is established.

Children with a poor self-image often are very little cheered when now and then they do succeed. Their perception of themselves as nonachievers and the idea that others perceive them in the same manner is a difficult cycle to break when success is infrequent. This may be explained with the analogy of people who are usually sick and suddenly start to feel well. Unlike the usually healthy people who think they will soon be well, sick people think that this good feeling surely cannot last. It is much the same with children. Even when the normal pattern of failure is broken occasionally with success, they still have the feeling that it cannot last and things will certainly go wrong soon.

The influence of a poor self-concept on the learning process can be tremendous. Brookover, et al. (1967) concluded from their extensive research on self-concept and achievement that the assumption that human ability is the most important factor in achievement is questionable, and that the student's attitudes limit the level of achievement in school. Students' perception of themselves as "learners" or "nonlearners" often has an effect on low academic achievement. Lecky (1945) demonstrated that low achievement is often due to children's definition of themselves as nonlearners because they resist learning when it is inconsistent for them, in their view, to learn. Children who feel that they cannot achieve experience a situation in which their actual ability to achieve is reduced or negated. On the other hand, children with a success-oriented outlook find that they can plunge into a project or take on a new challenge with little past experience and more often than not be successful. Wattenberg and Clifford (1962) reported that the best predictor of beginning reading achievement was children's perceptions of themselves in kindergarten.

In summary, the consequences of a poor self-concept can be devastating. Children with a poor self-image often display little interest in their expanding world. They often fail deliberately and perform poorly as both a protective device and an attempt to live up to perceived expectations. Children with a poor self-concept are little cheered by occasional successes. They often view themselves as nonlearners and perform poorly academically while possessing average or above-average intelligence. The consequences of negative feelings toward oneself are tremendous. They are associated with high anxiety, underachievement, behavior problems, learning difficulties, and delinquency. The establishment of a stable, positive self-concept is too important to be left to chance. The role of movement in self-concept development must be reexamined. Statements such as the following made by the American Alliance of Health, Physical Education, Recreation (1968), although admirable, are vague and provide little insight into how movement has an impact on the developing self:

Another prime goal in all physical education instruction is the development of a strong self concept or feeling of respect for the mind and body, and confidence in one's ability to function effectively. Individuals who feel good about themselves—who are active and involved, who can act effectively and with grace—are more at ease socially and more self-assured in whatever they try to do. (p. 3)

## THE INFLUENCE OF MOVEMENT ON SELF-CONCEPT

The way children feel about their bodies and the ease and efficiency with which they move play an important role in the types of activity they actively seek to engage in. If children are able to handle their bodies well, to move with a degree of success, they will experience positive reinforcement of their self-image. Cratty (1967) feels that almost without exception the children who have difficulty handling their bodies have a poor self-concept.

The playground, gymnasium, and play environment of children provide excellent media for positive self-concept development. Although it is certainly not the only way in which self-concept may be influenced, research is beginning to show clearly that it is a very basic one for most children. Little research has been conducted in the area of movement and self-concept. It has long been considered a "sloppy" area in which to do study, for a variety of reasons. First, it is difficult to isolate the possible variables that influence the self. Second, the criterion measures of self-concept that are used are often suspect in terms of their validity. Third, the manner of construction of numerous tests has often been "weird," according to McCandless (1976). Research in the area of movement and self-concept is now beginning to reflect a concern for these difficulties and to deal effectively with them within the scope of the particular investigation. Quality investigations into the effects of movement on the self-concept of children are just coming into view. Martinek and Zaichkowsky (1977) found that children given a chance to share in the decision-making process concerning the conduct of a physical education class actually developed more positive self-concepts. Erhartic (1977) and Martinek and Zaichkowsky (1977) also found that there is little correlation between children's motor abilities and their self-concept.

Wallace and Stuff (1973) administered a perceptual-motor training program conducted by classroom teachers over a one-year period for thirty minutes per day. The most frequently reported change by the teachers was in behavior areas. The data from the rating scales that were dispensed revealed a significant positive change in self-concept.

Exceptional children were studied by Johnson et al. (1968) in a clinical physical education program. A specially constructed self-concept scale was administered before and after the six-week hour-per-day program. The results of the experiment revealed that the discrepancy between ideal self and actual self decreased in several areas. The children showed a great desire to work in groups and an increased willingness to be with certain family members.

Clifford and Clifford (1967) reviewed the effects of the Outward Bound Program in Colorado. The stated purpose of the program was to build physical stamina and push each individual to his or her physical limit. Self-concept measures dealing with ideal self (what I would like to be) and actual self (what I am) were administered before and after the month-long program. At the conclusion of the program, the gap between ideal self and actual self scores was lessened with a positive change occurring in the actual self-concept.

Collingswood and Willett (1971) working with obese teenage boys, found that a specially constructed gymnasium and swimming program had positive affects on self-concept. Postsession scores of self-image were significantly increased, and the ideal self versus actual self discrepancy significantly decreased.

In a study to investigate the influence of competitive and noncompetitive programs of physical education on body image and self-concept, Read (1968) found significant differences in self-concept scores between those identified as consistent winners and consistent losers. The consistent winners had significantly higher self-concept scores than did the consistent losers. The subjects who were neither consistent winners nor losers did not drastically change in body image or self-concept.

The implications gleaned from these few but important studies are that well-conceived and properly implemented movement programs can have an effect on self-concept development. Yamamoto (1972) believes that for the teacher interested in learning the feelings of pupils toward themselves, a very good first step is in the observation of gross and fine motor performance in the gym, on the playground, in competitive games, and when writing.

## MOVEMENT AND THE DEVELOPING SELF

Children who have difficulty performing the many fundamental skills basic to proficient performance in games and sports encounter repeated failure in their everyday play experiences. As a result, they often encounter difficulties in establishing a stable view of themselves as worthy beings. Taylor (1980) stated that "one of the best and easiest pathways to a strong self-concept is through play. Play offers opportunities to assist the child in all areas of development. Its importance can be found in how he [the child] perceives himself, his body, his abilities and his relationships with others." (p. 133) The question now becomes a matter of: (1) What can we do? And (2) how can we utilize the movement activities of children and aid them in the formation of a stable, positive self-concept?

During the past several years, this author has conducted a motor development program designed to make positive contributions to the self-concept of children from ages 4 to 12 years. The "Challenger's" program caters to children who are experiencing difficulty in their everyday play world. A large percentage of the children are referred to the program because of problems in school adjustment, peer relations, self-confidence, and emotional instability. The others do not possess any apparent difficulties in these areas. The results of the informal research with the children have shown positive increases in self-concept as measured by the Piers-Harris Children's Self-Concept Scale (Piers, 1969) in a significant majority of the children taking part in the four-day-per-week program. Throughout the operation of the Challenger's program, a concentrated effort has been made to apply common-sense principles through movement to the enhancement of the developing self. The following paragraphs are a delineation of these principles. A film strip was developed by the author through a grant from Phi Delta Kappa, Phi Lambda Theta, and Delta Kappa Gamma education organizations depicting the efforts of the Challenger's program in enhancing self-concept (Gallahue, 1974).

## Success

The most important thing that we can do is to help children develop a proper perspective on success and failure in their daily lives. Because of the egocentric nature of children, it is very difficult for them to accept both success *and* failure. Success is that feeling of "I can," "I did it," or "Look at me" that we love to see in children. It is the sense of accomplishment that accompanies mastering a new skill, executing a good move, or making a basket. Failure is that feeling of "I can't," "I don't know how," or "I am always wrong." It is the feeling of frustration and hopelessness that often follows failure to master a skill or execution of a poor move.

We need to help children develop a balance between success and failure. We need to bolster their sense of self-worth so that when things go poorly and they fail to achieve at something, they will not be completely defeated. This backlog of successful experiences will help develop that "I can" attitude. Success is very important, particularly at the initial stages of learning. We need only look at ourselves and our tendency to continue those activities we are successful in. This basic principle of learning theory is applicable to both children and adults. We need to take the importance of success into consideration when working with young children, by using teaching methods that emphasize success.

The use of a problem-solving or movement-exploration approach to the learning of new movement skills enables all children to experiment and explore their movement potentials. It enables the children to become involved in the *process* of learning instead of being solely concerned with the *product*. In other words, it is a child-centered approach that allows for a variety of solutions or "correct" answers. Both the teacher and the children are more concerned about individual solutions to the problem than finding one best way. The astute teacher of young children recognizes the fact that there is no best way of performing at this level of development. The astute teacher is more interested in helping children gain greater knowledge of their bodies, how they move, and fostering more mature patterns of movement. For example, the teacher may structure a movement problem or challenge such as, "How can you balance on three body parts?" or "Who can balance on three body parts?" The number of possible solutions is great and so is the range of difficulty. As a result, several solutions are possible and all children gain increased knowledge of how they can move and balance their bodies. The teacher, through a question or challenge, also avoids imposing a predetermined model of what the performance should be and how it should look.

Individualizing instruction is another way of emphasizing success for each child. Individualized instruction takes into account the uniqueness of each learner and provides all with opportunities to achieve at their own particular level of ability. Although it is often difficult to put into practice because of large classes, limited staff, time, and facilities, teachers should try to individualize whenever possible. The typical nursery school program does a tremendous job of individualizing instruction through incorporation of an open classroom approach with a variety of interest centers. Too often, however, on entering the first- or second-grade classroom, children are faced with the rigid structure of the traditional classroom and gymnasium program that assumes all children to be at the same level in their interests, abilities, and motivation for learning. The unquestionable fact is that all children are not "typical" first-graders. Within any given class, the children can be functioning at levels passing through both ends of the spectrum of that particular grade level in cognitive, affective, and motor abilities. Greater attention to recognizing individual needs and interests and abilities will do much to strengthen the success potential of each child.

Traditional methods of teaching movement are valuable, especially at higher skill levels, but the teacher often requires that all students perform at a certain level or emulate a particular model of performance. Some children may have considerable difficulty accomplishing the desired level of parformance. Teacher dominated methods are often limited in providing success-oriented experiences for everyone. Although these methods should be a part of the movement activity program, they should not be stressed too early in the learning process. They should attempt to allow for individual differences in readiness rates, and abilities for learning new movement skills.

Movement programs that make use of problem-solving approaches and recognize the value of individualizing instruction whenever possible make positive contributions to self-concept development. But what actually is involved in using these success-oriented approaches?

Through the use of developmentally appropriate movement experiences that are challenging and properly sequenced, we can help children. We can also help in the formation of a good self-image by helping them establish reasonable expectations of their abilities and through communication of our expectations (Figure 15.1).

## Developmentally Appropriate Activities

We must recognize that children are not miniature adults ready to be programmed to the whims and wishes of adults. They are growing, developing, and emerging beings with needs, interests, and capabilities that are quite different from those of adults. Too often, we fall into the trap of trying to develop miniature athletes out of

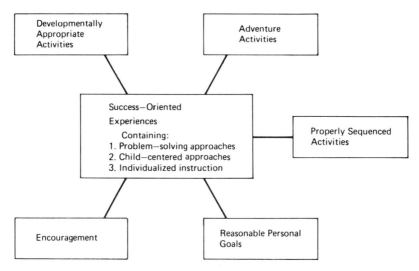

**Figure 15.1** Five important factors to consider when utilizing success-oriented experiences to enhance self-concept development.

6- and 7-year-olds without first developing the children's fundamental movement abilities. Too often, we force children to specialize in the development of their movement abilities at an early age. They become involved in competitive athletics before they are ready to handle the physical and emotional demands that competition can bring. Competition is not an evil or something to be excluded from the lives of children, but it must be kept within the proper perspective. Coaches and parents need to be fully cognizant of the children they are dealing with and the fact that winning is *not* everything, as proponents of that often-quoted phrase "Winning isn't everything, it's the only thing" philosophy would have us believe. Parents and coaches must have as their objective the balanced, wholesome, and healthful development of children under wise leadership, through the avenue of competition. The needs, interests, and capabilities of each child must be carefully considered. Developmentally appropriate activities must be sought out as a means of aiding children in establishing a realistic concept of their abilities.

## Adventure Activities

We can also have an impact on the self-concept of children in the area of adventure or pseudo-dangerous activities. Children need to experience the thrill offered by climbing, balancing, and crawling through objects. They need the feeling of mastery that comes from succeeding at activities that challenge their courage and imagination. They need to experience the adventure of hanging by their knees, balancing on a beam, climbing a ladder, riding a horse, or crawling through a tunnel.

The teacher, through voice inflection and the use of the child's imagination, can also help to create an atmosphere of challenge and adventure. Imaginary obstacles may be put in the path of successful completion of an activity. Such things as "sharks" beneath the balance beam, which has been transformed into a "narrow log" across a "shark-infested pond," or a story play depicting a bear hunt, or trip to the circus stimulate children's imaginations. Through adventure activities, both real and imagined, children have an opportunity to learn more about their own bodies and have the thrill of successfully overcoming a challenge.

## Sequencing of Tasks

A third factor involved in using a success-oriented approach to enhancing self-concept is the sequencing and difficulty of a movement task. The proper sequencing of movement activities is crucial in determining a child's sense of success or failure. For example, it seems perfectly logical to first learn a tripod or frog stand followed by a headstand, and then to learn a handstand, rather than

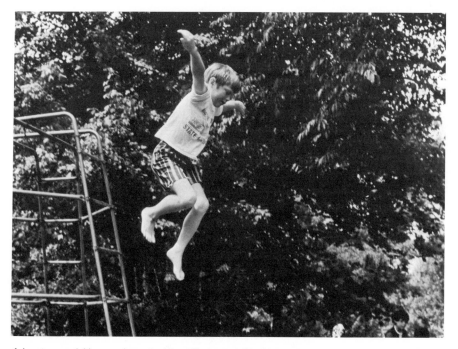

Adventure activities are important in self-concept development.

proceeding in the reverse order. Yet we often do just that when as adults we try to make miniature athletes out of 6- and 7-year-old children. Too often, parents and teachers neglect the development of fundamental movement abilities before proceeding to higher-level skills. Instead of looking at the development of movement skills from the point of view of the child, we all too often look at movement from our point of view, namely as athletes. We skip the basics and go directly to high-level skill development. It is much better to begin at a lower level where the chances for experiencing success are greater, and then to proceed to develop skill upon skill in a logical sequential progression. Success at the initial stages of learning will not only encourage continued performance, but will tend to generate success at later stages. Children who attempt a difficult task without the proper basic skills may not succeed and may give up entirely. It is important that we analyze movement activities that children engage in and determine logical sequences for accomplishing them.

Exactly scorable tasks such as archery or bowling may be difficult to deal with in the initial stages of learning unless modifications and provisions are made for success-oriented experiences. Cratty (1968) states that "tasks which have performance limits, e.g., a bullseye in archery, will be more likely to produce feelings of failure when projected goals are not achieved" (p. 30). It would be better, in

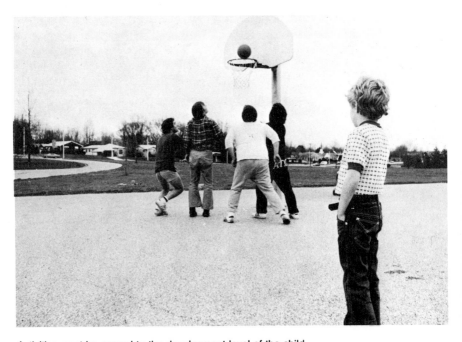

Activities must be geared to the development level of the child.

archery for example, to eliminate the target during the initial stages of learning, or to enlarge it or move it closer in order to maximize the opportunities for success.

Caution should also be taken not to introduce competition too early in the learning process. Because competition necessitates there being a winner and a loser, it gives too accurate an indication of relative success or failure during the early phases of learning. It may be better to postpone competitive situations until the child can make a sound appraisal of his or her ability.

## Reasonable Expectations

A fourth area in which we can have an influence on children's developing self is in helping them establish reasonable expectations of their abilities. This is especially true with young children because of their black and white world of good or bad, right or wrong, that allows little room for anything but these two extremes. It is important that we help children develop an attitude about personal success that is based on the extent to which they feel they have reached some goal, and not on the absolute scores obtained. Children need to learn how to set reasonable goals for themselves, and we can help them by providing goals that are not so high that attaining them is unrealistic, but high enough to ensure quality effort and a reasonable chance for success. For example, lowering the basket or reducing the size of the basketball will provide children with more opportunities for success than insisting on the use of a regulation ball and putting the standard at the regulation 10-ft height. It must be remembered, however, that once reasonable success through quality effort is ensured, new goals need to be established. This must be done in order to keep the activity challenging. Frost (1972) reinforces this by stating that "when tasks are too easy and success too cheap little development takes place. When tasks are too difficult and achievement impossible, frustration and reinforcement of a negative self-concept are likely to follow" (p. 21).

## Encouragement

A fifth area of influence that we have on the developing self is through communication of *our expectations* to the child. We must communicate how we feel about the child's accomplishments. Self-concept development is based in part on what we think others think of us. For children, these "significant others" center around the home and school. It is important to use positive encouragement in order to communicate our feelings about their accomplishments, whether they be large or small. Praise and positive encouragement must be used judiciously because children will soon "read" it as being meaningless if it is inappropriately used. We can communicate our feelings to children by praise for a job well done, with a pat on the back, or a smile. We need to communicate the feeling of "you are loved" and "you are worthwhile." One way to encourage these feelings is to recognize that it is often not so much what we say to children that influences their feelings about themselves as it is the way in which we treat them. Children value themselves to the degree that they are valued. The way we feel about our children actually builds in (or builds out) self-confidence and a sense of self-worth. Children build their picture of themselves from the words, attitudes, body language, and judgments of those around them.

By providing children with a nurturing climate of acceptance and experiences of success, negative attitudes can be changed to high self-esteem. It is important that when we do make a specific statement about something that disturbs us or that we do not like about a child's behavior, we should restrict our comments to the *behavior* instead of making generalized criticisms of the child *as a person*. For example, it is much better to say "I am worried about your difficulties with sharing" rather than "nobody likes a stingy person." Similarly, it is dangerous to label children as "stupid," "bad," or "motor moron." They often believe the labels that are attached to them and inadvertently act out their expected role. We should not link a personal lack of worth with undesirable behavior. We should not make children feel that they are personally worthless just because their schoolwork, sports abilities, or something else does not meet our expectations.

There is no place for devastating remarks in teacher–child communication. A teacher shuns comments that casually destroy children's self-concept. The teacher's role is not to injure but to prevent injury and to heal. Positive encouragement on the playground, in the classroom, and at home plays an important role in helping children develop a stable positive self-concept.

## ASSESSING SELF-CONCEPT IN CHILDREN

The accurate assessment of self-concept has been a problem plaguing psychologists for years. The validity of a vast majority of measures of self is questionable, and the reliability of the information is often subject to criticism (Wylie, 1974). In spite of these obvious limitations, a number of self-report measures have become available in recent years. The basic assumption underlying any self-report measure is that the respondent is the only individual qualified to reveal his or her feelings and that these responses provide an accurate and truthful indication of how that person feels.

The problems that surround self-concept assessment in children are many. Zaichowsky et al. (1980) have indicated that "attitudes toward the self do not become generalized until about 8 years of age. Up until that time they are more a function of the immediate situation" (p. 157). This, coupled with the additional problems of reading level, comprehension, and the testing environment makes it questionable whether the assessment of self-concept prior to age 8 or 9 can be of any real practical, let alone research, value. Nevertheless, a variety of self-concept measures suitable for use with children have been devised. A list of selected self-concept measures may be found at the end of this chapter. Caution is advised, however, in the use and interpretation of data obtained from these instruments.

## Summary

Self-concept is an important aspect of the affective development of children. The concept that children have of themselves is based on their feelings about themselves and what they think others think of them. Their self-concept is in the developmental stages and is profoundly influenced by all that happens to them in their daily life experiences. It is important that we as teachers and parents make an effort to ensure the development of a positive, stable self-concept in our children, because once it is firmly established, it becomes increasingly difficult to make radical changes. Combs and Snygg (1959) have alluded to the stability of self-concept beyond its developmental stages:

> Once established in a given personality, the perceived self has a high degree of stability. The phenomenal self with the self-concept as its core represents our fundamental frame of reference, our anchor to reality; and even an unsatisfactory self-organization is likely to prove highly stable and resistant to change. This stability has been repeatedly demonstrated in modern research. (p. 130)

Because of the importance of vigorous play in the lives of children and the high value placed on physical ability by children and adults, movement can serve as an important facilitator of a positive self-concept. We must, however, be sure to apply sound principles of growth and development to this important task. We need to provide children with success-oriented experiences that minimize the failure potential.

In order to do this, we must be sure to employ developmentally appropriate movement experiences that are within the ability level of the individual. We must be sure that the learning of new movement tasks is properly sequenced, based on sound progressions from the simple to the complex. We must also help children establish reasonable goals for their performance within the limits of their abilities. We must be sure also to provide encouragement and to incorporate adventure activities into their lives.

Although movement is only one avenue by which a positive self-concept may be fostered, we must recognize that it is an important one for most children. The development of a positive self-concept is too important to be left to chance and we must do all that we can to assure its proper development.

## CHAPTER HIGHLIGHTS

1. The child's self-concept begins developing at birth. Movement plays an important role in its development.
2. Teachers' expectations have a significant impact on self-concept development.
3. Little evidence exists to support the notion of self-concept differences

between boys and girls. However, girls have been less dependent on being good in sports and physical activities for self-concept reinforcement.

4. A negative self-concept can have devastating effects on all aspects of the child's life.
5. Significant others play an important role in self-concept reinforcement.
6. Once formulated, a negative self-concept is difficult to alter without special efforts by parents, teachers, and friends in a nonthreatening environment.
7. Self-concept has been shown to be enhanced in children participating in a success-oriented physical education program.
8. Children on athletic teams that are identified as consistent winners tend to have higher self-concepts than children on teams identified as consistent losers.
9. Success-oriented experiences play an important role in developing positive self-concepts in children.
10. Developmentally appropriate activities, adventure activities, properly sequenced experiences, and positive reinforcement are all important factors in self-concept development.
11. Self-concept is difficult to measure, and especially so in children.
12. There are serious questions concerning the reliability and validity of children's self-concept scales.
13. Attitudes toward oneself do not become generalized until about 8 years of age.

## CRITICAL READINGS

Canfield, J., and H.C. Wells: *100 Ways to Enhance Self-Concept in the Classroom,* Englewood Cliffs, N.J.: Prentice-Hall, 1976.

Felker, D.: Building Positive Self Concepts, Minneapolis, Minn.: Burgess, 1974.

Wylie, R.: *The Self Concept: A Critical Survey of Pertinent Research Literature,* Lincoln, Nebraska: University of Nebraska Press, 1974.

Yawkey, T.D. (ed.): *The Self-Concept of the Young Child,* Salt Lake City, Utah: Brigham Young Press, 1980.

## SELECTED MEASURES OF SELF-CONCEPT IN CHILDREN

Creelman, M.B.: "The CSC Test: Self-Conceptions of Elementary School Children," unpublished doctoral dissertation, Western Reserve University, 1954.

Martinek, T., and L.D. Zaichkowsky: *Manual for the Martinek-Zaichkowsky Self-Concept Scale for Children,* Psychologists and Educators, Inc., Jacksonville, Ill., 1977.

Piers, E.V.: *Manual for the Piers-Harris Children's Self-Concept Scale,* Counselor Recordings and Tests, Nashville, Tenn.: 1969.

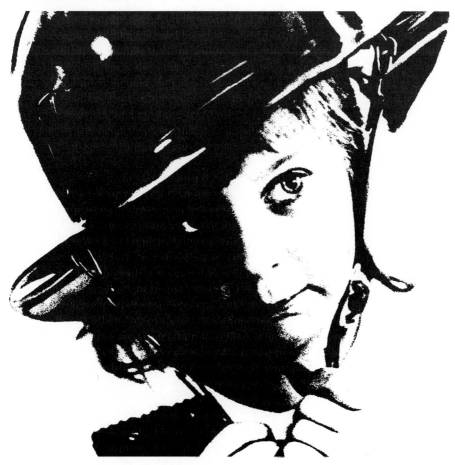

# 16

# Children's Play, Toys, and Play Spaces

For children, play is essentially a learning medium, but for too many years it has often been viewed as a frivolous pastime. It seems unnecessary among knowledge-able people to assert that play is valid as a learning medium as well as for its own inherent values, especially with the attention that the writings of Piaget (1957), Erikson (1963), and others have commanded in recent years and with the implications for developing cognitive and affective structures through play. Frank (1968), however, has noted that "within recent years there has been a strong movement to restrict the play of children, young and older, to adult-imposed patterns in order to promote formal learning, especially preparation for school" (p. 433). We must, therefore, reassert the validity and the necessity for play in child development.

The greatest values of play in education are that it is interesting to children, holds their attention, arouses their enthusiasm, is fun, and contributes to the developing self. As a result, a primary distinction between the terms *work* and *play* is that play is engaged in simply for its own sake. Play does, however, through proper guidance, have numerous residual benefits that make it a desirable medium through which myriad psychomotor, cognitive, and affective competencies may be developed. Play is an effective learning medium because of the importance placed on it by children and its potential influence on all aspects of behavior. It is time that the validity of children's play be recognized. In order to do this, we must pay more than lip service to its values. We must become sensitive to the play of children, and in doing so must become familiar with the types of toys and play spaces that are conducive to children's optimal growth. This chapter will focus on three important aspects of children's lives, namely, play, toys and play spaces.

## PLAY

The meaning of the word *play* is elusive and has various connotations to many people. Ellis (1973), in the excellent book *Why People Play,* explores in detail the questions as to what play is and why people play. Play is usually considered to be pleasant and voluntary. With reference to children, the definition of play offered by Galambos (1970) is perhaps the most appropriate for our discussion of motor development. Galambos considers play to be "direct, spontaneous activity by which children engage with people and things around them. It is imaginative, usually active; youngsters perform it with all their senses and use their hands or their whole bodies" (p. 61).

The following is a discussion of why children play and the developmental aspects of play. It should be read carefully in order to gain greater insight into the child's world of play.

### Why Children Play

To children, play is serious business, and it is this seriousness of purpose that gives it its educational value. Play is the way in which children explore and experiment with the world around them as they build up relations with that world, others, and themselves. Children at play are discovering how to come to terms with their world, to cope with the tasks of life, to master new skills, and to gain confidence in themselves as worthwhile individuals. Play provides a medium through which

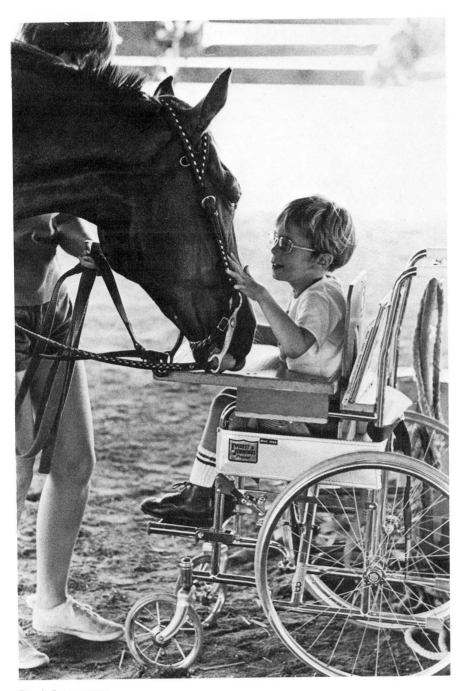

Play is for everyone.

children can learn through trial and error. It provides a means through which they can experience an endless number of real-life situations in miniature with a minimum of risks, penalties, and pain for mistakes. It is an excellent way in which to learn how to cope with the "real" world.

Play provides an avenue through which children gradually learn the difference between *mine* and *yours*. It permits children to first discover themselves and then to reach out to others in their rapidly expanding world. Through play, children learn basic patterns of living. Their imagination and love for creative drama enable them to assume various roles, feelings, attitudes, and emotions.

Play is also necessary for the mental health of children. Children engage in play wholeheartedly, discarding all self-consciousness and restraint. They reveal their true nature through play and often provide the parent and teacher with subtle indicators of their emotional well-being. Immature children who have had limited play experiences often need to be taught how to play in a meaningful and constructive manner. These children exhibit their lack of ability to play through their wandering, constant boredom, and pleas that "there is nothing to do." Aggressive behavior is often exhibited through destructive play and is typified by children who always manage to break their toys or inevitably end up in a wrestling match with their peers. Children who are emotionally disturbed often prefer to play with things rather than interact with other children and are demanding of adult attention and approval of their play. Children who are well adjusted find it easy to slip into and out of various roles in dramatic play.

Play helps meet children's emotional needs to belong and to have status within a group and a feeling of personal worth. As a result, they will generally play at things in which they do well (much the same as adults) and experience a reasonable degree of success.

Through active play, children learn to move for movement's sake as well as for learning's sake. Directed play experiences can serve as an effective means by which they may develop and refine a variety of fundamental movement abilities. It also serves as a facilitator for enhancing physical fitness and motor abilities. The natural drive by most children to be active needs to be continually nurtured by both parents and teachers.

## Developmental Aspects of Play

When viewing the play behavior of children, it is apparent that there is a predictable sequence of emergence of developmental aspects. The play of the infant and toddler is considerably different from that of the primary grade child. Increased complexity of the neuromuscular apparatus plus higher-order cognitive functioning and increased affective competencies makes for characteristic forms of play at various ages. However, when observing play, one runs the risk of interpreting it within the context of one's own interests and understandings, and failing to see it in its

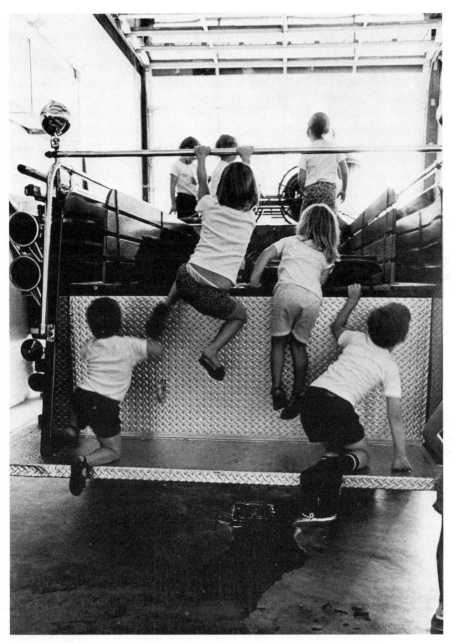

Play is adventure.

complete form. As a result, a narrow view of play is often developed. For example, a teacher primarily interested in the motor development of children may view play from the perspective of gross motor activities, games, and sport. Teachers interested primarily in cognitive development often view play from the quiet activity aspect of problem solving and experimentation with new equipment, materials, and ideas. Persons primarily concerned with the affective domain often view play from the functions that it serves as a socializing agent, without regard to either its active or its quiet forms. In actuality, play incorporates all aspects of development, whether motor, cognitive, or affective. We must, therefore, view play in light of its total contribution to the growth and development of children.

Play during the first year of life does not look much different from normal daily activity. The infant is constantly involved in using all of his or her senses and, when awake, appears to be in almost constant motion. The play of infants is centered around their own bodies, the bodies of others, and concrete objects. It involves the exploration and repetition of perceptual cues and is purposeful. Through play, the infant comes to grips with his or her world and develops a host of cognitive, affective, and psychomotor competencies. For example, the ever-popular game of peekaboo is enjoyed by all infants and may be viewed from a cognitive standpoint as a learning activity in which the child learns, through experience, the complex ideas of permanence, consistency, and reliability of objects, and that objects can reappear once they have disappeared. Peekaboo also has implications for affective development in that it provides a medium for the infant to learn to trust the world, to shape it, and to make things happen. From a psychomotor standpoint, it provides practice in controlling the musculature of the hands and proper sequencing of events in time.

The play of infants involves coming into contact with shapes, textures, colors, and sounds. A great deal of time is spent in looking, listening, grasping, sucking, teething, and exploring. In short, the play of infants is a sensorimotor experience that involves the broadening use of all of the senses in order to come to better know and to function better in the immediate world.

The toddler rapidly expands beyond the play of infancy. It is a time of reaching out into the world through ceaseless, joyful movement in an effort to order his or her world. The play of toddlers is primarily egocentric; that is, it is confined to the individual and does not involve interaction in a constructive manner. Toddlers use their newly acquired mobility to explore space. They spend a great deal of time trying out their movement potentialities. They crawl, climb, scoot, walk, run, roll, and jump. They attempt to order their world by classifying objects and searching for patterns. They enjoy play with small manageable toys, lining them up, stacking them, and exploring them with their mouths. They play at classifying objects according to size, shape, color, and function. Toddlers also spend a great deal of time testing the limits of their world through imagination, imitation, and dramatic play. The imitative play world of toddlers enables them to make sense of experience through dramatizing it in action. Toddlers enjoy loading and unloading objects of various sizes into containers and by doing so are developing concepts of volume and permanence. Stroking different-textured objects is a favorite quiet play activity of toddlers, and they often have a favorite cuddly toy or blanket. This may be viewed as an attempt by the child to find warmth and security at a time when many demands for more mature behavior are being made, such as with developing the self-help skills of feeding and toiletry.

The play of the preschooler is an elaboration of the earlier forms of play and also involves new aspects. Children at this age enjoy using and "mastering" a wide variety of materials. They thoroughly enjoy working with paints, sand, clay, water, and blocks. The use of these materials begins by being purely exploratory and then becomes more systematic, organized, and takes on concrete form. The imitative play of the toddler gives way during these years to highly involved sociodramatic play, with a more mature grasp of what is real and what is fantasy. They enjoy acting out social situations, dressing as grown-ups, and travel play with cars, fire engines, and airplanes. Preschool children enjoy active play. They love to run and jump, throw and catch, and need little encouragement for active movement. They enjoy building things and progress from blocks to more advanced forms of construction.

Primary grade children enjoy many of the same activities as preschoolers, but exhibit increasing ability to work with others in small groups. They are more interested in active games and table games with rules and regulations. They enjoy art and making designs in two- and three-dimensional form. Primary grade children enjoy drawing, painting, and molding as an expressivn of their creativity. Their imagination, however, is often less vivid than preschoolers, and care must be taken by adults to nurture it. Primary grade children enjoy discovery play, problem solving, and generally like vigorous movement activities.

There is considerable overlap between the play of toddlers, preschoolers, and elementary school children. Older children will often retreat to earlier forms of play in order to reestablish their security, and self-confidence. Younger children likewise will often attempt the more sophisticated forms of play behavior of an older brother or sister, only to find that they do not possess the necessary gross or fine motor coordinations, nor the cognitive or affective capacity, for successfully engaging in that form of play. We return to the principle of *readiness* as the primary determinant of what, when, and how children play. We should view each child as an individual and structure play situations that are appropriate for that particular person.

Three hierarchical stages in the development of play behavior have been proposed by Reilly (1974), who views the development of play as having exploratory, competency, and achievement stages. The *exploratory stage* roughly comprises the eary childhood years. Every new thing that the young child comes into contact with evokes curiosity, exploration, and play. The *competency stage* is characteristic of the elementary school child. This represents a time for mastery over the environment. Practice, persistence, and the quest for mastery are

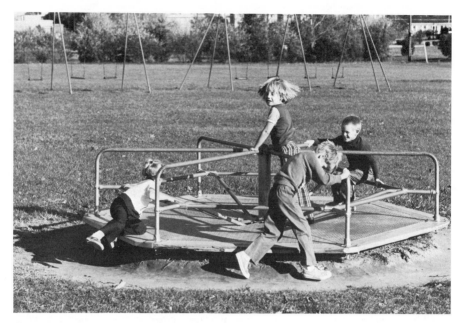

Play is thrilling.

characteristic of the competency stage. The *achievement stage* of play places the individual within the competitive realm and achievement of the expectancies children have for themselves as well as those others may hold for them.

Reilly's concept of the developmental aspects of play behavior is congruent with the Phases of Motor Development (Figure 16.1). The rudimentary movement phase corresponds nicely with the exploratory stage. Fundamental movement pattern development and refinement are congruent with the mastery stage, and the sport-related movement phase parallels Reilly's achievement stage.

## TOYS

One of the most visible differences between today's modern schools and traditional classrooms is the number of objects made available for the purpose of helping children learn. Traditionally schools have transmitted facts and concepts in an abstract way, by means of words, in an atmosphere removed from the everyday environment. In an effort to see that every child receives a socially useful and personally satisfying education, it has become apparent that this is not the only way for children to learn. For many it is not the best way, and for some, no way at all. Many children can learn better through activities that look suspiciously like play. Activities that involve toys, games, and puzzles, manufactured and self-made; tools

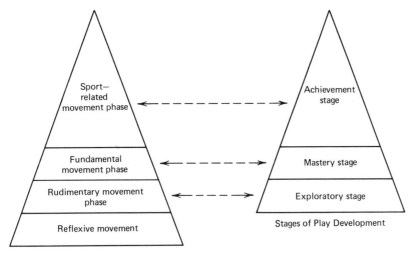

**Figure 16.1** Relationship between the development of play skills and the phases of motor development.

and materials; expressive media; models and replicas from the physical and social environment, concrete items that children can touch, handle, manipulate, and interact with are all being utilized with increasing frequency as an effective learning medium. In such ways they lay a solid foundation for abstract learning. This new emphasis is disturbing to many parents and some educators. "Why," they say, "the children are only playing. They can do that at home!" Such persons should be led to understand the many specific learning purposes for such "play" activities.

Toys and expressive media are often useful as tools for the various types of diagnosis that teachers make about the developmental stage, educational needs, and emotional health of their students. It is important, for example, for teachers to discover the maturational level of children entering the preschool or elementary grades. Observation of their skills in using materials and their interaction with the materials and other children is revealing and valid to the knowledgeable observer. Toys such as building blocks are a good example. They give children power to construct and manipulate their world within their own frame of reference. Their building may be free in form and unstructured, or realistic and elaborated. In watching such activities, as well as in talking with children, the teacher receives clues to many of their perceptual, cognitive, and emotional needs.

The therapeutic value of letting children express themselves in activities like finger painting, clay modeling, pounding, playing with dolls and other people figures, and role playing with the help of costumes or puppets, has been commonly accepted. They are useful in determining whether the child's need to relieve anxieties and to express concerns is temporary or results from a more deep-seated problem involving motor or perceptual difficulties or the expression of hostilities, fears, or other symptoms of psychological and social maladjustment.

Another use of tangible objects in the educational process, which teachers can apply with most children, is developmental. To determine whether a child's lack of readiness for academic work is due to age or to lack of stimuli in the home environment, object-oriented activities (toys) are a valuable aid. They encourage the desired learning in the cognitive, psychomotor, or affective area, or in a combination of these.

On the cognitive level, immature children must be encouraged to furnish their mind with the concrete experiences that are the necessary foundation for the increasing complexity and level of abstraction of their thoughts. Being deprived of these opportunities at home or at school may make it impossible for them to develop to their full potential for abstract thinking. Remediation by furnishing an environment rich in stimuli can do much to overcome the original deprivation. But the child's way of thinking may have been so affected that he or she will respond most easily to ideas demonstrated in a concrete way. An effective teaching strategy for such children is to give them solid, manipulable objects designed to demonstrate the desired concepts. Word games, cut-out letters, puzzles, and Cuisenaire rods are examples. Older children do better when ideas are presented with examples from their own experience. Such a presentation does not handicap the learning of children who are able to handle abstracts; it simply helps reinforce the concepts for them.

The development of movement abilities depends in large part on the availability of objects for children to interact with. They need things that can be folded, bent, nailed, glued, cut, sewed, stretched, bounced, poured, twisted, punched, tied, blown into, and crushed; surfaces that can be painted, carved, attached to, and washed; items to look at, listen to, sniff, taste, fondle, and stroke; and objects to climb, swing on, sit on, stamp on, jump over, and crawl through.

The ways that toys contribute to learning in the affective area are also many and varied. Games and toys help children learn to discriminate between and interrelate with their environment and with other people. The skills they develop as they interact give them a feeling of being able to cope, and of being in control of themselves and their surroundings. Becoming familiar with objects from the outside world, such as toy trucks, buildings, and household equipment, helps broaden their concepts in realistic terms. Trying out other roles, through dolls, puppets, and toys or real objects similar to those adults use or wear, also helps children explore and discover their own identity, and provides a safe way to try out more mature or different real-life roles.

Toys are big business. According to Toy Manufacturers of America, there are approximately 150,000 different toys on the market, with about 5000 new toys being introduced each year. Parents buy toys for a variety of reasons, ranging from tradition to providing toys that they never had. Some people buy toys and use them as bribes or rewards; hence toys are often used as a substitute for love and attention, to ease guilt, or to mold the child in the parents' image. For whatever purpose they are purchased, toys occupy many hours of the child's play and should be carefully selected.

Table 16.1 presents a list of appropriate types of gross and fine motor toys for children from infancy through the primary grades. It must be remembered that play materials must be safe, durable, and interesting to children.

## War Toys

When reviewing Table 16.1 it should be noted that there are no war toys (guns, etc.) listed. It is my feeling that the use of toy guns is not a form of play to be encouraged by adults. The purchase of commercially manufactured toy guns is discouraged because of their realism. One need only to visit a local toy store to see guns that smoke, "bang," look like machine guns, shotguns, and even the M14 rifle used in Vietnam. The use of guns purchased from the toy store serves no useful purpose. Many will argue with this, claiming that toy guns provide children with an avenue to work out their aggressions, and that they will outgrow their need for violent expression. It does seem ludicrous, however, that in a society that claims to abhor killing and violence, we go to such great lengths to ensure realism in the toy guns made for children. If children truly outgrow their need for violent expression, why, then, are the television channels and movie theaters filled with realistic scenes of violence and killing?

Children have a right and need to express themselves through fantasy play. Such things as "cops and robbers," "war," and "cowboys and indians" are forms of fantasy play that have been engaged in by children for generations. Children have a right to work out their aggressions, and they should be permitted to do so but in a manner that does not encourage or promote *realism*. Perhaps the use of a fantasy gun (such as a stick or the index finger) in this form of fantasy play would reduce the realism created by a commercially purchased toy gun.

Guns themselves are not an evil. It is the way that we condone and use them in our society. Whether in real life or play, shooting someone is not a form of behavior to be viewed as the norm for society, even though it takes place during war and is an aspect of law enforcement. The use of toy guns should be discouraged among children.

## Toy Safety

The Child Protection and Toy Safety Act was passed by the U.S. Congress in 1969. This law prohibits the sale of toys that may prove harmful to children. Any toy that presents an electrical, thermal, or mechanical hazard, or that may endanger the safety of children through sharp or protruding edges, fragmentation, explosion, strangulation, asphyxiation, electrical shock, or fire is not to be sold. The Bureau of

**Table 16.1 Appropriate Play Materials for Young Children**

### Infants (0 to 1 Year)

1. Teething ring
2. Rattles
3. Hedgehog
4. Textured ball
5. Ball rattle
6. Mirror
7. Shapes
8. Crawligator
9. Crib mobile
10. Buttons on a cord

### Toddlers (1 to 2 Years)

1. First blocks
2. Nesting boxes
3. Peg board
4. Stacking toys
5. Snap toys
6. Cuddly toys
7. Stepstool
8. Soft throwing toys
9. Washable doll
10. Bells and music box
11. Squeaky toys
12. Push and pull toys
13. Sand toys
14. Sturdy picture books
15. Simple inlay puzzles (3 to 6 pieces)

### Preschoolers (3 to 5 Years)

1. Picture books
2. Dress-up clothes
3. Shape, size, and texture toys
4. Miniature toys
5. Cardboard boxes
6. Blocks
7. Dolls and puppets
8. Furniture
9. Puzzles (8 to 20 pieces)
10. Painting and coloring materials
11. Pots and pans
12. Large balls
13. Climbing equipment
14. Balancing equipment
15. Striking toys
16. Beanbags
17. Woodworking equipment
18. Wading pool
19. Record player and records
20. Musical instruments
21. Blunt scissors, paste, and paper
22. Modeling clay
23. Simple storybooks
24. Floating bath toys

### Elementary Grades (6 to 10 Years)

1. Large and small balls
2. Climbing rope or ladder
3. Climbing frame
4. Balance beam
5. Tumbling mat
6. Jump rope
7. Bicycle
8. Tinker toys
9. Flash cards
10. Playing cards
11. Sports equipment
12. Building toys
13. Storybooks
14. Chalkboard
15. Science toys
16. Globe
17. Dolls and puppets
18. Playhouse
19. Water toys
20. Workbench and tools

Product Safety, a division of the Food and Drug Administration, prevents such products from entering the market and is responsible for recalling unsafe toys from the market.

Toy manufacturers have the responsibility to design toys in such a way that the materials used and the methods of construction make the toy as childproof as possible. That is, the toy should require a minimum of education of the user to make it safe. Ideally, no imaginable use or abuse of the toy by a child should make it unsafe.

The following is a listing of examples of toys that have been deemed unsafe by the Food and Drug Administration:

1. Sharp or protruding objects.
   *Dolls of Pliable Plastic.* The doll can be bent into positions in several directions. By doing so, however, sharp wires, serving as joints, protrude from the ends of the doll's hands and feet. This could puncture a child seriously.
   *Large Ring Darts.* The darts are 1 ft long and weigh about ½ lb. The child could easily lose an eye or receive puncture wounds on the body.
2. Fragmentation.
   *Clackers.* Not long ago "clackers" were introduced to the toy market. This created great fun for children of all ages. However, these are quite dangerous because the clackers may chip or fragment from being struck together. These flying pieces could cause serious eye injury.
3. Explosive toys.
   *Cap Guns.* These are a potential cause of deafness to children. Noises reaching 130 decibels are safe. At a distance of 2 ft, the noise produced indoors could be exposing themselves and others to a continuous sound level roughly fifteen times louder than that considered safe for continuous sound.
4. Strangulation.
   *Crib Mobiles.* Stuffed animal characters are often suspended from the side of the infant's crib and over the crib. When one of the figures is pulled, the plastic bracket that supports the mobile often breaks near its base, sending the entire assembly into the crib. The strings could cause strangulation, and the broken bars could cause serious injury.
5. Asphyxiation.
   *Fringed Balloon Squeakers.* The balloon is blown up and let go. As the air escapes from the balloon, it makes a loud noise because of a metal noisemaker lodged in the mouthpiece of the balloon. If the child does not take the balloon out of the mouth and allows the air to escape into the mouth, the noisemaker, because of the air pressure, acts as a missile and

may shoot down the child's mouth. This could become lodged in the throat, causing asphyxiation.

6.  Burns caused by electrical toys.

    *Ovens.* A toy stove was recently introduced on the market. The stove reached temperatures of 200°F on the sides of the oven. On top it reached 300°F, and the inside of the oven rose to an unbelievable 660°F. Most kitchen ranges rise to temperatures under 180°F on the noncooking surfaces. A child could easily receive serious burns from such a toy.

7.  Toxicity.

    *Rhythm Bandset.* One such set includes toy musical instruments, one of which is a pair of maracas. The maracas may come apart, and they contain pellets made of lead, which is poisonous. The chance of inhaling the tiny pellets into the lungs also makes them a serious hazard to children.

8.  Flammability.

    *Foam Balls.* A popular brand foam ball was tested against the flammability standard set by the 1969 Child Protection and Toy Safety Act. Under the specified conditions, the ball not only ignited within the time limits specified for contact with a candle flame, but it smoked profusely while it burned and shed drops of burning substances.

When a toy is determined to be unsafe for children's usage, it can be banned, according to the decision by the Division of Children's Hazards. When a toy is banned, it means that the item cannot be sold in interstate commerce. It is also considered illegal to sell banned items that are already on store shelves.

## Choosing Toys

Even though the Food and Drug Administration attempts to prevent the sale and use of toys determined to be unsafe, much of the burden of protecting children from the dangers of toys still rests with parents and teachers. A good deal of caution needs to be exercised in the purchase of toys. The following are among the most important questions to ask yourself when buying a toy for a child.

1.  Is it safe?
2.  Is it appropriate to the developmental level of the child?
3.  Is it durable?
4.  Is it fun (for the child)?
5.  Will it stimulate the child's imagination?

A good toy is one that does not do all of the playing for the child or "have all the fun." Many top companies list the approximate age range of interest in the toy and its potential benefits on the box or package. This information should be read carefully but used only as a general guide for purchasing the right toy for the particular child. A great deal of money is spent on toys, and we should be careful to get the most for our money. All too often a youngster will open an expensive new toy and proceed to play with the box rather than the toy. If the toy does not stimulate the interest or imagination of the child, no amount of encouragement will get him or her to play with it. Answering the five questions outlined above will do much to ensure the purchase of toys that children will play with, learn from, and enjoy.

The following is a partial list of safety recommendations to take into consideration when selecting toys for children.

1. Toys should fit the child's age and physical skill.
2. For children under 3 years of age, avoid toys with small or easily removable parts (loose nuts, bolts, removable eyes, projections, needles, nails, etc.).
3. Look for toys that do not shatter or break easily.
4. Wait until a child is at least 8 years old before giving him or her chemistry sets, bow and arrows, and sharp-edged toys that might come into contact with the hands, clothes, or other parts of the body and cause bruises, cuts, punctures, or fractures.
5. Only electrical toys with the Underwriters Laboratory (U.L.) seal should be purchased. This seal means that the toy is required to have a safety device that prevents the child from putting his hands in the heated area when the toy is hot. Cooking, melting, and molding toys should be used by older children and only under adult supervision.
6. All toys should be sturdy and durable.
7. Look for areas where the fingers can become pinched in slots, holes, on the underside of the wheels, and in wind-up mechanisms.
8. Darts, archery sets, or spring-loaded guns with rubber suction cups that can be removed may cause punctures. Avoid such toys.
9. Avoid crib or playpen toys that are suspended on strings.
10. Avoid purchasing helmets or play eyeglasses that can shatter. These could result in serious head and eye injuries.

## PLAY SPACES

The play environment provided for children should be conducive to all aspects of their development. It should be safe, attractive, and provide for a wide variety of stimulating and interesting activities. All too often, however, the indoor and the outdoor play spaces for a variety of reasons limit or discourage gross motor activities. As a result, there has, over the past several years, been a tremendous emphasis on the cognitive and affective aspects of the toys, games, and play equipment found in the indoor and outdoor play space. If we subscribe to the notion that the balanced development of children in the motor as well as the cognitive and affective areas of behavior is important, we must then see to it that children's play environments also stimulate gross motor activity. Children have a basic need to be active. Through the proper design of play environments, as well as the use of appropriate methods of teacher interaction, this need for activity will be successfully channeled to promote children's learning to move, and hence learning through movement.

## Indoor Play Spaces

Historically, the indoor play space found in most nursery schools has been one of children's "interest centers." The environment has been designed around a variety of areas that are geared to the children's needs, abilities, and interests. The following is a list of the various interest centers typically found in nursery schools. It should be noted that inclusion of any or all of these areas into the indoor play space depends primarily on budgetary considerations and the availability of space.

1. *Block Area.* The block area requires plenty of space and should be carpeted, if possible, to reduce the noise factor.
2. *Housekeeping Area.* This interest center should be equipped with a toy sink, stove, refrigerator, table, and chairs. Dolls, doll beds, and dress-up clothing are also found in this area. The housekeeping area provides for considerable dramatization and role playing.
3. *Book Area.* To be effective, this should be in a quiet part of the room. Books may be kept on shelves and/or a table. If possible, the area should be carpeted in order that children may sit comfortably on the floor if they so desire.
4. *Creativity Area.* Easels with paint and paper should be available for children who want to paint.
5. *Science Area.* This should be where materials can be easily displayed and seen by the children. Room to spread out leaves, stones, shells, and other "collector's" items should be provided in this area. Magnets, magnifying glasses, a terrarium, and an aquarium might also be added. Space should also be provided for pets brought into the room.
6. *Water and Sand Area.* Ideally, a table with built-in sections for sand and water is the best kind of equipment for this activity. Also included should be shovels, small buckets, things that float, things that sink, funnels, straws, and soap.
7. *Music Area.* The music area is a must in any program. A record player, records, cassette tape recorder, a variety of musical instruments, and a piano will make this an ideal area.
8. *Carpentry Area.* The carpentry area should include a workbench with an attached vise. An assortment of tools, nails, and wood should be available.
9. *Nesting Area.* In this area the children should have an opportunity to

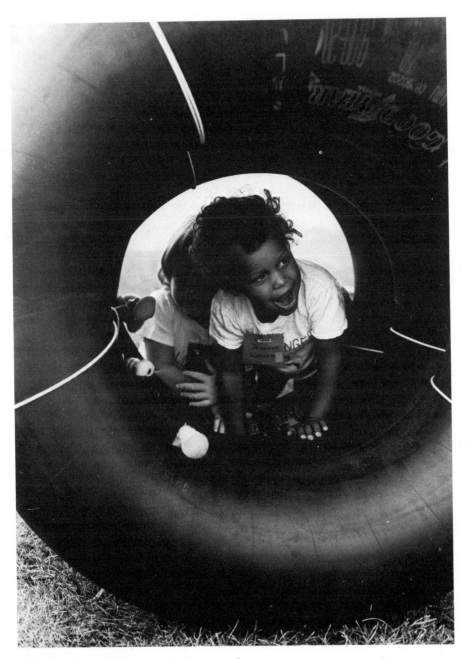

Inner tubes tied together make excellent tunnels.

"escape" from the hustle-bustle of the classroom. Nesting cubes, an old refrigerator carton, or collapsible tunnel makes an ideal nesting area.

**10.** *Movement Center.* A movement center is an essential part of the indoor play space for preschool children and is discussed in detail in the following section.

**The Indoor Movement Center.** Contrary to popular belief, an indoor movement center requires little space. The author has developed several movement centers in nursery schools in an area no larger than 8 by 10 ft. The key to success in developing an indoor movement center is to first establish the specific objectives that you want the children to achieve through participation in this activity area. Then, taking the space limitations and safety factors into consideration, carefully design and construct the movement center around the objectives. For example, you may have as one of your primary objectives "to provide the children with opportunities to enhance their movement abilities in a variety of fundamental stability, locomotor, and manipulative abilities." Therefore, the movement center should contain equipment that will encourage practice in a variety of stability, locomotor, and manipulative activities. The following is a partial list of equipment, which may be purchased or made by hand, that is appropriate for use in an indoor movement center.

1. Stability.
    (a) Balance beam.
    (b) Balance board.
    (c) Bounding board.
    (d) Newspaper mats.
    (e) Coffee-can stilts.
    (f) Ladder.
    (g) Inner tubes.
2. Locomotion.
    (a) Collapsible tunnel.
    (b) Carpet squares.
    (c) Ankle jump.
    (d) Cubes.
    (e) Portable climbing equipment.
    (f) Climbing rope.
3. Manipulation.
    (a) Beanbags.
    (b) Hoops.
    (c) Yarn balls.
    (d) Automobile tires.
    (e) Targets.
    (f) Suspended balls.

The indoor movement center should also include a variety of sensory stimuli. Play equipment consisting of various textures, colors, and geometric shapes is encouraged. The use of mirrors, for children to observe their movements, and portable equipment that may be used both indoors and outdoors is also recommended.

## Outdoor Play Spaces

The opportunity for active movement in the outdoor play space should go well beyond the traditional recess period characterized by mass confusion, boredom, and fighting. The outdoor play area should first of all be designed for children in such a way that it stimulates their interest, imagination, and large muscle development. As simple as this sounds, one need only look at the majority of outdoor play spaces at the nursery school and elementary school levels to see that they are *not* designed for children. All too often the outdoor play space is constructed with its primary objectives being to amuse children and require minimum upkeep instead of to encourage children's motor development. As a result, a typical outdoor play space, unfortunately, often consists of acres of blacktop and galvanized swing sets, teeter-totters, and slides.

"Outdoor equipment and structures should be selected to invite creative expression and imaginative interpretation by the children," according to Haase (1968, p. 10). The outdoor equipment should be abstract or neutral in its sculptural form in order to stimulate the child's imagination. It should stimulate a variety of locomotor, manipulative, and stability activities. Although individualistic in nature, outdoor play materials and equipment should encourage social contact. They should also stimulate imagination and cognitive processes through media that invite physical exploration and enjoyment.

In planning an outdoor play space the following questions must be answered.

1.  Is it safe?
2.  Is it of *real* interest to children?
3.  Is it developmentally appropriate?
4.  Is it practical?
5.  Is it economically feasible?
6.  Can it be easily supervised?
7.  Can it be maintained with a minimum of maintenance?
8.  Can it be made available to the general public?

The outdoor play area should provide children with a variety of large and small muscle activities. It should contain a wide selection of equipment that promotes its use in a manner that is creative, challenging, and developmentally appropriate. The outdoor area should provide:

1. Large muscle activities to enhance all areas of children's motor development.
   (a) Locomotion.
   (b) Manipulation.
   (c) Stability.
2. Experiences with various media.
   (a) Art.
   (b) Woodwork.
   (c) Dirt.
   (d) Sand.
   (e) Water.
3. Places for seclusion and quiet activities.
   (a) Tunnels.
   (b) Nesting cubes.
4. Opportunities to observe nature.
   (a) Animals.
   (b) Gardens.
   (c) Trees and shrubs.
5. Opportunities to dramatize real-life experiences.
   (a) Playhouse.
   (b) Junk car.
   (c) Boat.

**The Outdoor Movement Center** The outdoor movement center is easily incorporated into the total outdoor play space. There should be ample space for children to move freely. Ideally, there will be a large grassy area and hillside for running, jumping, sliding, rolling, and climbing. There will also be a hard surface area for riding wheel toys and activities with balls. Trees should be an integral part of the movement center, not only to provide shade but to encourage climbing. A variety of equipment that encourages gross motor activities should also be located in the outdoor play space. This equipment may be used in addition to or in conjunction with the equipment found in the indoor movement center. Climbing, striking, and balancing equipment should be an integral part of the outdoor area. The following is a partial list of suggested types of equipment designed to encourage the development of these abilities (Figure 16.2).

1. Climbing equipment.
   (a) Teepee tower.
   (b) Cargo net climber.
   (c) Climbing frames.
   (d) Barrel pyramid.
   (e) Climbing towers.

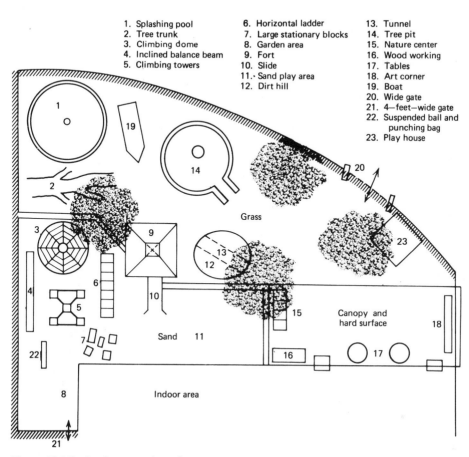

1. Splashing pool
2. Tree trunk
3. Climbing dome
4. Inclined balance beam
5. Climbing towers
6. Horizontal ladder
7. Large stationary blocks
8. Garden area
9. Fort
10. Slide
11. Sand play area
12. Dirt hill
13. Tunnel
14. Tree pit
15. Nature center
16. Wood working
17. Tables
18. Art corner
19. Boat
20. Wide gate
21. 4—feet—wide gate
22. Suspended ball and punching bag
23. Play house

**Figure 16.2** Design for an outdoor play space.

2. Striking equipment.
   (a) Tetherball frames.
   (b) Striking frames.
   (c) Rebound nets.
3. Balancing equipment.
   (a) Inclined balance beams.
   (b) Bouncing buddy.
   (c) Telephone poles.
   (d) Barrels.
   (e) Spools.

**Summary**

The rapidly expanding world of children is one in which play, toys, and play spaces are in central focus for their learning to move and learning through movement. As a result, it is important to have a clear understanding of what constitutes play, why children play, and the developmental aspects of play. The toys that we provide for children to play with and their play environment are important to their total balanced development.

The selection of children's toys should be a matter for considerable thought and careful attention by parents and teacher. A variety of questions should be answered prior to the purchase of any toy, whether it be for active or quiet play, large or small, inexpensive or expensive.

The indoor and outdoor play environment for children should be carefully designed. It should be conducive to gross motor development as well as to social interaction and cognitive growth.

Play, toys, and play spaces are important to children. This fact alone should be ample reason to see to it that the learning experiences within children's environments respond to their interests, needs, and developmental capabilities.

## CHAPTER HIGHLIGHTS

1. The evolution of play behavior follows a developmental sequence.
2. Play is the work of children. It is a primary means by which children come to grips with their world.
3. Toys can play an important role in both gross and fine motor development if properly selected and introduced into the child's environment.
4. Toys can promote cognitive and affective development as well as motor development.
5. War toys are of dubious value to the child, particularly the use of realistic toy guns.
6. The Child Protection and Toy Safety Act prohibits the sale of toys that may be harmful to children.
7. Care should be taken in the selection and purpose of toys. Guidelines are available from toy manufacturers and child development experts.
8. The play environment for children should be designed with care in order to maximize its utilization, developmental potential, and lasting enjoyment.
9. Indoor play spaces can be designed that require a minimum of space and provide for a maximum of vigorous physical activity.
10. Outdoor play spaces should be designed for the children they are intended to serve and should follow a set of predetermined guidelines that have been established by individuals knowledgeable in child development, play behavior, and motor development.

## CRITICAL READINGS

Ellis, M.J.: *Why People Play,* Englewood Cliffs, N.J.: Prentice-Hall, 1973.

Herkowitz, J.: "The Design and Evaluation of Playspaces for Children," in M.V. Ridenour (ed.), *Motor Development: Issues and Application,* Princeton, N.J.: Princeton, 1978, pp. 115–138.

Kritcherisky, S., and E. Prescott: *Planning Environments for Young Children,* Washington, D.C.: NAEYC, 1977.

NAPECW and NCPEAM: "Learning How to Play," *Quest,* Monograph 26, Summer 1976.

Riggs, M.L: "A Preschool Laboratory Gym," *Journal of Physical Education and Recreation, 50, 39*–41, February 1979.

## CHAPTER 17

# Education of Young Children

Traditionally, the education of young children has been assumed almost entirely by the family. The quantity and quality of learning experiences engaged in by children have been left to the discretion of parents. Little consideration has been given, until recently, to education outside of the home for the vast majority of preschool children. Many have scoffed at the Soviet practice of education by the State for children beginning at the age of 2 years instead of our more conservative and "acceptable" practice of beginning formal education at around age 5 or 6. This early education of children was often looked on as something that could not and would not be tolerated in our society. We looked at the education of young children as being the sole responsibility of the home, except in extreme cases. In recent years, however, there have been three major developments that have resulted in a dramatic reassessment of this position: (1) the marked change in the social structure of our society, (2) the rapidly changing economic structure of our society, and (3) the increased professional interest in the contribution of early learning to later development. A closer look at each of these factors will help us to more fully appreciate their significance.

North American society is currently experiencing tremendous changes in the role of women in society. Many women are no longer satisfied with only keeping a home and devoting a good portion of their life to the important but often frustrating task of raising children. Instead, they are returning to school, seeking full- or part-time employment, or searching for other expressions of fulfillment outside the home.

Our rapidly changing economic structure has often made it extremely difficult for many families to "survive" without two incomes. The present inflationary spiral has significantly reduced the amount of spendable income for many. The reduction of spendable income is coupled with the fact that many families find it "necessary" to have the luxuries so skillfully advertised by the media. These factors have played an important role in the tremendous increase in the number of children enrolled in some form of day care or nursery school program.

The dramatic growth of interest in the contribution of early experiences to the later development of young children is the third factor that has led to increased interest in early childhood education. Jean Piaget was among the first to stress the importance of early experience for future development. His stress on the importance of perceptual-motor experiences as a facilitator of cognitive development as well as physical development has been a prime factor in stimulating this interest. The late start by the United States into the Space Age brought about by the "Sputnik Era" of the 1950s stimulated many to begin viewing the potential of the early years as important determiners of later behavior. The 1970 White House Conference on Children and Youth was a first national look into the education of young children. The conference stressed the need for nursery schools, day care centers, and kindergartens to be open to *all* children from all walks of life under the qualified direction of a person trained in early childhood education.

Nursery schools, day care centers, and other organizations are now concerned with the care and education of a large number of our nation's young children for all or part of their day, and the number is increasing daily. The responsibility of programs for preschoolers for the motor, cognitive, and affective development of children has been a topic of considerable debate during recent years. As a result we have witnessed a rapid increase in the types as well as the number of programs available.

## THE MOTOR DEVELOPMENT DILEMMA

Movement is of central importance to young children and their optimal development. Contributions to the motor development of children are certainly a worthy goal of any early childhood educational program. Enhancing children's ability to move efficiently and effectively, with control and with joy, should be as important to the teacher of young children as are their affective and cognitive development. Realization that the balanced motor development of children also has implications for both these areas should amplify the importance of gross motor development. The fact is, however, that the vast majority of educators are: (1) poorly informed as to why motor development is important, (2) poorly informed as to what forms of physical activity to include in their programs, and (3) inadequately prepared as to how to go about such a task. As a result, the movement education of children is often taken for granted or dealt with solely through loosely supervised free play. Although free-play activities can and should play a part in the school experience, it is not enough to assume that the purchase of expensive pieces of indoor and outdoor play equipment will effectively aid in the development and refinement of the children's movement abilities. Too often children are turned loose on various forms of equipment and expected magically to develop efficient forms of movement

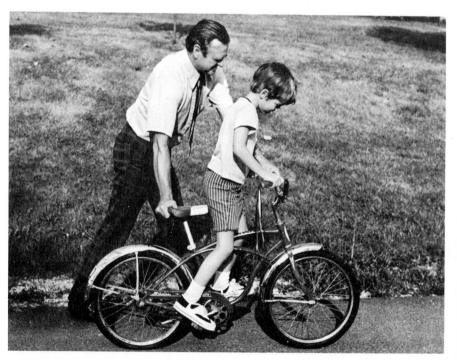

The education of young children has traditionally been the responsibility of the home.

behavior on their own. Only through wise guidance, thoughtful interaction, and careful planning can we assure the proper development of children's movement abilities.

The following is a discussion of five types of programs available for young children. The extent to which movement plays a role in each of these programs depends on individual teachers, their expertise, and their commitment to the *total* development of children.

## PROGRAMS FOR YOUNG CHILDREN

The number and types of programs available for preschool children has increased tremendously. Data from the 1980 census indicate that the number of children under 5 years of age is on the increase, even though the general population under 14 was predicted to drop by 1980. There were 55 million children under 14 years of age in the United States, according to the 1970 census report. A total of 18,013,000 were under 5. In 1980 these figures have been estimated to be 52,736,000 children under 14, with 19,881,000 under 5 years of age (White House Conference on Children, 1970). Also the number of working mothers with children under age 6 has increased significantly from 12.8 to 30.4 percent between 1948 and 1969. Over 56 percent of mothers with children in the home were gainfully employed by 1980 according to statistics released by the U.S. government.

The rise in the number of preschool children, coupled with the high percentage of working mothers, makes it abundantly clear that millions of children are cared for by persons other than the parents, relatives, or babysitters.

Over 8.7 percent of the total population in the United States is made up of children under 6 years of age (White House Conference on Children, 1970). The need for their care, supervision, and education is apparent, and many communities are rising to meet this need.

During the past several years a variety of programs have emerged. Each of these programs represents a particular philosophical outlook and attempts to provide for the particular developmental needs of children. The brief review of the major types of programs in existence throughout North America today is designed to provide the reader with a broader perspective of the nature and scope of programs for young children. Although each program differs in its purposes and content, all have a place in our society and can make a positive contribution to the development of young children. Table 17.1 provides a brief overview of the major types of preschool programs.

### Day Care Centers

The day care center or day nursery, as it was previously termed, has come into wide use in recent years. Day care centers are established primarily to serve the needs of working mothers. Upon their inception, they were often places where children could be safely "stored" for the day, with general assurance that their basic physical needs would be met. Little was done beyond serving their needs for basic physical care and ensuring that they were returned home in more or less the same condition in which they came. Today, however, many day care centers are broadening their scope and beginning to hire trained professionals who are developing sound programs that deal with the affective and cognitive growth of children.

The typical day care center is open on weekdays from 7 A.M. until 6 P.M. There are no set hours of attendance for the children; they come and go based on their parent's schedule. A great number of children require full-day care. Most of these children are from families with two working parents or only one parent, or from broken homes or low-income families.

The cost of quality day care is high. The cost is high because of the number of hours involved per week, the high demand for the low supply of quality centers, and the limited number of trained professionals. Many communities and county governments, as well as church-affiliated organizations, have seen fit to aid in the support of the many children in day care centers from low-income families. Communities far-sighted enough to help share the burdens of the disadvantaged home by making quality day care available are aiding society greatly. Their early concern for good care may help alleviate later delinquency, emotional problems, and frustrations, and do much to help children develop into happy, healthy, contributing members of society. The day care center is in a unique position to have a tremendous positive effect on the lives of children and will pay dividends in the future.

The continued upgrading of day care programs through hiring trained professionals and meeting state certification requirements is an important community matter. Day care centers need to concern themselves more with the development of children and must cease to view their purpose as simply a "storage place" for children. The opportunities are great and so are the responsibilities. The early years are too important to be left to chance, and quality day care can go a long way toward ensuring for our society a large segment of the care and nurturing it requires.

## Head Start Child Development Programs

These programs are a relatively recent phenomenon in American society. They were established as a result of the Economic Opportunity Act of 1964, which authorized the establishment of programs for economically deprived preschool children. Head Start Child Development Programs were designed to help prepare children for public school as a part of the federal government's war against poverty.

The 1960s became known to many as the decade of the disadvantaged. Head Start programs were one means by which the government made vast attempts at breaking the poverty cycle and alleviating cultural deprivation. The culturally

**Table 17.1 Types of Preschool Programs**

| Program | Ages | Description |
|---|---|---|
| Day care center | 8 weeks to 6 years | Usually a full-day program between 7 A.M. and 6 P.M. Programs vary greatly in quality and trained leadership. |
| Head Start Child Development Programs | 4 to 6 years | Federally supported compensatory program designed to provide enrichment experiences for culturally deprived children: half-day sessions, medical and dental programs, and hot meals. Trained staff, volunteers, and parent help. |
| Nursery schools | 2 to 5 years | Generally privately supported but some publicly supported programs. Half-day session. "Traditional" and "modern" approach. Trained staff, volunteers, and aids. |
| Parent cooperatives | 2 to 5 years | Formed by parents. Program developed and staffed by parents. Cost is minimal and quality varies greatly. |
| Home day care | 2 to 6 years | Private facilities often need to be licensed. Babysitting service for groups of three to ten children. Half or full day. |
| Kindergarten | 5 to 6 years | Publicly and privately supported. Certified teachers staff the program. Geared to preparing children for the first grade. |

deprived have been defined as "individuals or a group of people who lack social amenities and cultural graces associated with middle-class society" (Leeper et al., 1974, p. 86).

Head Start is an all-inclusive program designed to meet the physical, mental, and emotional needs of young children in an effort to prepare them for success in school. The program involves medical and dental services, social and psychological services, and nutritional care. Parents and local community volunteers are encouraged to take an active role whenever possible, performing many of the nonprofessional duties.

The program itself stresses development of language skills, personal health, self-concept, curiosity, and self-discipline. Head Start programs broaden the range of children's experiences and help them learn how to cope with their environment. They attempt to help children overcome some of the deficiencies of their environment by providing early enrichment experiences in order to help them more effectively meet the demands of school.

Children are selected on the basis of a minimum family income, where the family lives (rural or urban), and the number of children in the family. The vast majority of children come from poverty-level homes.

In a good Head Start program, classes are kept small. Children receive individual help, and the school is well staffed. Parents and community volunteers share in the decision making. Home and school are closely correlated in the program in an effort to help the home as well as the individual child better share in the responsibilities and benefits of our society.

The Head Start program has had a tremendous impact on early childhood education: (1) national attention has been focused on preschool education, especially that of culturally disadvantaged children, (2) the philosophy of early education of the young has undergone radical changes, (3) facilities and materials for young children have been vastly expanded, and (4) it has been documented that young children learn faster and earlier than previously thought to be true. Head Start has truly had a lasting impact on our society. It is through the early enrichment of countless young lives that the poverty cycle can be broken and the culturally disadvantaged can become valued, contributing members of society.

## Nursery Schools

The nursery school is not to be confused with the day care center. Unlike the day care center, nursery schools are established primarily to enhance the cognitive and affective development of children. They operate for only a portion of the school day. The children generally attend for 2 to 3 hours daily or every other day for the same period of time. The nursery school is the first in the series of units that make up elementary education. Public nursery schools generally begin at age 4 years. When operated privately, they often include children 2 to 4 years of age.

The nursery school is an educational experience that has been the primary form of preschool education for over fifty years. At their inception, nursery schools were primarily conducted as laboratory schools by colleges and universities. They were used extensively as training and testing grounds for teachers and materials. The early laboratory schools served a valuable purpose in enhancing our insight into the nature and characteristics of preschool children. Many laboratory schools continue to serve as valuable information gathering and research centers.

Today, nursery schools are conducted on both public and private bases throughout North America, the premise being that early experiences offered in the proper setting by trained professionals will have a positive effect on children's development. Today's nursery school serves the needs of 2- to 4-year-old children by providing them with experiences based on what is known about their development needs. It shares with parents the responsibility for promoting meaningful learning during a period when growth is rapid and significant.

The typical nursery school is an active one in which the open classroom concept is extensively employed. The children generally work in small groups at various interest centers such as the doll corner, carpentry corner, block area, and reading and puzzle corner. The teacher acts as a stimulator or motivator for involvement, encouraging experimentation and exploration of new ideas and ways of doing things.

Nursery school programs vary greatly but may be classified into two general types. The first type is what is sometimes termed the *traditional nursery school*. The traditional nursery school emphasizes the development of affective competencies. The learning of social skills such as sharing, taking turns, working constructively with others, and accepting simple responsibilities is an important aspect of the traditional program. Formal means of instruction are frowned on, and informal play experiences are the primary mode of instruction. The teacher establishes an environment conducive to learning and social interaction. Play experiences are utilized as a means of learning socialization skills. Less emphasis is placed on the formal development of cognitive abilities, although considerable cognitive development often occurs as a byproduct of a good program.

The *modern nursery school* is the second type of nursery school program. Unlike the traditional nursery school, greater emphasis is placed on the development of cognitive abilities. A more complete balance between affective and cognitive development is sought. Sometimes teachers in the modern nursery school view motor development as an integral part of their program.

The program in the modern nursery school utilizes a portion of the day for directed activities and the remainder for relatively free activities. The concepts that children learn in the directed aspect of the program are reinforced during play by the teacher's directing the child's attention to factors in the environment that may otherwise be missed or minimized.

## Parent Cooperatives

The parent cooperative has become a popular form of preschool education in recent years. The cooperative is formed by parents and is often completely staffed by them. Parents are regularly required to participate in the program and to plan and supervise its activities. The parent cooperative enables children to attend a preschool program for a minimum cost. The quality of cooperatives varies greatly, depending on the parents' commitment to the program, their ability to work constructively with groups of children, and the number of people involved.

Some cooperatives are able to hire a qualified professional to provide leadership, guidance, and training. Programs that are fortunate enough to enlist the aid of a trained professional often blossom into excellent programs. On the other hand, a great many parent cooperatives flounder for lack of leadership. Problems often arise in scheduling, planning, staffing, and providing continuity when the duties are rotated between parents.

## Home Day Care

The number of home care facilities has increased rapidly during the past few years. Home care programs are those in which a mother will generally care for from three to ten children in her home. Several states require licensing of home care facilities, but the quality of such programs runs from excellent to terrible. The home care program often is primarily one of babysitting for a group of children for either half or full days.

The licensing requirements of many states for home care are quite rigid. These regulations have been established in order to help, as much as possible, to ensure a safe and hygienic environment for the children.

## Kindergarten

Kindergartens have been in existence for over a century. The first public kindergarten was established in St. Louis, Missouri, in 1873. Many kindergartens operate on a private basis. The first private one was established in Watertown, Wisconsin, in 1855. The number of children attending both public and private kindergartens has been increasing steadily for the past twenty years. Many states include kindergarten programs as a portion of the total public school program. In states that do not have public kindergartens, several licensed and privately operated church-related kindergarten programs exist.

Kindergarten is that part of the school program that enrolls 5-year-old children for one year prior to entering the first grade. Kindergartens are generally half-day programs designed to prepare children for the first grade. They are operated by licensed teachers and one or two assistants. The program is generally individualized in order to meet each child's needs within a group setting as much as possible. The atmosphere of the kindergarten is one of little pressure in which exploration and investigation experiences are encouraged. The purpose of such a program is to help children learn to inquire and wonder, learn self-direction, self-selection, and the discovery of meaning. The kindergarten program helps children form the basis for lifelong habits of disciplined, joyful learning.

The objectives of the kindergarten are:

1. To recognize the value and dignity of all people.
2. To emphasize the importance of self-worth and realization of one's goals.
3. To develop an appreciation of different social, cultural, and ethnic groups.
4. To promote emotional stability in a world of rapid change, opportunities, and responsibilities.
5. To encourage independent thinking and to foster creativity within each individual.

6. To provide experiences geared to the needs and ability levels of each child.

7. To foster positive attitudes toward learning and school.

8. To develop basic readiness skills necessary for success in school.

9. To encourage the development and refinement of fundamental movement abilities.

10. To enlarge the concept of reliable citizenship, at both individual and group levels.

The kindergarten is an exciting first step into the world of learning for most children. It is an integral part of the elementary school that makes available the type of experience best suited to the immediate needs of children. It provides an atmosphere in which children develop new skills and ideas, increase their fund of information, and gain a better understanding of their neighborhood and community. It is a place where they learn to plan and think through simple tasks. They learn to share and do their part in taking responsibility for themselves and their work. Kindergarten is a happy place filled with eager faces, bright smiles, and active bodies. It helps to prepare children for the challenges forthcoming in the elementary school.

## MOVING TO LEARN, LEARNING TO MOVE

The directed play experiences of young children can serve as a primary vehicle by which they learn about themselves and their environment. Play and work are not opposites, as is often thought. For children, play is their way of exploring and experimenting while they gain information about themselves and their world. Through directed play experiences that have been carefully structured and pre-planned (but that avoid teacher domination), children learn to come to grips with their world, to cope with life's tasks, to master fundamental movements, and to gain confidence in themselves as individuals, moving effectively and efficiently through space. These early years serve as a time when children are intently involved in the process of *learning to move* and *moving to learn*. Although it is not possible to separate these two processes, it is important that the differences implied by the terms be understood.

Learning to move involves the continuous development of children's fundamental movement abilities. Preschoolers have passed through the period of infancy and are no longer immobilized by the confines of their crib or playpen. They can now move through their environment (locomotion), impart force to objects (manipulation), and maintain their equilibrium in response to the force of gravity (stability). The development of effective patterns of movement permits them to move about freely and in control of their bodies. Children involved in learning to move are constantly exploring, experimenting, practicing, and making a variety of spontaneous decisions based on their perceptions of the moment and past experiences. They are involved in a continuous process of sorting out their many daily experiences in order to gain increased knowledge about their body and its potential for movement.

While involved in learning to move, children are simultaneously involved in moving to learn, a process that involves utilizing movement as a means to an end rather than as an end in itself. Children involved in moving to learn use their bodies to gain increased knowledge about themselves and their world. Their basic inability to concpeutalize at a sophisticated level makes it difficult for them to learn through formal means of education. As a result, movement becomes one of the primary agents by which they grasp fundamental cognitive and affective concepts of direction, space, time, peer relations, and self-assurance. Movement serves as a medium by which they can increase their fund of knowledge in all aspects of their behavior and is not limited to the physical self.

The balanced motor development of children can and must become a concern of the teacher of young children. The important contributions of movement to learning to move and learning through movement should be carefully studied by all. Figure 17.1 presents a schematic representation of the different types of preschool programs and the obligation of these programs to the development of the total child. The extent to which any program incorporates meaningful movement depends on the specific program, its educational goals, and the expertise of the teacher.

## Summary

Parents, teachers, psychologists, and pediatricians are becoming increasingly aware of the critical need for children to move about freely in order that they may grow and develop their potential. The literature on child growth and development is replete with information indicating that the child's experiential background in movement plays an important role in the total developmental process.

Teachers should be concerned with developing a variety of fundamental movement and sport skill abilities. This may be accomplished by structuring the environment and providing opportunities for the performance of movement activities, with a judicious degree of teacher direction and interaction. For individuals untrained in this area of education, it may be difficult initially to structure movement experiences and provide the proper degree of guidance, but with practice and study, successful experiences will be forthcoming.

Teachers need to develop a keen awareness of the importance of directed movement experiences in the lives of children and to become knowledgeable as to how to implement successful programs in this area. It is time that the so-called frivolous play experiences of children be viewed in the light of their potential educational value. Motor development must be put into proper perspective in the education of children, for it truly plays an integral part in their total growth and development.

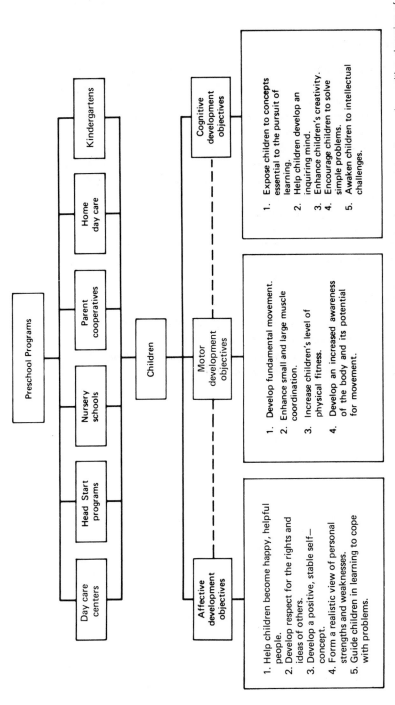

**Figure 17.1** Preschool programs are responsible for the development of children in the affective, psychomotor, and cognitive domains of behavior. The extent to which children develop in these areas depends on the type of program offered and the expertise of the teacher.

## CHAPTER HIGHLIGHTS

1.  The changing complexion of North American society has created a situation where over half of all preschoolers are involved in some form of education or care outside the home.
2.  In most preschool programs a movement education program is absent or takes the form of loosely supervised free play.
3.  Free play is of value to the developing child, but it cannot take the place of a planned program of developmentally appropriate movement experiences.
4.  A variety of preschool programs are available to young children. Each type has a different emphasis and all have a place in our society.
5.  The directed play experiences of preschool and elementary school children can do much to enhance their movement abilities.
6.  Movement can serve as an effective avenue for moving to learn as well as for learning to move.

## CRITICAL READINGS

Cohen, D.: *The Learning Child,* New York: Pantheon, 1972.
Jones, E.: "Teacher Education: Entertainment or Interaction?" *The Journal of the National Association for the Education of Young Children,* March 1978.
Riggs, M.L.: *Jump to Joy,* Englewood Cliffs, N.J.: Prentice-Hall, 1980.

## CHAPTER 18

# Developmental Physical Education: A Curricular Model

Throughout the discussions in the preceding chapters, we have continually focused on the developmental stages that children pass through in their acquisition of motor, cognitive, and affective abilities. The thesis of this entire text has focused on the process of motor development and factors that impinge on its normal sequential progression in the development of movement abilities. If the phases and stages of motor development presented in Chapter 3 and elaborated on throughout this text are to have any real meaning, we should be able to construct a curricular model congruent with these phases. This curricular model should be able to serve as a "blueprint for action." In other words, it should make up the basic structure around which the daily lesson is planned and carried out by the teacher in the gymnasium or on the playing field. What has been discussed in the preceding chapters is of little value if we cannot bring order to it and make practical application of it to the lives of children. The value of theory and research that fails to foster models for implementation is limited at best. Curricular models not based on sound research and theory are little better. It is, therefore, the purpose of this chapter to propose a developmentally based curricular model for implementing the physical education program during the preschool and elementary school years.

## CURRICULAR MODELS IN PHYSICAL EDUCATION

Curricular rationales take many forms. Bain (1978) has identified six curricular rationales that are in use today by physical education teachers: (1) movement forms, (2) movement analysis, (3) human movement disciplines, (4) developmental stages, (5) motor learning tasks analysis, and (6) student motives and purposes. The movement analysis and developmental stage models are most often found at the elementary school level and are the most common choices for curriculum development. These two approaches were debated by Tanner (1979) and Gallahue (1979) and are summarized in an article by Ward and Werner (1981).

The developmental model is an approach to physical education that aims to educate children in the use of their bodies so that they can move more efficiently and effectively in a wide variety of fundamental movements and be able to apply these basic abilities to a wide variety of movement skills that may or may not be sport-related. At the heart of the developmental model is the focus on developmentally appropriate movement experiences that promote increased proficiency at all levels. Games, sports, dances, and the like, serve as a vehicle for improving skill.

The movement analysis approach to physical education is defined as "that approach to physical education which teaches children to move skillfully with a knowledge of how they move and a meaningfulness in their movement" (Ward and Werner, 1981, p. 61). The movement analysis model is exemplified by movement education programs that place emphasis on understanding and application of the movement concepts originally proposed by Laban and Lawrence (1947). These movement concepts are important but, like the content areas of physical education, should serve as a vehicle by which appropriate movement abilities are developed and refined. The developmental model for teaching physical education presented here recognizes the validity of both the developmental stage and movement analysis curriculum rationales. It places the child rather than content areas or movement concepts, at the center of the curricular process.

In order to facilitate presentation of the developmental model, we will first review the three categories into which movement may be classified and the appropriate movement skill themes that may be extracted from each category. Then we will discuss the three major content areas of physical education and the three movement concepts of movement education. We will then look at the stages in the process of motor skill learning and the implications for emphasizing indirect or direct methods of teaching. A developmental model will be presented for both the preschool and the primary grades, and the upper elementary and middle school grades. No attempt will be made to provide a scope and sequence chart, lesson plans, or suggestions for developmentally appropriate activities. The reader is instead referred to *Developmental Movement Experiences for Children* by Gallahue (1982) and to the suggested additional readings at the end of this chapter.

## CATEGORIES OF MOVEMENT AND MOVEMENT SKILL THEMES

The three categories of movement as they relate to motor development have been discussed extensively. Briefly, a *category of movement* is a classificatory scheme based on common underlying principles of movement. The terms locomotion, manipulation, and stability are used here to represent these underlying principles. Although others have used the term nonlocomotor rather than stability as a category of movement, I have chosen to give recognition to the term stability as a movement category. Doing so is not arbitrary or without support from others. O.W. Smith and P.C. Smith (1966), and more recently Riggs (1980) have all chosen to classify movement behavior into the categories of locomotion, manipulation, and stability. These three categories serve as the organizing centers of the developmental physical education curriculum during the preschool and elementary school years and as the basis for the formation of movement skill themes (Figures 18.1 and 18.2).

A developmental *skill theme* is a particular fundamental movement or sport skill around which a specific lesson or series of lessons is organized. In the developmental curriculum a category of movement serves as the organizing center of each unit of the curriculum, while skill themes serve as the organizing centers of

| Fundamental Stability Movements Stressed | Fundamental Locomotor Movements Stressed | Fundamental Manipulative Movements Stressed |
|---|---|---|
| Bending | Walking | Throwing |
| Stretching | Running | Catching |
| Twisting | Jumping | Kicking |
| Turning | Hopping | Trapping |
| Swinging | Skipping | Striking |
| Inverted supports | Sliding | Volleying |
| Body rolling | Leaping | Bouncing |
| Landing | Climbing | Ball rolling |
| Stopping | | Punting |
| Dodging | | |
| Balancing | | |

**Figure 18.1.** Selected fundamental movement themes.

the daily lesson plan. Each category of movement is briefly reviewed here, and a few examples of possible skill themes are given.

## Stability

Stability refers to the ability to maintain one's balance in relationship to the force of gravity even though the nature of the application of the force may be altered or parts of the body may be placed in unusual positions. The classification of stability extends beyond the concept of balance and includes various axial movements and postures in which a premium is placed on controlling one's equilibrium. Stability is the most basic form of human movement. It is basic to all efficient movement and permeates the categories of locomotion and manipulation. Bending, stretching, pivoting, dodging, and walking on a balance beam are examples of skill themes that may be incorporated into the daily lesson plan at the fundamental or sport skill phase of development.

## Locomotion

Locomotion refers to changes in the location of the body relative to fixed points on the ground. To walk, run, hop, jump, slide, or leap is to be involved in locomotion. The movement classification of locomotion develops in conjunction with stability, not apart from it. Fundamental aspects of stability must be mastered before efficient forms of locomotion may take place. The vertical jump, rebounding, and high jumping are examples of skill themes that may be incorporated into the daily lesson plan at the fundamental or sport skill phase of development.

| Sport Skill Themes | Locomotor Skills Stressed | | Manipulative Skills Stressed | | Stability Skills Stressed |
|---|---|---|---|---|---|
| Basketball sport skills | Running Sliding Leaping Jumping | | Passing Catching Shooting Dribbling Rebounding | Tipping Blocking | Selected axial movement skills Pivoting      Blocking Dodging      Cutting Guarding Picking Faking |
| Combative sport skills | Steping Sliding Hopping(karate) | | Dexterity (fencing) Striking (kendo) | | All axial movement skills Dodging and feinting Static balance skills Dynamic balance skills |
| Dance skills | Running Leaping Jumping | Hopping Skipping Sliding Stepping | Tossing Catching | | All Axial Movement skills Static balance postures Dynamic balance postures |
| Disc sport skills | Stepping Running Jumping | | Tossing Catching | | All axial movement skills Static balance postures Dynamic balance postures |
| Football sport skills | Running     Jumping Sliding Leaping | | Passing Catching Carrying | Kicking Punting Centering | Blocking      Pivoting Tackling Dodging |
| Gymnastic skills | Running     Leaping Jumping     Hopping Skipping    Landing | | | | Inverted supports Rolling, landing All axial movement skills Static balance tricks Dynamic balance tricks |
| Implement Striking sport skills (tennis, squash, racketball, hockey, lacrosse, golf) | Running Sliding Leaping Skating Walking | | Forehand Backhand Striking Driving Putting Chipping | Lob Smash Drop Throwing Catching Trapping | Dynamic balance skills Turning Twisting Stretching Bending Dodging Pivoting |
| Skiing sport skills | Stepping Walking Running Sliding | | Poling | | All axial movement skills Dynamic balance skills Static balance skills |
| Soccer sport skills | Running Jumping Leaping Sliding | | Kicking Trapping Juggling Throwing Blocking | Passing Dribbling Catching Rolling | Tackling      Feinting Marking      Turning Dodging |
| Softball/baseball skills | Running     Jumping Sliding Leaping | | Throwing Catching | Pitching Batting Bunting | Selected axial movement skills Dynamic balance skills Dodging |
| Target sport skills | | | Aiming Shooting | | Static balance skills |
| Track and field skills | Running     Horizontal Hopping    jumping Vertical    Leaping jumping    Starting | | Shot put Discus Javelin | Hammer Pole vault Baton passing Throwing | All axial movement skills Dynamic balance skills |
| Volleyball sport skills | Running     Jumping Sliding     Diving Sprawling Rolling | | Serving Volleying Bump | Dig Spike Dink Block | Dynamic balance skills Selected axial movements |

**Figure 18.2.** Selected sport skill themes.

## Manipulation

Manipulation is concerned with giving force to objects and absorbing force from objects by the use of the hands or feet. The tasks of throwing, catching, kicking, trapping, and striking are included under the category of manipulation. Manipulation also refers to the fine motor controls required for tasks such as buttoning, cutting, printing, and writing. The scope of this book, however, has been limited to gross motor aspects of manipulation. Large muscle manipulative abilities tend to develop somewhat later than stability and locomotor abilities. This is due, in part, to the fact that most manipulative movements incorporate elements of both stability and locomotion. Throwing a ball, passing a football, and pitching a baseball are examples of skill themes within the manipulative category of movement.

## CONTENT AREAS OF PHYSICAL EDUCATION

Fundamental movements and sport skills within the three categories of movement outlined above may be developed and refined through the three major content areas of physical education: *games and sports, rhythms,* and *self-testing activities.* The learning of particular games, rhythms, or self-testing activities is a means of developing stability, locomotor, and manipulative abilities appropriate to the developmental level of the child. Teachers must not lose sight of this goal. Every activity used in the program should be selected with an awareness that it can contribute to developing and refining certain movement abilities. For children, their primary objective may be fun, but for teachers of movement the objectives should involve the children's learning to move and learning through movement. The possibility of fun as the motivation to learn is a byproduct of any good educational program, and is an important objective. This point cannot be overemphasized, but when fun becomes the primary objective of the program for the teacher, then it ceases to be a physical education program and becomes a recreation period.

## Games and Sports

Games and sports are used as a means of enhancing movement abilities appropriate to the child's developmental level. They are often classified into three subcategories that proceed from the simple to the complex as follows.

1. Low organized games and relays.
2. Lead-up games.
3. Official sports.

## Rhythms

Rhythms are an important content area of the movement program. They are generally categorized into four subcontent areas:

1. Rhythmic fundamentals.
2. Creative rhythms.
3. Folk and square dance.
4. Social dance.

## Self-Testing

Self-testing is the third major content area of the program. This area represents a wide variety of activities in which children work on their own and can improve their performance through their own efforts. Self-testing activities may be classified in a variety of ways. The following is a common classification scheme for typical self-testing activities.

1. Fundamental movement activities.
2. Sport skill activities.
3. Physical fitness activities.
4. Stunts.
5. Tumbling.
6. Small (hand) apparatus.
7. Large apparatus.

Achieving effectiveness and efficiency in each of the three categories of movement at either the fundamental or the sport skill phase is the primary reason for incorporating games, rhythms, and self-testing activities in the program. The degree to which this is achieved depends on the particular developmental level of the children and the teacher's expertise in structuring developmentally appropriate movement experiences. Games, rhythms, and self-testing activities serve only as the *vehicle* by which these experiences are applied.

## MOVEMENT CONCEPTS OF MOVEMENT EDUCATION

Fundamental movements and sport skills within the three categories of movement may be elaborated upon and dealt with in terms of movement concepts. The development of particular movement concepts, namely, *effort, space,* and *relationships,* is the central focus of many movement education programs and is omitted from most traditional physical education programs. In a developmental curriculum, movement concepts are included and represent an emphasis of the program along with the three content areas discussed in the preceding section. The primary focus of the developmental curriculum is on fundamental movement and sport skill development through implementation of skill themes. These skill themes are applied to the understanding and application of movement concepts and the content areas of physical education.

A brief explanation of the three movement concept areas in relationship to movement skill development follows and is also highlighted in Table 18.1.

**Table 18.1   The Movement Concepts of Movement Education**

| Program (How the body moves with varying amounts of —) | Space (Where the body moves at different—) | Relationships (Moving with—) |
|---|---|---|
| —Force<br>strong<br>light | —Levels<br>high/medium/low | —Objects (or people)<br>over/under<br>in/out<br>between/among |
| —Time<br>fast<br>slow<br>medium<br>sustained<br>sudden | —Directions<br>forward/backward<br>diagonally/sideward<br>up/down<br>various pathways<br>(curved, straight,<br>zig-zag, etc.) | in front/behind<br>lead/follow<br>above/below<br>through/around |
| —Flow<br>free<br>bound | —Ranges<br>body shapes (wide<br>narrow, curved,<br>straight etc.)<br>body spaces (self-<br>space, and general<br>space)<br>body extensions<br>(near/far, large/<br>small with & without<br>implements) | —People<br>mirroring<br>shadowing<br>in unison<br>together/apart<br>alternating<br>simultaneously<br>partner/group |

## Effort

The concept of effort deals with *how* the body moves. Children during the preschool and primary grade years need to learn about the concept of effort. Effort may be subdivided into three categories, with the possibility for a wide variety of movement experiences combined with locomotor, manipulative, and stability movements.

1.  *Force.* Refers to the degree of muscular tension required to move the body or its parts from place to place or to maintain its equilibrium. Force may be heavy or light or in between these two extremes.
2.  *Time.* Refers to the speed at which movement takes place. A movement may be fast or slow, gradual or sudden, erratic or sustained.
3.  *Flow.* Refers to the continuity or coordination of movements. A movement may be smooth or jerky, free or bound.

## Space

The concept of space deals with *where* the body moves. Children need to understand where their body can move in space as well as how it can move. The following movement concepts of space can be directly related to all locomotor, manipulative, and stability movements.

1. *Level.* Refers to the height at which a movement is performed. A movement may be performed at a high, medium, or low level.
2. *Direction.* Refers to the path of movement. Movement may occur in a forward, backward, diagonal, up, down, left, or right direction, or it may be in a straight, curved, or zigzag pattern.
3. *Range.* Refers to relative location of ones body (self-space/general space) and how various *extensions* of the body (wide/narrow, far/near, long/short, large/small) are used in movement.

## Relationships

The concept of relationships deals with both *how and where* the body moves in harmony with objects and other people. The concept of relationships is important for children to understand and experience through the medium of movement.

1. *Objects.* Refers to stationing oneself in different positions to objects. Object relationships may be over/under, near/far, on/off, behind/in front, alongside, front/back, underneath/on top, in/out, between/among, and so on.
2. *People.* Refers to moving in various forms *with* people. People relationships include solo, partner, group, and mass movement.

## LEVELS OF MOTOR SKILL LEARNING

The content areas and the movement concepts just discussed may be implemented in a variety of ways. The teacher must, however, be aware that individuals tend to pass through typical learning levels as they develop and refine new movement skills. These levels are based on two developmental concepts. First, that the acquisition of movement abilities progresses from the simple to complex. Second, that children proceed gradually from general to specific in the development and refinement of their abilities. Based on these two concepts and fortified with the models of Fitts and Posner (1967), Gentile (1972), and Lawther (1977), it is possible to view learning a skill as a phenomenon that occurs in the following sequence (Figure 18.3).

1. Exploration.
2. Discovery.
3. Combination.
4. Selection.
5. Refined performance.

When involved in developing new stability, locomotor, or manipulative skills that are to be used in games, and sports, rhythm, or self-testing activities, we all generally go through the following sequence of learning experiences.

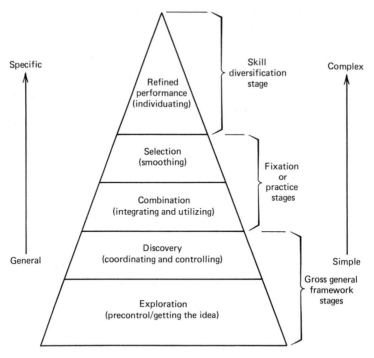

**Figure 18.3.** Levels of motor skill learning.

1.  We *explore* the movements involved in the task in relative isolation to one another. The learner does not have control of movement but gets used to the task and forms a gross general framework of the pattern or skill.
2.  We *discover* ways and means of executing each of these movements better through indirect means such as the observation of others performing, pictures, films, or books. During this aspect of achieving a gross general framework, the learner begins to gain control and to coordinate the task. It becomes relatively automatic.
3.  We *combine* the isolated movements with others and experiment with them in various ways. This is a practice stage in which separate tasks are integrated, elaborated upon, and begin to be utilized in varying ways.
4.  We *select* "best" ways of combining each of these movements through a variety of lead-up games, informal means of competition, and presentation. This aspect of practice is more specific and detailed than the previous stage, with more attention given to smoothing out the whole of several skill-related tasks.

5.   We *refine* the selected movements to a high degree and perform the particular activity through formal or informal means of competition or through leisure-time pursuits. This is often called the automatic or skill diversification stage, and is rarely reached in elementary or middle school physical education classes.

This sequential progression of skill learning is similar for adolescents and adults as well as for children, although it may not be as apparent. This is because the adolescent and adult are generally at the sport skill phase and may spend less time with exploration, discovery, and the combination of new skills, and more time in the selection and performance aspects of the sequence. Preschool and primary grade children at the fundamental movement pattern phase of development spend a great deal of time exploring, discovering, and combining new movements and less time with the selection of best ways of moving and the refined performance of activities.

Intermediate grade children typically at the general movement skill level spend the bulk of their time combining skills and less time with all others. Those at the specific movement skill level spend the greater portion of their time on more direct forms of combination and selecting best ways of executing skills. Those at the specialized level are involved primarily in refined performance activities and in continuing to select best ways of moving.

The teacher who is aware that the emphasis given to certain types of movement experiences depends on the child's level of development will structure the environment and utilize teaching approaches that provide appropriate types of learning. Figure 18.4 illustrates how teachers may utilize various forms of indirect and direct teaching approaches that are best suited to the developmental level of their students in order to facilitate the development of fundamental and sport skill abilities.

## Facilitating Exploration

Exploration represents the first level of the skill learning hierarchy. In order to take advantage of this level, the teacher focuses on indirect teaching approaches that encourage exploration. The movement exploration technique of teaching movement helps children enhance knowledge of their bodies and its potential for movement in space. Children are encouraged to explore and experiment with the movement potentials of their bodies. Accuracy and skill in performance are not stressed. This is accomplished by the teacher's refraining from establishing a model of performance for the particular movement being explored. Instead, the children are presented with a series of movement questions or challenges posed by the teacher and are given an opportunity to solve these problems as they see fit. Any *reasonable* solution to the problem is regarded as correct. At this time, there is no ''best'' method of performance that the teacher attempts to elicit from the children. The

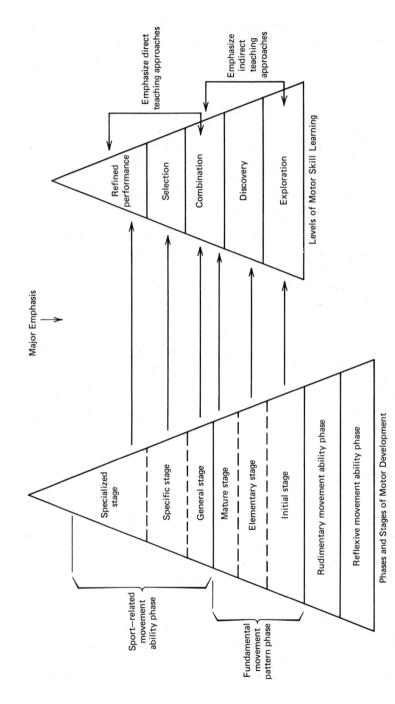

**Figure 18.4.** Interaction between the phases of motor development and the levels of motor skill learning.

teacher is more concerned with their creative involvement in the learning process.

Movement exploration experiences are not particularly concerned with the product of the movement act other than with acceptable execution of fundamental movements. However, the process of learning that children are involved in during the act is of great importance. In other words, the teacher is not particularly concerned with whether the ball goes in the hoop, the distance David can jump, or whether Jennifer can execute a handstand with "perfect" form, but is interested in their achieving some degree of success within the level of their own particular abilities. The teacher also places importance and value on the ability to think and act as an individual.

This is not to imply that success or goal-directed behavior is not important. On the contrary, movement exploration techniques are particularly appropriate for young children because they structure the environment for success simply by considering all reasonable solutions to the problems posed by the teacher as correct. Success and goal-directed behavior are individual standards that do not require children to emulate a model of performance or to compete with their peers, but permit success within the limits of one's own abilities. In doing so, the child is continually encouraged to explore and experiment with endless variations that influence the performance of all locomotor, manipulative, and stability movements in both the content areas (games, rhythms, and self-testing activities) and the movement concept areas (effort, space, and relationships).

## Facilitating Discovery

Discovery represents the second classification of the learning hierarchy. Movement experiences that incorporate discovery may be included in the lesson by the teacher in an indirect manner similar to the use of movement exploration techniques. The directed discovery or limitation method of teaching is often used when the child is in the process of discovery. The use of this technique requires that the teacher not establish a model for "correct" performance at the outset of the experience. Problems are stated in the form of questions or challenges that are posed by the teacher. These questions result in emphasis being placed on movement pattern development rather than on skill development. Both the movement exploration and the limitation methods utilize problem-solving techniques as a common tactic in developing the child's movement abilities. Gilliom (1970) has defined problem solving as:

> original thinking, an individual's technique of productive thinking, his techniques of inquiry, which is characterized by (1) a focus on an incomplete situation, (2) the freedom to inquire, and (3) the desire to put together something new to him, on his own, to make the incomplete situation into a complete one. (p. 21)

It is the method employed by the child in the solution of the problems posed by the teacher that causes exploration and guided discovery to be considered separately here. The limitation or guided discovery technique incorporates an observation phase into the total experience instead of accepting all solutions as correct and not providing a performance model as with movement exploration. The observation phase takes the form of observing the solutions of fellow students, the teacher, or individuals on film in relation to the problem presented. Only after the students have had an opportunity to solve the problem within the limits of their own understanding and ability is the observation phase utilized.

Instead of problems being entirely open-ended, as with movement exploration, there is a gradual funneling of questions in such a manner that they lead the children to discover for themselves how to perform the particular movement under consideration. There is no best way to move at this stage of development, and it allows for the performance of several "best" ways. At the end of the process of attempting solutions to the problem at hand, the children have an opportunity to evaluate their interpretations in light of the solutions of others. They are then given an opportunity to reassess their solutions in light of the performance of others (Figure 18.5).

## Facilitating Combination

Combination represents a transitional category in the hierarchical sequence of learning experiences. Movement experiences that use a combination of movement patterns or skills are incorporated into the lesson by the teacher through the use of both indirect and direct styles of teaching.

Indirect combination is a logical extension of the movement exploration and guided discovery approaches. These experiences differ only in that activities

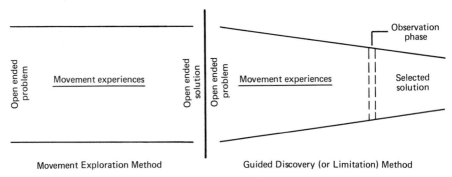

**Figure 18.5.** Differences between movement exploration and the guided discovery (limitation method) teaching techniques, both of which utilize indirect methods.

involving stability, locomotion, and/or manipulation are combined through the problem-solving approaches used at the exploration and discovery stages of learning.

Direct combination experiences follow a more traditional approach to developing and refining combinations of stability, locomotor, and/or manipulative movements. Direct, or traditional, teaching approaches involve establishing a model for correct performance through explanation, and demonstration of the skills to be learned before they are practiced by the students. The children then duplicate the movement characteristics of the model as nearly as possible within the limits of their abilities in a short practice session or drill. The class is generally stopped, and the model is presented again along with general comments concerning problems that the class as a whole may be encountering. The class is then involved in an activity that incorporates these skills. The teacher circulates among the students and aids those individuals who may still be having difficulty executing the skills with a general level of proficiency. Direct combination experiences require a model for performance to be established before the movement experience begins, while indirect experiences do not. The task and the command styles of teaching as proposed by Mooston (1981) are two of the most commonly used teacher-directed methods (Figure 18.6).

## Facilitating Selection

Selection represents the fourth level of the learning hierarchy. In order to take advantage of this level of experience, the teacher aids the students in making conscious decisions concerning the best methods of performing the numerous combinations of stability, locomotor, or manipulative skills. Rather than merely refining combinations of fundamental movements, children at both the general and specific sport skill stages begin to select preferred ways of moving in a wide variety of sport, game, and dance activities. Selection experiences follow the same direct progression of explanation, demonstration, and practice, followed by general and specific correction and drill that is used with direct combination experiences. Selection experiences, however, use more advanced activities than those found in the combination stage. These experiences generally take the form of advanced lead-up activities to dual, team, and individual sports, not low organized games and sport skill practice. Lead-up activities combine two or more selected skills into an approximation of the official sport. Advanced lead-up activities used during this period incorporate numerous elements of the official sport. They are modified primarily in terms of the time, equipment, and facilities required and are a close approximation of the final desired combination of specialized movement skills that will be performed in the official sport.

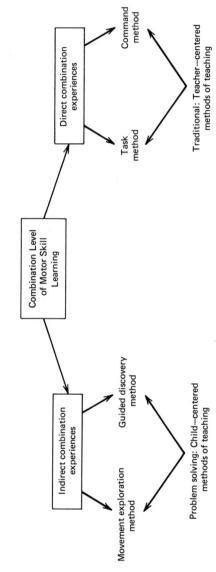

**Figure 18.6.** At the combination level of motor skill learning, the teacher often utilizes both indirect and direct methods of teaching.

## Facilitating Refined Performance

Refined performance is the fifth and final level of the motor skill learning hierarchy. Individuals at this stage are ready to pit their skills and abilities against those of others. Refined performance experiences have no place in a developmentally sound physical education curriculum for the preschool and elementary school child and must not be confused with appropriate forms of informal and low-level competition. Refined performance as used here refers to the actual implementation of activities from the selection stage in interscholastic, intercollegiate, intramural, or informal recreational activities. As the performance becomes more refined, greater stress is placed on accuracy and form in performing in a single, best way.

To be involved in the movement experiences that stress refined performance is to be at the specialized skill stage of development. The job of the preschool and elementary school teacher is to provide children with a series of experiences that contribute to fundamental movement pattern and general sport skill development that forms the basis for specialized skill development in later years.

## A DEVELOPMENTAL CURRICULAR MODEL

Unfortunately, programs stressing specialized skill development for young children abound throughout North America. Specialized skill development places primary emphasis on refined performance and little emphasis on the other aspects of the learning sequence outlined here. There is nothing inherently wrong with skill specialization, but we must ask ourselves whether skill specialization in the preschool and elementary school is really in the best interests of most children. If it is considered to be in the children's best interest, it should only *supplement* the regular program in the form of after-school activities. Specialized skill development should never overshadow, replace, or serve as the primary purpose of the regular physical education program. The regular program in the nursery and elementary school should stress the development and refinement of fundamental movement patterns and a wide variety of sport skills instead of dealing with specialized skill development through refined performance experiences.

We must involve children in a series of coordinated movement experiences that go beyond the learning of isolated skills and the in-school playing of specific sports that they would probably learn on their own through some form of organized activity outside of the school, such as the YMCA, YWCA, Boys' or Girls' Clubs, or the Police Athletic League. As Broer (1973) has stated, "If physical education is to make a real contribution to the total education of each student it must do more than give him a few isolated skills, most of which can be used only in specific recreational situations (p. 8).

The developmental model of physical education is based on the proposition that the development of children's movement abilities occurs in distinct but often overlapping *phases* (reflexes, rudimentary movement abilities, fundamental movement patterns, and sport-related abilities) in each of the *categories of human movement* (stability, locomotion, and manipulation) and that this is achieved through participation in *skill themes* that are applied to the various *content areas* of physical education (self-testing, games and sports, and rhythmics) and *movement concepts* of movement education (effort, space, and relationships) at the appropriate *level of motor skill learning* (exploration, discovery, combination, selection, or refined performance) that is recognized through the implementation of various *indirect* (movement exploration and guided discovery) and *direct* (command and task) teaching approaches (Figure 18.7).

## Preschool and Primary Grades

Developmental teaching recognizes that preschool and primary grade children are involved in developing and refining fundamental movement patterns in the three

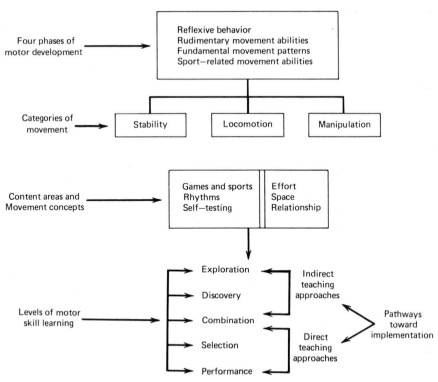

**Figure 18.7.** Outline of a sequentially based model for the motor development and physical education of the individual.

categories of movement. These categories are the organizing centers of the curriculum and formation of skill themes at this level. This can be done because each pattern of movement found under these three categories can be dealt with in relative isolation from the others (see Figure 18.1). These fundamental movements are the basis for sport skill movements. They are developed and refined at the exploration, discovery, and combination stages of learning *primary* through indirect styles of teaching that make use of games, rhythms, and self-testing activities and the application of effort, space, and relationship concepts to aid in their development (Figure 18.8).

## Upper Elementary and Middle School Grades

When the developmental model is applied to the upper elementary and middle school grades, the focus of the curriculum changes from the fundamental movement phase to the sport-related movement phase of development. During this phase of development, children are constantly combining various stability, locomotor, and manipulative patterns of movement in a wide variety of sport skills. Because of this, it becomes impossible to implement movement skill themes that focus on only one category of movement. Instead, at this level, skill themes are viewed in the context of the sport area to which they are being applied. The game of softball, for example, becomes a *sport skill theme* and involves combinations and elaborations of fundamental manipulative abilities (throwing, catching, striking), locomotor abilities (base running, and sliding) and stability abilities (twisting, turning, and stretching). The teacher at this level places attention on developing sport skills related to a particular sport skill theme. This is applied to the various content areas and *knowledge concepts* (rules, strategies, understandings, and appreciation) of physical education. The teacher recognizes that the children's major learning focus at this level is on the combination of skills and selection of "best" ways of performing; therefore, the teacher uses direct teaching methods as his or her *primary* approach to teaching (Figure 18.9).

## Summary

For too many years teachers of physical education, as well as the general population, have had only a vague notion of why the balanced motor development and movement education of children are important. The developmental model presented here is based on the Phases of Motor Development. Movement experiences and teaching methodologies are used that recognize the developmental level of the child. The use of games, rhythms, and self-testing activities as well as concepts of effort, space, and relationships is viewed as a means to achieving increased skill rather than as an end in itself. Learning to move is too important to be left to chance or to the whims of untrained persons. The individual with

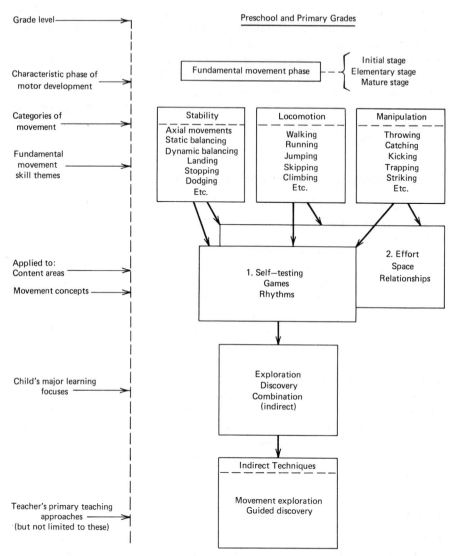

Grade level ⟶ Preschool and Primary Grades

Characteristic phase of motor development ⟶

Fundamental movement phase — Initial stage / Elementary stage / Mature stage

Categories of movement ⟶

| Stability | Locomotion | Manipulation |
|---|---|---|
| Axial movements | Walking | Throwing |
| Static balancing | Running | Catching |
| Dynamic balancing | Jumping | Kicking |
| Landing | Skipping | Trapping |
| Stopping | Climbing | Striking |
| Dodging | Etc. | Etc. |
| Etc. | | |

Fundamental movement skill themes ⟶

Applied to: Content areas ⟶

Movement concepts ⟶

1. Self–testing
Games
Rhythms

2. Effort
Space
Relationships

Child's major learning focuses ⟶

Exploration
Discovery
Combination
(indirect)

Indirect Techniques

Movement exploration
Guided discovery

Teacher's primary teaching approaches ⟶
(but not limited to these)

**Figure 18.8.** Implementing the developmental curricular model at the preschool and primary grade levels.

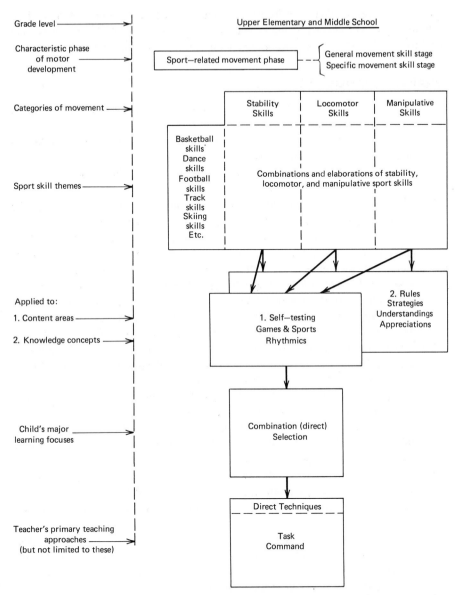

Grade level ───────────►| Upper Elementary and Middle School

Characteristic phase
of motor ───────────►| Sport—related movement phase {General movement skill stage
development | Specific movement skill stage

Categories of movement ───►| Stability | Locomotor | Manipulative
Skills | Skills | Skills

Sport skill themes ───────►| Basketball skills / Dance skills / Football skills / Track skills / Skiing skills / Etc.

Combinations and elaborations of stability, locomotor, and manipulative sport skills

Applied to:
1. Content areas ─────────►| 2. Rules Strategies Understandings Appreciations
2. Knowledge concepts ───►| 1. Self—testing Games & Sports Rhythmics

Child's major ──────────►| Combination (direct) Selection
learning focuses |

Teacher's primary teaching | Direct Techniques
approaches ────────────►| Task
(but not limited to these) | Command

**Figure 18.9.** Implementing the developmental curricular model in the upper elementary grades and middle school.

knowledge of (1) the Phases of Motor Development, (2) how children learn, and (3) how to implement developmentally appropriate programs for children can serve a vital role in developing children's movement abilities and physical abilities.

## CHAPTER HIGHLIGHTS

1. There are a variety of curricular rationales for organizing the physical education curriculum.
2. If research and theory concerning motor development cannot be brought to a practical level, it is of little use.
3. If curricular models are not based on sound research and theory, they have little value.
4. The developmental stage and movement analysis rationales are among the most popular curricular models at the elementary school level.
5. A fundamental movement theme or a sport skill theme is the focal point of the daily lesson and is composed of one or more movement skills from the locomotor, manipulative, and/or stability categories of movement.
6. The content areas of physical education (games and sports, rhythms, and self-testing activities) and the movement concepts of movement education (effort, space, and relationships) are of secondary importance to the development of skilled movement and serve as a means to that end.
7. When learning a new skill, we all pass through a series of levels of motor skill learning that focus on particular aspects of skill development (exploration, discovery, combination, selection, refined performance).
8. Indirect teaching approaches involving problem-solving techniques encourage exploration, discovery, and the indirect combination of movements.
9. Direct teaching approaches involving command and task teaching techniques are best suited for combining skills, selecting best ways to move, for refining the performance of movement skills.
10. A developmental curricular model can be constructed for children at the preschool and primary grade level that encourages development and refinement of fundamental movement abilities through the incorporation of indirect teaching techniques.
11. A developmental curricular model can be constructed for children in the upper elementary and middle school grades that encourages development and refinement of a wide variety of sport-related movement abilities, through the incorporation of direct teaching techniques.
12. The developmental curricular model emphasizes indirect styles of teaching at the preschool and primary grade level and direct styles of teaching at the upper elementary and middle school levels. This does not mean, however, that one is limited to the use of these techniques; it simply means that the *emphasis* switches from indirect to direct techniques. Individuals progress in their development of abilities according to particular levels of readiness.

## CRITICAL READINGS

Bruner, J.S.: "The Act of Discovery," *Harvard Educational Review,* 31, 1, 1961.

Lawther, J.D.: *The Learning and Performance of Physical Skills,* Englewood Cliffs, N.J.: Prentice-Hall, 1977, Chapters, 1, 4.

Schurr, E.: *Movement Experiences for Children,* Englewood Cliffs, N.J.: Prentice-Hall, 1980, Chapter 3.

Ward, D., and P. Werner: "Analysis of Two Curricular Approaches in Physical Education," *Journal of Physical Education and Recreation,* 52, 60–63, 1981.

*K-12 Physical Education:* Winnipeg, Canada: Manitoba Department of Education, 1981, Part One.

Whiting, H.T.A.: *Concepts In Skill Learning,* London: Lepus Books, 1975, Chapters 1-4.

# 19

# Assessing Children's Motor Behavior

There is no lack of tests that purport to measure the motor abilities of children. Wade (1981) has conservatively estimated that there are at least 250 assessment instruments, 91 of which have been published. The problem lies not in the quantity of instruments available but in their *quality*. The vast majority of tests have little or no rationale for development, and are based on quantitative measures (i.e., how far, how fast, how many), rather than on qualitative measures (how the child moves). Furthermore, the majority of these assessment instruments fail to compare individuals to their *own* previous performance but instead establish performance criteria based on the performances of their chronological peers. Tests of this nature, although potentially reliable, objective, and relatively easy to administer, reveal little about the motor "development" of the child. They may be valuable, however, in that they describe the status of the child at that particular time in terms of the criterion measures and in comparison with his or her peers. However, if we view the term development as the process of change over time and are interested in assessing this change, there is little to be gained from administering a battery of tests that merely describe the quantity of an individual's performance at a given point in time. Tests of this nature have little to do with development and may be more properly labeled as performance tests.

There are essentially two types of assessment instruments available to assess the motor behavior of children: product-oriented instruments and process-oriented instruments. Product, task-oriented, or descriptive measures, as they are often termed, are by far the most prevalent. They are probably best exemplified by the devices designed by Apgar (1953), Frankenburg and Dodds (1967), Bayley (1969), Brazelton (1973), Roach and Kephart (1966), and Bruininks (1978). Each of these assessment instruments will be briefly described and critiqued in the following sections. The process-oriented assessment instruments designed by McClenaghan (1976) Seefeldt, and Haubenstricker (1976), and others will also be discussed.

## PRODUCT-ORIENTED ASSESSMENT INSTRUMENTS

There is an abundance of descriptive performance tests designed to screen children and to assess their current level of ability as measured by a variety of behavioral events. Screening tests are designed to provide a relatively quick and simple means of differentiating normal infants or children from those who may not be developing normally. Behavioral assessment instruments, on the other hand, tend to be more varied in intent and design. They may attempt to distinguish between normal and abnormal behavior, predict later abilities, or measure individual differences.

### Screening Tests

Three widely used screening devices are the Apgar screening technique used at birth, the Denver Developmental Screening Test used from infancy through early childhood, and the Purdue Perceptual Motor Survey used from early childhood through childhood.

**Apgar.** Virginia Apgar (1953) developed the Apgar screening technique as a quick and reliable method of assessing the newborn one minute after birth. Supplemental ratings can be made at three, five, and ten minutes after birth. The newborn is evaluated on five items and given a score of 0, 1, or 2 on each for a total of up to 10, depending on its condition. A score of 0 is given if the sign to be observed is absent, a 1 if all of the conditions are not met for a score of 2. Ten is the highest score possible for the five-test total. Infants are rated on (1) heart rate, (2) respiratory effort, (3) irritability, (4) muscle tone, and (5) color. Table 19.1 provides a summary of the five items and how they are scored.

Apgar scores appear to be quite reliable. The test was standardized by Apgar and James (1962) on 27,715 infants. The standardization showed that infants with the lowest Apgar scores had the highest mortality rates and that the device was useful in predicting infant mortality. Self and Horwitz (1979) indicated that Apgar scores are directly related to the type of delivery. Breech deliveries have the lowest average scores, followed by caesarian section deliveries, with spinal anesthesia and natural childbirth deliveries receiving the highest scores. Yang et al. (1976) did note, however, that maternal drug dosage is directly related to Apgar scores. Yang found that the more drugs the mother is given, the lower is the infant's five-minute Apgar score.

The Apgar system has been helpful in screening newborns in need of special attention. It is quick, easy to administer, appears to be highly reliable, and has been used successfully for almost a quarter of a century as a diagnostic tool for the physician.

**Denver Developmental Screening Test.** The Denver Developmental Screening Test (DDST) developed by Frankenburg and Dodds (1967) is a helpful device used to screen infants and young children. It has been successfully used to detect evidence of retarded development in order that effective intervention techniques may be implemented at an early age. Both gross and fine motor skills are evaluated along with language and personal-social skills. The 105 items on the test are scaled according to their normal developmental order of appearance in children. Table 19.2 provides a brief overview of the test and some of the items assessed.

Although the DDST has been roundly criticized for underscreening, it does offer the advantage of indicating the age at which 25, 50, 75, and 90 percent of the population pass each item. Benchmarks of behavior for each of the items assessed are displayed with bar graphs on a screening chart that illustrate the overlapping but sequentially based skills of infancy and early childhood. Seldom are more than 20 of the 105 items administered in order to provide a profile of the child's developmental level.

The DDST has been standardized on a sample of 1036 children ranging in age from 2 weeks to 6 years that has been criticized as unrepresentative (Buros, 1971). Furthermore, Herkowitz (1978) has stated that:

> So—although easy to administer, and capable of being used by relatively untrained testers—the DDST is not so reliable or valid as its authors had hoped. Its use for children under 30 months old should be discouraged because of questionable reliability at that age. (p. 168)

**Table 19.1  Scoring the Apgar Screening Test**

| Item tested | Scoring | | |
| --- | --- | --- | --- |
| | *2* | *1* | *0* |
| Heart rate | 100–140 bpm | Under 100 | No heartbeat |
| Respiratory effort | Regular breathing and lusty crying | Irregular or shallow breathing | No breathing |
| Reflex irritability (measured by a slap to the soles of the feet) | Lusty crying when soles of feet are slapped | No crying but grimace or movement when soles of feet are slapped | No reaction when soles of feet are slapped |
| Muscle tone | Spontaneously flexed arms and legs resist attempts at extension | Spontaneously flexed arms and legs offer little resistance from attempts at extension | Completely flaccid |
| Color[a] | Entirely pink | Some pink | Other than pink |

[a] This is the most controversial item in the test. Few infants receive at 2 at one minute, and the item is, of course, invalid with dark-skinned babies.

403

**Table 19.2  Sample Items from the Denver Developmental Screening Test**

| Area Tested | Sample Items Measured |
|---|---|
| Gross motor (31 items measured) | Rudimentary stability abilities: control of head, neck, trunk, rolling over, sitting, standing with support, pulling to stand, cruising, standing alone, walking |
| | Fundamental manipulative abilities: kicking, throwing, tricycle riding, catching |
| | Fundamental locomotor abilities: jumping in place, long jumping, hopping |
| | Fundamental stability abilities: balancing on one foot, heel—toe walk |
| Fine motor (30 items measured) | Rudimentary manipulative abilities: reaching, grasping, and releasing, cube stacking, scribbling, copying, draw-a-person |
| Language (21 items measured) | Vocalizing, laughing, squealing, sound localization, imitation of speech sounds, rudimentary language, combining words, following directions, recognizing colors, defining words |
| Personal-social (22 items measured) | Smiling, feeding, drinking from cup, imitating housework, helping in house, removing garment, putting on clothing, washing and drying hands, playing interactive games, separating from mother easily, dressing without supervision |

The usefulness of the DDST is questionable. It should only be used as a gross screening measure that may provide some clues to the developmentally delayed child. It should not, at this time, be considered as a valid or reliable instrument for research or placement purposes.

**The Purdue Perceptual-Motor Survey.** The Purdue Perceptual-Motor Survey (PPMS) developed by Roach and Kephart (1966) is *not* a test. It is a behavioral assessment *survey* that provides the examiner with an opportunity to observe a broad spectrum of behaviors. In fact, Roach and Kephart note that "at its present level of development the survey should be regarded merely as an instrument which allows the examiner to observe a series of perceptual-motor behaviors and to isolate areas which may need further study" (p. 10—11). The survey is based on Kephart's theory that all learning is based on the sensorimotor experiences of childhood.

The PPMS is designed for children from 6 to 10 years of age but is often used with both younger and older children in an effort to gain some clues concerning possible perceptual-motor problems. Table 19.3 outlines the various components of the survey and how they are measured.

**Table 19.3   Test Items from the Purdue Perceptual-Motor Survey**

| Items Assessed | Method |
| --- | --- |
| Balance and posture | Walking forward, backward, sideways on walking board; performing a series of eight tasks evaluating ability to jump, hop, and skip while maintaining balance. |
| Body image and differentiation | Identification of body parts, imitation of movement, obstacle course activities, Kraus-Weber Test, angels-in-the-snow. |
| Perceptual-motor match | Making circle, double circle, lateral line, and vertical line on chalkboard; performing eight rhythmic writing tasks. |
| Ocular control | Ocular pursuits of both eyes, right eye, left eye, and convergence are tested. |
| Form perception | Seven geometric forms—circle, cross, square, triangle, horizontal, diamond, vertical diamond, and divided rectangle—are drawn on sheet of paper. |

The PPMS has been used successfully for several years to discriminate between children who are experiencing problems in their motor development and those who are not. As a survey, however, interpretation and generalization of results are limited. Standardization of the PPMS was conducted on only 200 children all from the same school and using Kephart's original scale rather than the one published later by Roach and Kephart (Buros, 1971). Reliability scores within subjects and between raters has been reported at .95 (Buros, 1971). The question of validity still has not been answered to the satisfaction of many. Several of the tasks on the PPMS require multiple skills, and some demonstrate the need for more cognitive than motor ability. Also, factor analytic studies have shown that items are not appropriately grouped. Factors do not remain stable through grades K to 4, nor do they develop at similar or even rates (Dunsing, 1969). Despite its many shortcomings, the PPMS may be of use by the teacher as an observational assessment survey that may offer some important clues to the perceptual and motor functioning of the child.

## Behavioral Assessment Tests

There are a wide variety of behavioral assessment tests available. Only a few are presented here. They represent, however, a sampling of the most widely used behavioral assessment tests in North America and provide a cross section of tests appropriate for use with neonates, infants, young children, and older children.

**Brazelton Neonatal Behavioral Assessment Scale.** The Brazelton Neonatal Behavioral Assessment Scale (BNBAS) was developed by Brazelton (1973) with the intention of scoring the infant's responses to his or her environment. The test is designed for use with normal neonates and is divided into twenty elicited neurological items and twenty-seven behavioral items. Table 19.4 provides an overview of the items measured on the BNBAS.

Scoring of the majority of the infant's behavior is done after administration of all the test items. The elicited neurological responses are scored on a four-point scale ranging from 0 to 3 points (0, absent; 1, low; 2, medium; 3 high) for intensity of response. The behavioral items are scored on a scale of 1 to 9 points. This scale represents the state of arousal of the infant. A 1, for example, signifies that the infant is sleeping, while a 9 indicates that the infant is actively crying. The ideal state of the infant for assessment lies somewhere between 1 and 9 and varies from item to item. The testing conditions as well as overall impressions of the neonate are also recorded along with general biographical data such as length, weight, and age in days.

Unfortunately, the Brazelton scale has not been standardized beyond the report by Heidelise et al. (1979), in which a homogeneous group of fifty-four healthy, full-term white newborns were assessed over a ten-day period. Brazelton himself (Brazelton et al., 1979) has recognized the problem of standardization based on his findings that newborns from different cultures behave differently. The problem, therefore, is to be able to identify a group of newborns that are in fact representative of the "population at large." To date, this difficult feat has not been accomplished. Interrater reliability of the BNBAS, however, has been reported to be quite high ranging from .85 to 1.00 (Horowitz and Brazelton, 1973; Heidelise et al., 1979), and its predictive validity is good, having been reported at 80 percent in a sample of forty-three children followed over a seven-year period (Tronick and Brazelton, 1975).

The Brazelton scale appears to be a useful device for identifying high-risk infants and for studying the effects of obstetrical medication, cross-cultural infant behavior, and caregiver intervention. It is a helpful measure for assessing the general, specific, and neurological behavior of the neonate.

**Bayley Scales of Infant Development.** The Bayley Scales of Infant Development (Bayley, 1969) are a revision of Bayley's (1935) earlier work, which attempted, through behavioral assessment, to measure the intellectual development of the child. Very little relationship was found between the infant's score on mental scales and later intelligence or later performance on mental scales. As a result, the current Bayley Scales of Infant Development (BSID) purport to assess only the child's developmental status from 1 month of age to 2½ years.

The BSID is divided into three separate scales. Table 19.5 presents a brief overview of these three scales and the general items measured. Space limitations do not permit a full description of each of the scales. The Mental Scale contains 163 items. The Motor Scale is made up of 81 items measuring progressive change in

**Table 19.4  Test Items for the Brazelton Neonatal Behavioral Assessment Scale**

| *Elicited Neurological Responses* | *Behavioral Responses* | |
| --- | --- | --- |
| | *Specific* | *General* |
| 1. Plantar grasp | 1. Response decrement to light (2,3)[a] | 1. Degree of alertness (4) |
| 2. Hand grasp | 2. Response decrement to rattle (2,3) | 2. General tonus (4,5) |
| 3. Anal colonus | 3. Response decrement to bell (2,3) | 3. Motor maturity (4,5) |
| 4. Babinski reflex | 4. Response decrement to pinprick (1,2,3) | 4. Cuddliness (4,5) |
| 5. Standing reflex | 5. Inanimate visual orientation response (focusing and following an object) (4) | 5. Consolability with intervention (6 to 8) |
| 6. Primary stepping reflex | | 6. Peak to excitement (6) |
| 7. Placing | 6. Inanimate auditory orientation response (reaction to an auditory stimulus) (4,5) | 7. Rapidity of buildup (1,2 to 6) |
| 8. Incurvation | | 8. Irritability (3,4,5) |
| 9. Reflex crawling | 7. Animate visual orientation (reaction to persons) (4) | 9. Activity (alert states) |
| 10. Glabulla reflex | | 10. Tremulousness (all states) |
| 11. Tonic deviation of head and eyes | 8. Animate auditory orientation (reaction to a voice) (4,5) | 11. Amount of startle (3,4,5,6) |
| 12. Nystagmus | | 12. Lability of skin color (all states) (1-6) |
| 13. Tonic neck reflex | 9. Animate visual and auditory orientation (reaction to a person's face and voice) (4) | 13. Lability of states (all states) |
| 14. Moro reflex | | 14. Self-quieting activity (6,5 to 4,3,2,1) |
| 15. Rooting reflex intensity | 10. Pull-to-sit (3,5) | 15. Hand-to-mouth facility (all states) |
| 16. Sucking reflex intensity | 11. Defensive movements (4) | |
| 17–20. Passive movements (right arm, left arm, right leg, left leg) | | |

[a]Numbers in parentheses represent the ideal state for assessment.

**Table 19.5   General Description of the Items Measured on the Bayley Scales of Infant Development**

| Scale | Items Assessed |
|---|---|
| Mental scale | Sensory-perceptual acuities<br>Object discrimination<br>Object constancy<br>Memory<br>Learning<br>Problem solving<br>Vocalization<br>Verbal communication<br>Generalizations and classificatons |
| Motor scale | Control of the body<br>Gross motor coordination<br>Fine motor coordination |
| Infant behavior record | Administered after the Mental and Motor Scales. Assesses the child's social development, interests, emotions, energy, and tendencies to approach or withdraw from situations |

gross motor abilities such as sitting, standing, walking, and stair climbing, and fine motor abilities. Materials for the Motor Scale are expensive and require special equipment.

The BSID has been standardized on 1262 children from 2 to 3 months of age (Self and Horwitz, 1979). Observer agreement of trained observers (i.e., minimum of six months training) for the Mental Scale was rated at 89.4 percent and 93.4 percent for the Motor Scale (Werner and Bayley, 1966). Werner and Bayley (1966) also achieved test-retest reliability ratings of .76 for the Mental Scale and .75 for the Motor Scale. Validity data for the BSID have never been published.

The BSID scales are probably the best standardized behavioral assessment techniques available for infants. They have had the most extensive use as a research instrument of any of the infant assessment scales and have proven to be helpful in determining the developmental status of individual infants at a given age. When administered and interpreted by a trained examiner, they can be a valuable research tool.

**Bruininks-Oseretsky Test of Motor Proficiency.** The Bruininks-Oseretsky Test of Motor Proficiency (BOT) was developed by Bruininks (1978) as an "individually administered test that assesses the motor functioning of children from 4½ to 14½ years of age" (p. 11). The BOT is based, in part, on the adaptation by Doll (1946) of the original Oseretsky Tests of Motor Proficiency, and is designed to assess the motor skills of children. The BOT is composed of eight subtests designed to measure important aspects of motor development. Table 19.6 provides an overview

**Table 19.6   Test Items from the Bruininks-Oseretsky Test of Motor Proficiency**

| Area Tested | Subtest | Items |
|---|---|---|
| Gross motor skills | 1. Running—Designed to measure running speed. | Shuttle run. |
| | 2. Balance (8 items)—Designed to measure static and dynamic balance abilities. | Static balance (3 items). Dynamic balance (5 items). |
| | 3. Bilateral coordination (8 items)—Designed to measure simultaneous coordination of upper and lower limbs. | Foot and finger tapping (3 items). Jumping in place (4 items). Drawing lines and crosses simultaneously (1 item). |
| | 4. Strength (3 items)—Designed to measure upper arm and shoulder girdle strength, abdominal strength, and leg strength. | Standing broad jump. Sit-ups. Knee push-ups (boys under 8 and all girls). Full push-ups (boys 8 and older). |
| Gross and fine motor skills | 5. Upper limb coordination (9 items)—Designed to measure gross and fine eye-hand coordination. | Ball bounce and catch (2 items). Catching tossed ball (2 items). Throwing a ball (1 item). Touching swinging ball (1 item). Precise upper limb movements (3 items). |
| Fine motor skills | 6. Response speed (1 item)—Designed to measure response to a moving object. | Yardstick drop (1 item). |
| | 7. Visual-motor control (8 items)—Designed to measure coordination of eye-hand movements. | Cutting (1 item). Drawing and copying (7 items). |
| | 8. Upper limb speed and dexterity (8 items)—Designed to measure hand and finger dexterity, hand speed, and arm speed. | Penny placing (2 items). Card sorting (1 item). Bead stringing (1 item). Peg displacing (1 item). Lines and dots (3 items). |

of the BOT. The gross motor skill and fine motor skill sections of the test may be administered separately and will yield separate composite scores. In order to arrive at a composite score for the entire battery of tests, a combination gross and fine motor skills test must be taken along with the separate gross motor items and separate the fine motor items. A short form of the BOT is also available.

The BOT has been standardized on a sample of 765 children carefully proportioned on the basis of age, sex, race, community size, and geographic location as indicated by 1970 census figures. Norms have been developed and test-retest reliability scores average .87 for the battery composite of the long form and .86 for the short form of the test (Bruininks, 1978). The validity of the BOT according to Bruininks (1978) "is based on its ability to assess the construct of motor development of proficiency" (p. 28). In terms of motor *proficiency* as measured by the performance of a given child on a given day, the BOT is indeed a valid test. It is, however, too much to assume that the BOT is a valid test of motor *development* if the term development is viewed as progressive change over time.

The relative merits and drawbacks of the BOT were debated at a meeting of the Motor Development Academy of the AAHPERD (Bruininks, 1981; Haubenstricker, et al., 1981; Broadhead, 1981). The test is not without fault or need for improvement. However, despite its limitations, it does seem to have good potential for assessing the motor proficiency of children. It should also be of value as a research tool, and an aid for identifying children with special needs.


## PROCESS-ORIENTED ASSESSMENT INSTRUMENTS

Few formalized tests exist that examine the process of movement. There is, however, a growing body of research oriented toward the quality of children's movement. What is needed now is careful longitudinal study of a variety of movement behaviors in order to generate developmental continuums. Roberton (1981) notes: "Motor development ought to be assessed by observing a child's movement and locating what is seen within a developmental sequence" (p. 3). The three-stage developmental sequence of fundamental movements presented in Chapter 11 offer a means by which the quality of a child's movements can be observed and his or her progress charted over time. It should be stressed, however, that several of the developmental sequences presented in Chapter 11, although based on careful observational assessment, are merely *proposed* developmental descriptions of fundamental movements. Only through film analysis and longitudinal study can these sequences be validated, or refuted. A description of the observational assessment instruments developed by McClenaghan (McClenaghan, 1976; McClenaghan and Gallahue, 1978b), and by Seefeldt and Haubenstricker (1976) follows.

## Fundamental Movement Pattern Assessment Instrument

The Fundamental Movement Pattern Assessment Instrument (FMPAI) designed by McClenaghan (1976) and later published by McClenaghan and Gallahue (1978b) is a carefully developed observational assessment instrument. It is used to classify individuals at the initial, elementary, or mature stage of development in five different movements (throwing, catching, kicking, running, and jumping). The developmental sequence for each of these movements is based on an exhaustive review of the biomechanical literature on each fundamental movement.

Validity of the FMPAI was established through the research base on which the developmental progressions of the five movement patterns were formulated and by the opinions of a panel of motor development experts. Interrater reliability for each of the assessed items ranged from a high of 95 percent agreement for throwing to a low of 80 percent agreement for running, with 94 percent, 91 percent, and 90 percent agreement for jumping, catching, and kicking, respectively. Subject performance reliability was rated at 88.6 percent on a retest five days after the original assessment.

The FMPAI is an easy-to-administer, easy-to-use, motor development test designed to measure the present status of children and to assess change over time. It attempts to view the quality of the child's movement, and is based on documented developmental sequences for acquiring selected fundamental movement abilities. The FMPAI does not, however, yield a quantitative score, nor can it be used for comparing one child with another. This instrument is intended instead to assess developmental changes over time, using observational assessment as a valid and reliable method of data collection and comparison within individuals.

## Developmental Sequence of Fundamental Motor Skills Inventory

The Developmental Sequence of Fundamental Motor Skills Inventory (DSFMSI) assessment instrument was developed by Seefeldt and Haubenstricker (1976) and Haubenstricker et al. (1981). The DSFMSI categorizes each of ten fundamental motor patterns into four or five stages. The fundamental movements of walking, skipping, hopping, running, striking, kicking, catching, throwing, jumping, and punting have been studied. These developmental sequences are based on combinations of longitudinal and cross-sectional data obtained from film analysis. Children are observed and matched to both visual and verbal descriptions of each stage. Individuals are classified along a continuum from stage one (immature) to stage five (mature).

Although reliability scores have not been reported, personal communication with one of the developers (Haubenstricker, 1980) has indicated that with training using specially designed films and a stop-action projector, interrater reliability is quite high.

## Other Process-Oriented Assessment Instruments

There are a few other useful process-oriented approaches to motor development assessment. Robertson's (1978c) method represents an expansion of stage theory and analyzes the components of movement within a given pattern. Her longitudinal study of the development of throwing abilities lends support for the concept of developmental stages and offers hope for validation of developmental sequences. The Ohio State University Scale of Intra-Gross Motor Assessment (OSU Sigma) developed by Loovis (1975) and the De Oreo Fundamental Motor Skills Inventory developed by De Oreo (1977) also represent promising efforts at observing the process of movement.

The ongoing research being conducted by Roberton and Halverson at the University of Wisconsin, and by Seefeldt, Haubenstricker, and Branta at Michigan State University, McClenaghan, at the University of South Carolina, and Gallahue, at Indiana University, is providing a great deal of the descriptive data on which future process-oriented motor development tests will be based. The mixed longitudinal data collection process is long and tedious. It requires considerable patience and years of effort before sound, validated developmental progressions can be formulated.

## Summary

There is an ever-increasing number of published and unpublished tests purported to be measures of motor development. The vast majority of these assessment instruments are product-oriented and provide information concerning the present status of the child in a variety of areas. These tests are descriptive and generally establish a standard of performance based on certain expectations for each chronological age.

Product-oriented assessment instruments can be of value to the motor development specialist if they are both valid and reliable. Unfortunately, the validity of many tests is suspect because of the lack of a sound rationale, or because of inadequate correlational attempts with other tests purporting to measure the same thing.

Product-oriented tests may be classified as either screening devices or behavioral assessment devices. The Apgar, Denver Developmental Screening Test, and Purdue Perceptual-Motor Survey are easy-to-use tools available for quick but gross classification of children. The Brazelton Neonatal Assessment Scale, Bayley Scales of Infant Development, and Bruininks-Oseretsky Test of Motor Proficiency are among the most widely used behavioral assessment instruments for neonates, infants, and children, respectively.

There are far fewer process-oriented tests than product-oriented tests, although there is great need to know more about the developmental progression of movement skill acquisition. The Fundamental Movement Pattern Assessment Instrument and the Developmental Sequence of Fundamental Motor Skills Inventory represent two initial attempts at assessing the quality, rather than the quantity, of movement.

## CHAPTER HIGHLIGHTS

1. Several hundred tests that purport to measure children's motor abilities exist.
2. The quality of the vast majority of motor assessment instruments is questionable.
3. The validity of many motor assessment instruments is highly questionable.
4. Most tests of motor abilities are based on quantitative measures of how far, how fast, or how many.
5. Most assessment instruments are scored on chronologically based criteria.
6. Many tests that purport to be motor *development* tests are really measures of motor *performance*.
7. Tests of motor behavior in children may be classified as product-oriented or process-oriented.
8. Product-oriented tests are sometimes referred to as task-oriented or descriptive measures.
9. Product-oriented tests may be classified as either screening or behavioral assessment instruments.
10. Screening tests are designed to differentiate normal from abnormal behaviors.
11. Behavioral assessment instruments attempt to distinguish, predict, and measure individual differences.
12. The Apgar, Denver Developmental Screening Test, and Purdue Perceptual-Motor Survey are three easy-to-administer screening devices designed for newborns, infants, and young children, respectively.
13. The Brazelton Neonatal Behavioral Assessment Scale, Bayley Scales of Infant Development, and Bruininks-Oseretsky Test of Motor Proficiency are three behavioral assessment devices designed for neonates, infants, and children, respectively.
14. Process-oriented tests of motor development are concerned with the quality of one's movements, are based on developmental references, and are scored in a diagnostic manner.
15. The Fundamental Movement Pattern Assessment Instrument and Developmental Sequence of Fundamental Motor Skills Inventory are process-oriented motor development tests that are reliable, appear to be valid, and are easy to administer.
16. The ongoing research of a variety of investigators is providing a basis for the development of motor development tests that view the quality of the child's movement.

## CRITICAL READINGS

Haubenstricker, J.: "A Critical Review of Selected Perceptual-Motor Tests and Scales Currently Used in the Assessment of Motor Behavior," in D.M. Landers and R.W. Christina (eds.), *Psychology in Motor Behavior and Sport—1977*, Champaign, Ill.: Human Kinetics, 1978, pp. 536−543.

Herkowitz, J.: "Assessing the Motor Development of Children: Presentation and Critique of Tests," in M.V. Ridenour (ed.), *Motor Development: Issues and Applications*, Princeton, N.J.: Princeton, 1978, pp. 175−187.

Herkowitz, J.: "Instruments Which Assess the Efficiency/Maturity of Children's Motor Pattern Performance," in D.L. Landers and R.W. Christina (eds.), *Psychology in Motor Behavior and Sport—1977*, Champaign, Ill.: Human Kinetics, 1978, pp. 529−535.

Roberton, M.A.: "Stability of Stage Categorizations in Motor Development," In D.M. Landers and R.W. Christina (eds.), *Psychology in Motor Behavior and Sport—1977*, Champaign, Ill.: Human Kinetics, 1978, pp. 494−505.

Self, P.A., and F.D. Horwitz: "The Behavioral Assessment of the Neonate: An Overview," in J.D. Osofsky (ed.), *The Handbook of Infant Development*, New York: Wiley, 1979, pp. 126−164.

# Bibliography

AAHPER: *What Every Parent Should Know About the New Physical Education*, Reston, Va.: AAHPERD, 1968.

AAHPER: *Annotated Bibliography of Perceptual-Motor Development*, Reston, Va.: AAHPERD, 1973.

AAHPER: *Testing for Impaired, Disabled and Handicapped Individuals*, Reston, Va.: AAHPERD, 1975.

AAHPER: *Youth Fitness Test Manual: Revised 1976 Edition*, Reston, Va: AAHPERD, 1976.

AAHPERD: *Health Related Physical Fitness Test, Manual*, Reston, Va.: AAHPERD, 1980.

Alexander, G.J., et al.: "Injection in Early Pregnancy Produces Abnormalities in Offspring of Rats," *Science*, 157, 459–460, 1967.

Ames, L.: "The Sequential Patterning of Prone Progression in the Human Infant," *Genetic Psychology Monographs*, 19, 409–460, 1937.

Anderson, K.L., et al.: "The Rate of Growth in Maximal Aerobic Power of Children in Norway," in J. Borms and M. Hebbelinck (eds.), *Medicine and Sport Science Series, Vol. II, Pediatric Work Physiology*, Basel, Belgium: S. Karger, 1978.

Apgar, V.: "A Proposal for a New Method of Evaluation of the Newborn Infant," *Current Researcher in Anesthesia and Analgesia*, 32, 260–267, 1953.

Apgar, V., and L.S. James: "Further Observations on the Newborn Scoring System," *American Journal of the Diseases of Children*, 104, 419–428, 1962.

Armstrong, D.B., et al.: "Obesity and Its Relation to Health and Disease," *Journal of the American Medical Association*, 147, 1007, 1951.

Armussen, E.: "Growth in Muscular Strength and Power," in G.L. Rarick (ed.), *Physical Activity: Human Growth and Development*, New York: Academic Press, 1973.

415

Astrand, P.O.: *Experimental Studies of Working Capacity in Relation to Sex and Age*, Copenhagen, Denmark: Munksgoard, 1952.

Astrand, P.O., and K. Rodahl: *Textbook of Work Physiology*, New York, McGraw-Hill, 1970.

Athletic Institute: *National Youth Sports Directors' Conference*, November 19–21, 1975, Proceedings Report, Chicago: Athletic Institute, 1975.

Bailey, D.A., et al.: "Size Dissociation of Maximal Aerobic Power During Growth in Boys," in J. Borms and M. Hebbelinck (eds.), *Medicine and Sport Science Series, Vol. II, Pediatric Work Physiology*, Basel, Belgium: S. Karger, 1978.

Bailey, R.A., and E.C. Burton: *The Dynamic Self: Activities to Enhance Infant Development*, St. Louis: Mosby, 1982.

Bain, L.: "Status of Curriculum Theory in Physical Education," *Journal of Physical Education and Recreation*, 49, 25, 1978.

Barness, L.W.: "Nutrition for the Low Birth Weight Infant," *Clinical Perinatology*, 2, 345–352, 1975.

Barrow, H.M., and R. McGee: *A Practical Approach to Measurement in Physical Education*, Philadelphia: Lea and Febiger, 1979.

Barsch, R.H.: *Achieving Perceptual-Motor Efficiency*, Seattle: Special Child Publications, 1965.

Bayley, N.: "The Development of Motor Abilities During the First Three Years," *Monograph of the Society for Research on Child Development*, 1, 1–26, 1935.

Bayley, N.: *Manual for the Bayley Scales of Infant Development*, New York: Psychological Corporation, 1969

Bee, H.: *The Developing Child*, New York: Harper & Row, 1975.

Behar, M.: "Prevalence of Malnutrition Among Preschool Children," in N.S. Scrimshaw and J.E. Gordon (eds.), *Malnutrition, Learning and Behavior*, Cambridge, Mass., MIT Press, 1968.

Bench, J., et al.: "A Comparison Between the Neonatal Sound-Evoking Startle Response and the Head-Drop (Moro) Reflex," *Developmental Medicine and Child Neurology*, 14, 308–314, 1972.

Bergel, R.: "Motor Performance and Physical Growth Components of Headstart and Non-Headstart Pre-School Children," Symposium papers, AAHPER Research Consortium, Reston, Va. 1, 53–56, 1978.

Bernard, J., and L.W. Sontag: "Fetal Reactivity to Tonal Stimulation: A Preliminary Report," *Journal of Genetic Psychology*, 70, 205–210, 1947.

Beumen, G., et al.: "Learning Effects of Repeated Measure Designs," in K. Berg and B. Erickson (eds.), *Children and Exercise IX*, Baltimore: University Park Press, 41–48, 1980.

Birch, H.G., and J.D. Gussow: *Disadvantaged Children*, New York: Harcourt, Brace & World, 1970.

Bloom, B.S., et al.: *Taxonomy of Educational Objectives: Handbook I: Cognitive Domain*, New York: David McKay, 1956.

Bolby, J: "The Nature of the Child's Tie to His Mother," *International Journal of Psychoanalysis*, 39, 350–373, 1958.

Bonica, J.J.: *Principles and Practices of Obstetric Analgesia and Anesthesia*, Philadelphia: F.A. Davis, 1967.

Bower, T.G.R.: "The Visual World of Infants," *Scientific American*, 215, 80–97, 1966.

Bower, T.G.R.: *Development in Infancy*, San Francisco: W.H. Freeman, 1974.

Bower, T.G.R.: *The Perceptual World of the Child*, Cambridge, Mass.: Harvard University Press, 1977.

Bower, T.G.R., et al.: "Demonstration of Intention in the Reaching Behavior of Neonate Humans," *Nature*, 228–234, 1970.

Brackbill, Y.: *Continuous Stimulation and Arousal Level in Infants: Additive Effects*, Proceedings, 78th Annual Convention, American Psychological Association, 5, 271–272, 1970.

Brackbill, Y.: "Obstetrical Medication and Infant Behavior," in J.D. Osofsky (ed.), *The Handbook of Infant Development*, New York: Wiley, 1979.

Brain, D.J., and I. Moslay: "Controlled Study of Mothers and Children in Hospital," *British Medical Journal*, 278–280, 1968.

Brazelton, T.B.: *Neonatal Behavior Assessment Scale*, Clinics in Developmental Medicine, No. 50, Philadelphia: Lippincott, 1973.

Brazelton, T.B., et al.: "Specific Neonatal Measures: The Brazelton Neonatal Behavior Assessment Scale," in J.D. Osofsky (ed.), *The Handbook of Infant Development*, New York: Wiley, 1979.

Broadhead, G.D.: "Motor Performance Assessment in a Special Education Context," Paper presented in the Motor Development Academy at the AAHPERD Convention, Boston, Mass. April 13, 1981.

Broer, M.: *Efficiency in Human Movement*, Philadelphia: W.B. Saunders, 1973.

Broer, M.R., and R.F. Zernicke: *Efficiency of Human Movement*, Philadelphia: W.B. Saunders, 1979.

Brookover, W.B., et al.: *Self Concept of Ability and School Achievement*, U.S. Office of Education, Cooperative Research Project, No. 2831, East Lansing: Michigan State University, 1967.

Brown, C.H., et al.: "The Effects of Cross Country Running on Pre-Adolescent Girls," *Medicine and Science in Sports*, 4, 1–5, 1972.

Brown, N.A., et al.: "Ethanol Embryotoxicity: Direct Effects on Mammalian Embryos in Vitro," *Science*, 206, 573–575, 1979.

Bruch, H.: "Energy Expenditure of Obese Children," *American Journal of Diseases of Children*, 60, 5, 1940.

Bruch, H.: *The Golden Cage—The Enigma of Anorexia Nervosa*, New York: Vintage Books, 1979.

Bruner, J.S., "The Act of Discovery," *Harvard Educational Review*, 31, 1, 1961.

Bruner, J.S.: *The Process of Education*, Cambridge, Mass.: Harvard University Press, 1965.

Bruner, J.S.: "Processes of Growth in Infancy," in A. Ambrose (ed.), *Stimulation in Early Infancy*, New York: Academic Press, 1969.

Bruininks, R.H.: *Bruininks-Oseretsky Test of Motor Proficiency*, Circle Pines, Minn.: American Guidance Service, 1978.

Bruininks, R.H.: "Assessing the Motor Performance of Children: An Overview of the Bruininks-Oseretsky Test of Motor Proficiency," Paper presented in the Motor Development Academy at the AAHPERD Convention, Boston, Mass., April 13, 1981.

Burnett, C.N., and E.W. Johnson: "Development of Gait in Childhood, Part II,"

*Developmental Medicine and Child Neurology,* 13, 207–212, 1971.

Buros, O.K. (ed.): *The Seventh Mental Measurement Yearbook,* Highland Park, N.J.: Gryphon Press, 1971.

Butler, R.N., et al.: "Cigarette Smoking in Pregnancy: Its Influence on Birthweight and Prenatal Mortality," *British Medical Journal,* 2, 127–130, 1972.

CAHPER—Canadian Association for Health, Physical Education and Recreation: *Manitoba Physical Fitness Performance Test Manual and Fitness Objectives,* Ottawa, Canada: CAHPER, 1980.

Caputo, A.J., et al.: "Primitive Reflex Profile: A Pilot Study," *Physical Therapy,* 58, 1061–1065, 1978.

Caputo, D.V., and W. Mandell: "Consequences of Low Birth Weight," *Developmental Psychology,* 3, 363–383, 1970.

Carmichael, L.: "Heredity and Environment: Are They Antithetical?" *Journal of Abnormal and Social Psychology,* 20, 245–260, 1925.

Carpenter, G.: "Mother's Face and the Newborn," in R. Lewin (ed.), *Child Alive,* New York: Doubleday, 1975.

Chess, S., and A. Thomas: "Temperament in the Normal Neonate," in J.C. Westman (ed.), *Individual Differences in the Child,* New York: Wiley, 1973.

Clarke, D.: "Predicting Certified Weight of Young Wrestlers," *Medicine and Science in Sports,* 6, 52–57, 1974.

Clarke, H.H.: *Physical Motor Tests in the Medford Boys Growth Study,* Englewood Cliffs, N.J.: Prentice-Hall, 1971.

Clarke, H.H.: "Joint and Body Range of Movement," *Physical Fitness Research Digest,* 5, 16, 1975.

Clifford, E., and M. Clifford: "Self Concepts Before and After Survival Training" *British Journal of Social and Clinical Psychology,* 6, 241–248, 1967.

Collingswood, T.B., and L. Willett: "The Effects of Physical Training upon Self-Concept and Body Attitude," *Journal of Consulting Psychology,* 2, 411–412, 1971.

Comalli, P.E., et al.: "Perception of Verticality in Middle and Old Age," *Journal of Psychology,* 47, 259–266, 1959.

Combs, A. W., and D. Snygg: *Individual Behavior,* New York: Harper & Row, 1959.

Congressional Report: "Alcohol Labeling and Fetal Alcohol Syndrome," *Hearing Before the Subcommittee on Alcohol and Drug Abuse,* 95–102, 1978.

Conway, E., and Y. Brackbill: "Delivery Medication and Infant Outcomes," *Monographs of the Society for Research in Child Development,* 35, 24–34, 1970.

Cooper, J.M., and W. Andrews: "Rhythm as a Linguistic Art," *Quest,* 65, 61–67, 1975.

Cooper, J.M., et al: *Kinesiology,* St. Louis: Mosby, 1982.

Coopersmith, S.: *The Antecedents of Self-Esteem,* San Francisco: W.H. Freeman, 1967.

Corbin, C.B. (ed.): *A Textbook of Motor Development,* Dubuque, Iowa: W.C. Brown, 1980.

Cratty, B.J.: *Social Dimensions of Physical Activity,* Englewood Cliffs, N.J.: Prentice-Hall, 1967.

Cratty, B.J.: *Psychology and Physical Activity,* Englewood Cliffs, N.J.: Prentice-Hall, 1968.

Cratty, B.J.: *Physical Expressions of Intelligence,* Englewood Cliffs, N.J.: Prentice-Hall, 1972.

Cratty, B.J.: *Perceptual and Motor Development in Infants and Children,* Englewood, Cliffs, N.J.: Prentice-Hall, 1979.

Cratty, B.J., and M. Martin: *Perceptual-Motor Efficiency in Children,* Philadelphia: Lea and Febiger, 1969.

Cruikshank, R.M.: "The Development of Visual Size Consistency in Early Infancy," *Journal of Genetic Psychology,* 58, 327−351, 1941.

Cumming, G.R., et al.: "Repeated Measurements of Aerobic Capacity During a Week of Intensive Training at a Youth's Track Camp," *Canadian Journal of Physiology and Pharmacology,* 45, 805−811, 1967.

Cumming, G.R., et al.: "Failure of School Physical Education to Improve Cardiorespiratory Fitness," *Canadian Medical Association Journal,* 101, 69−73, 1969.

Cumming, G.R., and W. Friesen: "Bicycle Ergometer Measurement of Maximal Oxygen Uptake in Children," *Canadian Journal of Physiology and Pharmacology,* 45, 937−946, 1967.

Cumming, G.R., and A. Hnatiuk: "Establishing of Normal Values for Exercise Capacity in a Hospital Clinic," in K. Berg and B. Erickson (eds.), *Children and Exercise IX,* Baltimore: Academic Press, 1980.

Cunningham, D.A., et al.: "The Cardiopulmonary Capacities of Young Hockey Players—Age 10," *Medicine and Science in Sports,* 8, 23−25, 1976.

Cunningham, D.A., et al.: "Reliability and Reproducibility of Maximal Oxygen Uptake Measures in Children," *Medicine and Science in Sports,* 9, 104−105, 1977.

Curry, N.L.: "Self Concept and the Educational Experience in Physical Education," *The Physical Educator,* 31, 116−119, 1974.

Daniels, J., and N. Oldridge: "Changes in Oxygen Consumption of Young Boys During Growth and Training," *Medicine and Science in Sports,* 3, 161−165, 1971.

Davids, A., et al.: "Anxiety, Pregnancy and Childbirth Abnormalities," *Journal of Consulting Psychology,* 25, 74−77, 1961.

Davidson, H.P.: "A Study of Reversals in Children," *Journal of Genetic Psychology,* 44, 452−465, 1934.

Davies, P., and A.L. Stewart: "Low Birth-Weight Infants: Neurological Sequelae and Later Intelligence," *British Medical Bulletin,* 31, 85−91, 1975.

Daw, S.F.: "Age of Boy's Puberty in Leipzig, 1727−49, as Indicated by Voice Breaking in J.S. Bach's Choir Members," *Human Biology,* 46, 381−384, 1974.

Deach, D.F.: "Genetic Development of Motor Skills in Children Two Through Six Years of Age," Unpublished doctoral dissertation, University of Michigan, 1951.

Dean, R.F.: "Effects of Malnutrition, Especially of Slight Degree, on the Growth of Young Children," *Courrier* 15, 78−83, 1965.

De Oreo, K.L.: "Dynamic and Static Balance in Preschool Children," Unpublished doctoral dissertation, University of Illinois, 1971.

De Oreo, K.L: "De Oreo Fundamental Motor Skills Inventory," Unpublished paper, Kent State University, 1977.

De Oreo, K.L: "Performance of Fundamental Motor Tasks," in C.B. Corbin (ed.), *A Textbook of Motor Development,* Dubuque, Iowa: W.C. Brown, 1980.

Delacato, C.: *Neurological Organization and Reading,* Springfield, Ill.: Charles C Thomas, 1966.

Delacato, C.: *Treatment and Prevention of Reading Problems,* Springfield, Ill.: Charles C Thomas, 1959.

DeMyer, W.: "Congenital Anomalies of the Central Nervous System," in D.B. Tower (ed.), *The Nervous System,* New York: Raven, 1975.

Dennis, W.: "The Effect of Restricted Practice upon the Reaching, Sitting, and Standing of Two Infants," *Journal of Genetic Psychology*, 47, 17−32, 1935.

Dennis, W.: "Does Culture Appreciably Affect Patterns of Infant Behavior?" *Journal of Social Psychology*, 12, 307−317, 1940.

Dennis, W.: "Causes of Retardation Among Institutional Children: Iran," *Journal of Genetic Psychology*, 96, 47−59, 1960.

Dennis, W., and P. Najarian: "Infant Development Under Environmental Handicap," *Psychology Monographs*, 71, 7, 1957.

DiNucci, J.M.: "Gross Motor Performance: A Comprehensive Analysis of Age and Sex Differences Between Boys and Girls Ages Six to Nine Years," in J. Broekhoff (ed.), *Physical Education, Sports and the Sciences*, Eugene, re.: Microform Publications, 1976.

Documenta, G.: "Scientific Tables," in K. Dierm, and C. Lentner (eds.), *Scientific Tables*, Barle, Switzerland: Ciba-Geigy Ltd, 1970.

Doll, E.A.: *The Oseretsky Tests of Motor Proficiency*, Circle Pines, Minn.: American Guidance Service, 1946.

Drillien, C.M.: "The Small-for-Dates Infant—Etiology and Prognosis," *Pediatric Clinics of North America*, 17, 9−23, 1970.

Dunsing, J.D.: "Perceptual-Motor Factors in the Development of School Measures: An Analysis of the Purdue Perceptual-Motor Survey," *American Journal of Optometry*, 46, 760−765, 1969.

Easton, T.A.: "On the Normal Use of Reflexes," *American Scientist*, 60, 591−599, 1972.

Eckert, H., "Age Changes in Motor Skills, in G.L. Rarick (ed.), *Physical Activity: Human Growth and Development*, New York: Academic Press, 1973.

Eckert, H.M., and G.L. Rarick: "Stabliometer Performance of Educable Mentally Retarded and Normal Children," *Research Quarterly*, 47, 619−621, 1975.

Egan, D.F., et al.: *Developmental Screening 0−5 Years*, London: Spastic International Medical Publications, 1969.

Eichenwald, H.P., and P.C. Frye: "Nutrition and Learning," *Science*, 163, 644−648, 1969.

Eichorn, D.H.: "Biology of Gestation and Infancy," *Merrill-Palmer Quarterly*, 14, 47−81, 1968.

Eichorn, D.H.: "Physical Development: Current Foci of Research," in J. Osofsky (ed.), *The Handbook of Infant Development*, New York: Wiley, 1979.

Eisenberg, R.B., et al.: "Habituation to an Acoustic Pattern as an Idea of Differences Among Neonates," *Journal of Auditory Research*, 6, 239−248, 1966.

Ekbolm, B.: "Effect of Physical Training on Adolescent Boys," *Journal of Applied Physiology*, 27, 350−355, 1969.

Ellis, M.J.: *Why People Play*, Englewood Cliffs, N.J.: Prentice-Hall, 1973.

Engen, T., et al.: "Olfactory Responses and Adaptation in the Human Neonate," *Journal of Comparative Physiological Psychology*, 56, 73−77, 1963.

Enos, W.F., et al.: "Pathogenesis of Coronary Disease of American Soldiers Killed in Korea," *Journal of the American Medical Association*, 158, 912−914, 1955.

Erhartic, M.: "Stability of Global Self-Concepts of Children from Three Different Elementary Schools During Their First Year in a Regionalized Junior High School," Unpublished doctoral dissertation, Boston University, 1977.

Erikson, E.: *Childhood and Society*, New York: Norton, 1963.

Eriksson, B.O., and K. Gunter: "Effect of Physical Training on Hemodynamic Response During Submaximal and Maximal Exercise in 11–13 Year Old Boys," *Acta Physiologica Scandinavica*, 87, 27–39, 1973.

Espenschade, A.S., and H.M. Eckert: *Motor Development*, Columbus, Ohio: Merrill, 1980.

Eveleth, P.B., and J.M. Tanner: *Worldwide Variation in Human Growth*, Cambridge, Mass.: Cambridge University Press, 1976.

Falls, H.B.: "Modern Concepts of Physical Fitness," *Journal of Health, Physical Education and Recreation*, 51, 25, 1980.

Fantz, R.L.: "Pattern Vision in Newborn Infants," *Science*, 140, 296–297, 1963.

Felker, D.W.: *Building Positive Self-Concepts*, Minneapolis, Minn.: Burgess, 1974.

Field, J.: "The Adjustment of Reaching Behavior to Object Distance in Early Infancy," *Child Development*, 47, 304–308, 1976.

Fiorentino, M.R.: *Reflex Testing Methods for Evaluating C.N.S. Development*, Springfield, Ill.: Charles C Thomas, 1963.

Fisch, R.O., et al.: Obesity and Leanness at Birth and Their Relation to Body Habitus in Later Childhood, *Pediatrics*, 56, 421–428, 1975.

Fitts, P.M., and M.I. Posner: *Human Performance*, Belmont, California: Brooks/Cole, 1967.

Fleishman, E.A., "Toward a Taxonomy of Human Performance," *American Psychologist*, 30, 1127–1149, 1975.

Ford, E.H.T.: *Human Chromosomes*, New York: Academic Press, 1973.

Frank, L.K.: "Play Is Valid," *Childhood Education*, 3, 433–440, 1968.

Frankenburg, W.K., and J.B. Dodds, "The Denver Developmental Screening Test," *Journal of Pediatrics*, 71, 181–191, 1967.

Frederick, S.D.: "Performance of Selected Motor Tasks By Three, Four and Five Year Old Children," Unpublished doctoral dissertation, Indiana University, 1977.

Freud, A.: *Normality and Pathology in Childhood: Assessment of Development*, New York: International Universities Press, 1965.

Freud, S.: *The Ego and the Id*, New York: Norton, 1962.

Frost, R.B.: "Physical Education and Self-Concept," *Journal of Physical Education*, 36, 1972.

Frostig, M.: *Move Grow and Learn*, Chicago: Follett, 1969.

Gad-Elmawla, E.K.G.: "Kinematic and Kinetic Analysis of Gain in Children at Different Age Levels in Comparison With Adults," Unpublished doctoral dissertation, Indiana University, 1980.

Galambos, J.W.: *Organizing Free Play*, Office of Child Development, Department of HEW, 1970.

Gallahue, D.L.: "The Relationship Between Perceptual and Motor Abilities," *Research Quarterly*, 39, 948–952, 1968.

Gallahue, D.L.: "Effect of Movement and Vision on Visual-Motor Adjustment to Optical Rearrangement," *Perceptual Motor Skills*, in press, 1982.

Gallahue, D.L.: *Yes I Can! Movement and the Developing Self* (film strip), Bloomington, Ind.: Phi Delta Kappa, 1974.

Gallahue, D.L.: *Developmental Movement Experiences for Children*, New York: Wiley, 1982.

Gallahue, D.L.: "Movement Education, Its Place in the Elementary School Physical Education Program," in *Proceedings of the Contemporary Elementary School Physical*

*Education Conference,* Georgia State University, Atlanta, Ga., 1979.

Gangirly, P.: "The Problem of Human Adaptation: An Overview," *Man in India,* 57, 1–22, 1977.

Gentile, A.: "A Working Model of Skill Acquisition with Application to Teaching," *Quest,* 17, 3–23, 1972.

Gentile, A.M.: "Developmental Aspects of Motor Learning," Paper presented at the Motor Development Academy at the AAHPER Convention, Boston, Mass., April 17, 1981.

Gerber, M., and R.F.A. Dean: "Gesell Tests of African Children," *Pediatrics* 20, 1055–1065, 1957.

Gesell, A.: *Infancy and Human Growth,* New York: Macmillan, 1928.

Gesell, A.: *The Embryology of Behavior,* New York: Harper, 1945.

Gesell, A., et al.: *The First Five Years of Life: A Study of the Preschool Child,* New York: Harper, 1949.

Gesell, A., and H. Thompson: "Learning and Growth in Identical Twins," *Genetic Psychology Monographs,* 6, 1–124, 1929.

Gesell, A., and H. Thompson: *Infant Behavior, Its Genesis and Growth,* New York: McGraw-Hill, 1934.

Getman, G.N.: *How to Develop Your Child's Intelligence* (a research publication), Lucerne, Minn.: G.N. Getman, 1952.

Gibson, E.J., and R.D. Walk: "The Visual Cliff," *Scientific American,* 4, 67–71, 1960.

Gilliam, T.B.: "What Volunteer Coaches and Youth Sport Administrators Should Know About Training, Conditioning, and Injury Prevention," Paper presented at the Second Annual Youth Sports Forum, Youth Sports Institute, Michigan State University, April 27, 1981.

Gilliam, T.B., et al.: "Physical Activity Patterns Determined by Heart Rate Monitoring in 6–7-Year-Old Children," *Medicine and Science in Sports and Exercise,* 131, 65–67, 1981.

Gilliom, B.C.: *Basic Movement Education for Children: Rationale and Teaching Units,* Reading, Mass.: Addison-Wesley, 1970.

Glassow, R.L., and P. Kruse: "Motor Performance of Girls Age 6–14 Years," *Research Quarterly,* 31, 426–431, 1960.

Goetzinger, C.P.: "Re-evaluation of Heath Rail Walking 1951 to 1967," *Journal of Educational Research,* 54, 187–191, 1961.

Goldstein, K.M., et al.: "The Effects of Prenatal and Perinatal Complications on Development at One Year of Age," *Child Development,* 47, 613–621, 1976.

Gordon, R.L.: "A Neurological Paradigm: An Analysis of Swimming and Walking Acquisition," Unpublished paper, School of HPER, The Ohio State University, 1981.

Graham, G., et al.: *Children Moving,* Palo Alto, Calif.: Mayfield, 1980.

Grieve, D.W., and R.J. Gaer: "The Relationship Between the Length of Stride, Step, Frequency, Time of Swing and Speed of Walking for Children and Adults," *Ergonomics,* 9, 379–399, 1966.

Gustafson, J.: "Teaching for Self-Esteem," *The Physical Educator,* 35, 67–70, 1978.

Guttridge, M.: "A Study of Motor Achievements of Young Children," *Archives of Psychology,* 244, 1–178, 1939.

Haase, R.: *Designing the Child Development Center,* U.S. Office of Education, Project Head Start, Washington, D.C.: U.S. Government Printing Office, 1968.

Hagberg, B.M.: Pre-, Peri-, and Postnatal Prevention of Major Neuropediatric Handicaps, *Neuropaediatrics,* 6, 331–338, 1975.

Hagstrom, J., and J. Morrill: *Games Babies Play,* New York: A&W Visual Library, 1979.

Haith, M.M.: "The Response of the Human Newborn to Visual Movement," *Journal of Experimental Child Psychology,* 3, 235–243, 1966.

Halverson, H.M.: "Studies of the Grasping Responses in Early Infancy," *Journal of Genetic Psychology,* 51, 437–449, 1937.

Halverson, H.M., et al.: "An Environmental Study of Prehension in Infants by Means of Systematic Cinema Records," *Genetic Psychology Monographs,* 10, 107–186, 1931.

Halverson, L.: "The Motor Development Academy," *Journal of Physical Education and Recreation,* 51, 38, 1980.

Halverson, L.E., and M.A. Roberton: "A Study of Motor Pattern Development in Young Children," Paper presented at the AAHPER Conference, Chicago, 1966.

Halverson, L.E., and M.A. Roberton: *Motor Development Laboratory Manual,* Madison, Wisc.: American Printing and Publishing, 1979.

Harbison, R.D., and B. Mantilla-Plata: "Prenatal Toxicity, Maternal Distribution and Placental Transfer of Telralydrocan-Malinol," *Journal of Pharmacology Experimental Therapeutics,* 180, 446–453, 1972.

Harrow, A.J.: *A Taxonomy of the Psychomotor Domain,* New York: David McKay, 1971.

Hasselmeyer, E.G.: "The Premature Neonates' Response to Handling," *American Nurses Association,* 11, 15–24, 1964.

Haubenstricker, J.: "A Critical Review of Selected Perceptual-Motor Tests and Scales Currently Used in the Assessment of Motor Behavior," in D.M. Landers and R.W. Christina (eds.), *Psychology in Motor Behavior and Sport—1977,* Champaign, Ill.: Human Kinetics, 1978.

Haubenstricker, J.: Inter-Rater Reliability of the Developmental Sequences of Fundamental Motor Skills, personal communication, October 1980.

Haubenstricker, J., et al.: "The Efficiency of the Briuninks-Oseretsky Test of Motor Proficiency in Discriminating Between Normal Children and Those with Gross Motor Dysfunction," Paper presented at the Motor Development Academy at the AAHPERD Convention, Boston, Mass., April 13, 1981.

Havighurst, R.: *Developmental Tasks and Education.* New York: Longmans, Green, 1952.

Havighurst, R.: *Human Development and Education,* New York: David McKay, 1953.

Havighurst, R.: *Developmental Tasks and Education,* New York: David McKay, 1972.

Havighurst, R., and R. Levine: *Society and Education,* Reading, Mass.: Allyn and Bacon, 1979.

Heath, S.R.: "The Railwalking Test: Preliminary Motivational Norm for Boys and Girls," *Motor Skills Research Exchange,* 1, 34, 1949.

Hebb, D.O.: *The Organization of Behavior,* New York: Wiley, 1949.

Heidelise, A., et al.: "Specific Neonatal Measures: The Brazelton Neonatal Behavior Assessment Scale," in J.D. Osofsky (ed.), *The Handbook of Infant Development,* New York: Wiley, 1979.

Held, R.: "Plasticity of Sensory-Motor Systems," *Scientific American,* 213, 84–94, 1965.

Held, R., and J. Blossom: "Neonatal Deprivation and Adult Rearrangement: Complementary Techniques for Analyzing Plastic Sensory-Motor Coordinations," *Journal of Comparative Physiological Psychology,* 54, 33−37, 1961.

Held, R., and A. Hein: "Movement-Produced Stimulation in the Development of Visually Guided Behavior," *Journal of Comparative Physiological Psychology,* 56, 872−876, 1963.

Held, R., and H. Mikaelian: "Motor Sensory Feedback Versus Need in Adaptation to Rearrangement," *Perceptual Motor Skills,* 18, 685−688, 1964.

Hellebrandt, F., et al.: "Physiological Analysis of Basic Motor Skills," *American Journal of Physical Medicine,* 40, 14−25, 1961.

Henry, F.M.: "Influence of Motor and Sensory Sets: Reaction Latency, and Speed of Discrete Movement," *Research Quarterly,* 31, 459−468, 1960.

Henry, F.M., and D. Rogers: "Increased Response Latency for Complicated Movements and a Memory Drum Theory of Neuromotor Reaction," *Research Quarterly,* 31, 448−468, 1960.

Hepner, R.: "Maternal Malnutrition and the Fetus, *Journal of the American Medical Association,* 169, 1774−1777, 1958.

Herkowitz, J.: "Instruments Which Assess the Efficiency/Maturity of Children's Motor Pattern Performance," in D.L. Landers and R.W. Christina (eds.), *Psychology in Motor Behavior and Sport—1977,* Champaign, Ill.: Human Kinetics, 1978.

Hershenson, M.: "Visual Discrimination in the Human Newborn," *Journal of Comparative Physiological Psychology,* 158, 270−276, 1964.

Hess, E.H.: "Imprinting," *Science,* 130, 133−141, 1959.

Hilgard, J.R.: "Learning and Maturation in Preschool Children," *Journal of Genetic Psychology,* 41, 36−56, 1932.

Hockey, R.V.: *Physical Fitness,* St. Louis: Mosby, 1973.

Hockey, R.V.: *Physical Fitness,* St. Louis: Mosby, 1981.

Hoepner, B.J.: "Comparison of Motor Ability, New Motor Skill Learning and Adjustment to a Rearranged Visual Field," *Research Quarterly,* 38, 605−614, 1967.

Holle, B.: *Motor Development in Children: Normal and Retarded,* St. Louis: Blackwell Scientific Publications, 1977.

Holt, J.: *What Do I Do Monday?* New York: Dutton, 1970.

Hooker, D.: *The Prenatal Origin of Behavior,* Lawrence, University of Kansas Press, 1952.

Horwitz, F.D.: "Infant Learning and Development: Retrospect and Prospect," *Merrill-Palmer Quarterly,* 14, 101−120, 1968.

Horowitz, F.D., and T.B. Brazelton: "Research with the Brazelton Neonatal Scale," in T. Brazelton (ed.), *Neonatal Behavioral Assessment Scale,* Philadelphia, Lippincott, 1973.

Houston, K.B.: "Review of the Evidence and Qualifications Regarding the Effects of Hallucinogenic Drugs on Chromosomes and Embryos," *American Journal of Psychiatry,* 126, 251−254, 1969.

Humphrey, J.: *Child Learning,* Dubuque, Iowa: W.C. Brown, 1974.

Hunsicker, P., and G. Reiff: "Youth Fitness Report, 1958−1965−1975," *Journal of Physical Education and Recreation,* 48, 32, 1977.

Hupperich, F.L., and P. Sigerseth: "The Specificity of Flexibility in Girls," *Research Quarterly,* 21, 25−33, 1950.

Jeffrey, W.E.: "Discrimination of Oblique Lines by Children," *Journal of Comparative Physiological Psychology,* 62, 154−156, 1966.

Johnson, L.: "Effects of 5-Day-a-Week Vs. 2- and 3-Day-a-Week Physical Education Classes on Fitness, Skill, Adipose Tissue, and Growth," *Research Quarterly*, 40, 93, 1969.

Johnson, M.L., et al.: "Relative Importance of Inactivity and Overeating in the Energy Balance of Obese High School Girls," *American Journal of Clinical Nutrition*, 4, 37, 1956.

Johnson, R.: "Measurement of Achievement in Fundamental Skills of Elementary School Children," *Research Quarterly*, 33, 94–103, 1962.

Johnson, W.R., et al.: "Changes in Self Concept During a Physical Education Program," *Research Quarterly*, 39, 560–565, 1968.

Jones, H.E., *Motor Performance and Growth*, Berkeley: University of California Press, 1949.

Jones, O.H.: "Caesarean Section in Present-Day Obstetrics," *American Journal of Obstetrics and Gynecology*, 126, 521–530, 1976.

Joslin, E.P., et al.: *Treatment of Diabetes Mellitus*, Philadelphia: Lea and Febiger, 1952.

Kallen, D.J. (ed.): "Nutrition, Development and Social Behavior," HEW Publication No. (NIH) 73–242, Washington, D.C.: U.S. Government Printing Office, 1973.

Karpovitch, P.V.: "Textbook Fallacies Regarding the Development of the Child's Heart," *Research Quarterly*, 8, 33–37, 1937.

Kaufman, D.A.: "Fundamentals of Fat," *The Physical Educator*, 32, 77–79, 1975.

Kemper, H.C.G., et al.: "Investigation into the Effects of Two Extra Physical Education Lessons per Week During One School Year upon Physical Development of 12- and 13-Year-Old Boys," in J. Borms and M. Hebbelinck (eds.), *Medicine and Sport Science Series, Vol. II, Pediatric Work Physiology*, Basel, Belgium: S. Karger, 1978.

Kennell, J.H., et al.: "Maternal Behavior One Year After Early and Extended Post-Partum Contact," *Developmental Medicine and Child Neurology*, 16, 172–179, 1974.

Kennell, J.H., et al.: "Parent-Infant Bonding," in J.D. Osofsky (ed.), *The Handbook of Infant Development*, New York: Wiley, 1979.

Keogh, J.F.: *Motor Performance of Elementary School Children* (Monograph), Los Angeles: University of California, Physical Education Department, 1965.

Kephart, N.C.: *The Slow Learner in the Classroom*, Columbus, Ohio: Merrill, 1971.

Kessen, W., et al.: "Human Infancy: A Bibliography and Guide," in P.H. Mussen (ed.), *Manual of Child Psychology*, New York: Wiley, 1970.

Klopper, P., et al.: "Maternal Imprinting in Goats," *Proceedings of the National Academy of Science*, 52, 911, 1964.

Knuttgen, H.G.: "Aerobic Capacity of Adolescents," *Journal of Applied Physiology*, 22, 655–658, 1967.

Kopp, C.B., and A.H. Parmelee: "Prenatal and Perinatal Influence on Infant Behavior," in J.D. Osofsky (ed.), *The Handbook of Infant Development*, New York: Wiley, 1979.

Kraft, R.E.: "Can the Movement Specialist Really Influence Self-Concept?" *The Physical Educator*, 35, 20–21, 1978.

Krahenbuhl, G.G., et al.: "Field Estimate of VO2 Max in Children Eight Years of Age," *Medicine and Science in Sports*, 9, 37–40, 1977.

Krathwohl, D.R., et al.: *Taxonomy of Educational Objectives, Handbook II: Affective Domain*, New York: David McKay, 1964.

Kraus, H., and R.P. Hirschland: "Minimum Muscular Fitness Tests In Children," *Research Quarterly*, 25, 178, 1954.

Krogman, W.M.: *Child Growth,* Ann Arbor: University of Michigan Press, 1972.

Laban, R., and F. Lawrence: *Effort,* London: Unwin Brothers, 1947.

Lamaze, F.: *Painless Childbirth: The Lamaze Method,* Chicago: Regency, 1970.

Landreth, C.: *The Psychology of Early Childhood,* New York: Knopf, 1958.

Langer, J.: Werners' Comparative Organismic Theory,'' in P.H. Mussen (ed.), *Manual of Child Psychology,* New York: Wiley, 1970.

Larson, R.L.: ''Physical Activity and the Growth and Development of Bone Structure,'' in G.L. Rarick (ed.), *Physical Activity: Human Growth and Development,* New York: Academic Press, 1973.

Lawther, J.D.: *The Learning and Performance of Physical Skills,* Englewood Cliffs, N.J.: Prentice-Hall, 1977.

Le Boyer, R.: *Birth Without Violence,* New York: Knopf, 1975.

Lecky, P.: *Self Consistency: A Theory of Personality,* New York: Island Press, 1945.

Leeper, S., et al.: *Good Schools for Young Children,* New York: Macmillan, 1974.

Leifer, A., et al.: ''Effects of Mother-Infant Separation on Maternal Attachment Behavior,'' *Child Development,* 43, 1203–1218, 1972.

Leighton, J.R.: ''Flexibility Characteristics of Males Ten to Eighteen Years of Age,'' *Archives of Physical Medicine and Rehabilitation,* 37, 494–499, 1956.

Lerner, P.M.: *Concepts and Theories of Human Development,* Reading, Mass.: Addison-Wesley, 1976.

Leuko, J.H., and S.L. Greendorfer: ''Family Influence and Sex Differences in Children's Socialization into Sport: A Review,'' in D.M. Landers and R.W. Christina (eds.), *Psychology of Motor Behavior and Sport—1977,* Champaign, Ill.: Human Kinetics, 1978.

Levanthal, A., and L.P. Lipsett: ''Adaptation, Pitch Discrimination and Sound Vocalization in the Neonate,'' *Child Development,* 35, 759–767, 1964.

Lewis, M.J., et al.: ''Pattern of Fixation in the Young Infant,'' *Child Development,* 37, 331–346, 1966.

Lipton, E.L., et al.: ''Autonomic Function in the Neonate,'' *Psychosomatic Medicine,* 23, 472–484, 1961.

Litch, S.: *Towards Prevention of Mental Retardation in the Next Generation,* Fort Wayne, Ind.: Fort Wayne Printing, 1978.

Lockhart, A., ''What's in a Name?'' *Quest,* 2, 9–13, 1964.

Logsdon, B.J., et al.: *Physical Education for Children: A Focus on the Teaching Process,* Philadelphia: Lea and Febiger, 1977.

Loovis, E.M., and W.F. Ersing: *Assessing and Programming Gross Motor Development For Children,* Lexington, Ky.: Wallace's, 1979.

Luedke, G.C.: ''Range of Motion as the Focus of Teaching the Overhand Throwing Pattern to Children,'' Unpublished doctoral dissertation, Indiana University, 1980.

Lugo, J.O., and G.L. Hershey: *Human Development, a Multi-Disciplinary Approach to the Psychology of Individual Growth,* New York: Macmillan, 1974.

Macek, M., and J. Vavra: ''Cardiopulmonary and Metabolic Changes During Exercise in Children,'' *Journal of Applied Physiology,* 30, 200–204, 1971.

Maier, H.W.: *Three Theories of Child Development,* New York: Harper, 1978.

Malina, R.M.: *Growth and Development: The First Twenty Years,* Minneapolis, Minn.: Burgess, 1975.

Malina, R.M.: "Secular Changes in Growth and Performance," in R.S. Hutton (ed.), *Exercise and Sport Science Reviews,* 6, 206–255, 1978.

Malina, R.M.: "Environmentally Related Correlates of Motor Development and Performance During Infancy and Childhood," in C. Corbin (ed.), *A Textbook of Motor Development,* Dubuque, Iowa: W.C. Brown, 1980.

Martin, T.P., and G.A. Stull: "Effects of Various Knee Angle and Foot Spacing Combinations on Performance in the Vertical Jump," *Research Quarterly,* 40, 324, 1969.

Martens, R., et al.: *Coaching Young Athletes,* Champaign, Illinois: Human Kinetics, 1981.

Martinek, T., and L.D. Zaichkowsky: *The Martinek-Zaichkowsky Self-Concept Scale for Children,* Jacksonville, Ill.: Psychologists and Educators, 1977.

Marx, J.L.: "Cytomegalovirus: A Major Cause of Birth Defects," *Science,* 190, 11984–1186, 1975.

Massicotte, L.R., and B.J. MacNab: "Cardiorespiratory Adaptations to Training at Specific Intensities in Children," *Medicine and Science in Sports,* 6, 242–246, 1974.

Mayer, J.: "Exercise and Weight Control," in *Exercise and Fitness,* Chicago: Athletic Institute, 1960.

Mayer, J.: *Overweight: Causes, Cost and Control,* Englewood Cliffs, N.J.: Prentice-Hall, 1968.

Maynard, R.: *Guiding Your Child to a More Creative Life,* New York: Doubleday, 1973.

McCandless, B.R.: *Children—Behavior and Development,* New York: Holt, Rinehart and Winston, 1967.

McCaskill, C.L., and B.L. Wellman: "A Study of Common Motor Achievements at the Preschool Ages," *Child Development,* 9, 141, 1938.

McClenaghan, B.A.: "Development of an Observational Instrument to Assess Selected Fundamental Movement Patterns of Low Motor Functioning Children," Unpublished doctoral dissertation, Indiana University, 1976.

McClenaghan, B.A., and D.L. Gallahue: *Fundamental Movement: A Developmental and Remedial Approach,* Philadelphia: W.B. Saunders, 1978. (a)

McClenaghan, B.A., and D.L. Gallahue: *Fundamental Movement: Observation and Assessment,* Philadelphia: W.B. Saunders, 1978.(b)

McGarrity, W.J., et al.: "Effect on Reproductive Cycle of Nutritional Status and Requirements," *Journal of the American Medical Association,* 168, 2138–2145, 1958.

McGraw, M.: *The Neuromuscular Maturation of the Human Infant,* New York: Hafner, 1934.

McGraw, M.: *Growth: A Study of Johnny and Jimmy,* New York: Appleton-Century, 1935.

McGraw, M.B.: "Later Development of Children Specially Trained During Infancy," *Child Development,* 10, 1, 1939.(a)

McGraw, M.B.: "Swimming Behavior of the Human Infant," *Journal of Pediatrics,* 15, 485–490, 1939.(b)

McGraw, M.B.: "Maturation of Behavior," in L. Carmichael (ed.), *Manual of Child Psychology,* New York: Wiley, 1954.

McNamera, J.J., et al.: "Coronary Artery Disease in Combat Casualties in Vietnam," *Journal of the American Medical Association,* 216, 1186–1187, 1971.

Mehlman, J.: "The Tonic Neck Reflex in Newborn Infants," *Journal of Pediatrics,* 16, 767–769, 1940.

Mercer, J.: *Labeling the Mentally Retarded,* Berkeley: University of California Press, 1973.

Meredith, H.V.: "North American Negro Infants: Size at Birth and Growth During the First Postnatal Year," *Human Biology,* 24, 290, 1952.

Meredith, H.V.: "Somatic Changes During Human Prenatal Life," *Child Development,* 46, 603−610, 1975.

Milinaire, C.: *Birth,* New York: Harmony, 1974.

Miller, S.: "The Facilitation of Fundamental Motor Skill Learning in Young Children," Unpublished doctoral dissertation, Michigan State University, 1978.

Mills, C.A.: "Climate Effects on Growth and Development, with Particular Reference to the Effects of Tropical Residence," *American Anthropology,* 41, 1−13, 1942.

Minuchin, D., et al.: *Psychosomatic Families—Anorexia Nervosa in Context,* Cambridge, Mass.: Harvard University Press, 1978.

Mitchell, J., and G. Blomquist: "Maximal Oxygen Uptake," *New England Journal of Medicine,* 284, 1018−1022, 1971.

Montague, M.F.A.: *Prenatal Influences,* Springfield, Ill.: Charles C Thomas, 1962.

Montoye, H.: *Introduction to Measurement in Physical Education,* Indianapolis, Ind.: Phi Epsilon Kappa Fraternity, 1970.

Moore, S., and S. Kilmer: *Contemporary Preschool Education,* New York: Wiley, 1973.

Mooston, M.: *Teaching Physical Education,* Columbus, Ohio: Merrill, 1981.

Morley, D., and M. Woodland: *See How They Grow-Monitoring Child Growth For Appropriate Health Care In Developing Countries,* New York: Oxford University Press, 1979.

Morison, R.: *A Movement Approach to Educational Gymnastics,* London: J.M. Dent and Sons, 1969.

Mrzena, B., and M. Macuek: "Uses of Treadmill and Working Capacity Assessment, in Preschool Children," in J. Borms and M. Hebbelinck (eds.), *Medicine and Sports Series, Vol. II, Pediatric Work Physiology,* Basel, Belgium: S. Karger, 1978.

Muller, P.F., et al.: "Prenatal Factors and Their Relationship to Mental Retardation and Other Parameters of Development," *American Journal of Obstetrics and Gynecology,* 109, 1205−1210, 1971.

Murray, J.L.: *Infaquatics: Teaching Kids To Swim,* West Point, N.Y.: Leisure Press, 1980.

Mussen, P., et al., *Child Development and Personality,* New York: Harper & Row, 1969.

Myers, C.B., et al.: "Vertical Jumping Movement Patterns of Early Childhood," Unpublished paper, Indiana University, Physical Education Department, 1977.

Naeye, R.L., et al.: "Urban Poverty: Effects of Prenatal Nutrition," *Science,* 166, 1026, 1969.

Nagel, C., and F. Moore: *Skill Development Through Games and Rhythmic Activities,* Palo Alto, Calif.: National Press, 1966.

National Center for Health Statistics: Washington, D.C.: U.S. Department of Health, Education and Welfare (ARA), 25, 76−1120, June 22, 1976.

National Foundation/March of Dimes: *Birth Defects, Tragedy and Hope, 1977.*

*Nora, J.J., and F.C. Fraser: Medical Genetics: Principles and Practices,* Philadelphia: Lea and Febiger, 1974.

Oscai, L.B.: "The Role of Exercise in Weight Control," in J.H. Wilmore (ed.), *Exercise and Sport Science Reviews, Vol. 1,* New York: Academic Press, 1973.

Oscai, L.B.: "Exercise and Weight Control," Symposium on Overweight and Obesity,

AAHPER Conference, Anaheim, Calif., March 30, 1974.

Oscai, L.B., et al.: "Effects of Exercise and of Food Restriction in Early Life on Adipose Tissue Cellularity," Abstract of the 21st Annual Meetings of the American College of Sports Medicine, Spring 1974.

Osofsky, J.D. (ed.): *The Handbook of Infant Development,* New York: Wiley, 1979.

Osofsky, J.D., and K. Conners: "Mother Infant Interaction: An Integrative View of a Complex System," in J.D. Osofsky (ed.), *The Handbook of Infant Development,* New York: Wiley, 1979.

Ounsted, M., and C. Ounsted: "On Fetal Growth Rate," *Clinics in Developmental Medicine,* London: William Heinemann Medical Books, 1973.

Owen, G.M., et al.: "A Study of the Nutritional Status of Preschool Children in the United States," USDHEW, 53 Part II, Supplement, 1974.

Parizkova, J.: *Body Fat and Physical Fitness,* The Hague, Netherlands: Martinus Nijkoff B.V.: Medical Division, 1977.

Parker, D.E.: "The Vestibular Apparatus," *Scientific American,* 243, 118−135, 1980.

Pasamanuck, B., and N. Knoblach: "Retrospective Studies on the Epidemiology of Reproductive Causality: Old and New," *Merrill-Palmer Quarterly,* 12, 7−26, 1966.

Payne, G.: "The Effects of Object Size, Experimental Design and Distance of Projection of Object Reception by Children in the First Grade," Unpublished doctoral dissertation, Indiana University, 1981.

Payne, G., et al.: *Head Start: A Tragicomedy with Epilogue,* New York: Behavioral Publications, 1973.

Pederson, E.J.: "A Study of Ball Catching Abilities of First-, Third-, and Fifth-Grade Children on Twelve Selected Ball Catching Tasks," Unpublished doctoral dissertation, Indiana University, 1973.

Peterson, K.L., et al.: "Factor Analyses of Motor Performance for Kindergarten, First and Second Grade Children: A Tentative Solution," Paper presented at the Annual Convention of the AAHPER, Anaheim, California, March 31, 1974.

Piaget, J.: *The Origins of Intelligence in Children,* New York: International Universities Press, 1952.

Piaget, J.: *The Construction of Reality and the Child,* New York: Basic Books, 1954.

Piaget, J.: *Play, Dreams and Imitation in Childhood,* London: William Heinemann Medical Books, 1957.

Piaget, J.: *The Psychology of the Child,* New York: Basic Books, 1969.

Piers, E.V.: *Manual for the Piers-Harris Children's Self-Concept Scale,* Nashville, Tenn.: Counselor Recordings and Tests, 1969.

Piers, M.W. (ed): *Play and Development,* New York: Norton, 1972.

Plummer, G.W.: "Anomalies Occurring in Children Exposed in Utero to Atomic Bomb in Hiroshima," *Pediatrics,* 10, 687−692, 1952.

Poe, A.: "Description of the Movement Characteristics of Two-Year-Old Children Performing the Jump and Reach," *Research Quarterly,* 47, 200, 1976.

Pratt, K.C.: "The Neonate," in L. Carmichael (ed.), *Manual of Child Psychology,* New York: Wiley, 1954.

Prechtl, H.F.R.: "Problem of Behavioral Studies in the New Born Infant," in D.S. Leckarman, et al. (eds.), *Advances in the Study of Behavior, Vol. 1,* New York: Academic Press, 1965.

Prechtl, H.F.R., and D.J. Beintema: *The Neurological Examination of the Full Term*

*Newborn Infant,* William London: Heinemann Medical Books, 1964.

*Profiles on Children, 1970. White House Conference on Children,* Washington, D.C., Superintendent of Documents, U.S. Government Printing Office, 1970.

Rarick, G.L.: *Physical Activity: Human Growth and Development,* New York: Academic Press, 1973.

Rarick, G.L.: "Motor Development, Its Growing Knowledge Base," *Journal of Physical Education and Recreation,* 51, 20, 1980.

Rarick, G.L., and A. Dobbins: "Basic Components in the Motor Performance of Children Six to Nine Years of Age," *Medicine and Science in Sports,* 17, 105–110, 1975.

Read, D.G.: "The Influence of Competitive–Non-Competitive Programs of Physical Education on Body Image and Self Concept," Unpublished doctoral dissertation, Boston University, 1968.

Reilly, M. (ed.): *Play as Exploratory Behavior,* Beverly Hills, Calif.: Sage, 1974.

Ridenour, M.V. (ed.): *Motor Development: Issues and Applications,* Princeton, N.J.: Princeton, 1978.

Riesen, A.H., and L. Aarons: "Visual Movement and Intensity Discrimination of Pattern Vision," *Journal of Comparative Physiological Psychology,* 52, 142–149, 1959.

Riggs, M.L.: *Jump to Joy,* Englewood Cliffs, N.J.: Prentice-Hall, 1980.

Roach, E.G., and N.C. Kephart: *The Purdue Perceptual Motor Survey,* Columbus, Ohio: Merrill, 1966.

Roberton, M.A.: "Stability of Stage Categorization Across Trials: Implications for the Stage Theory of Overarm Throw Development," *Journal of Human Movement Studies,* 3, 49–59, 1977.

Roberton, M.A.: "Longitudinal evidence For Developmental Stages in the Forceful Overarm Throw," *Journal of Human Movement Studies,* 4, 167–175, 1978. (a)

Roberton, M.A.: "Stability of Stage Categorization in Motor Development," in D.M. Landers and R.W. Christina (eds.), *Psychology in Motor Behavior and Sport—1977,* Champaign, Ill.: Human Kinetics, 1978.(b)

Roberton, M.A.: "Stages in Motor Development," in M. Ridenour (ed.), *Motor Development: Issues and Applications,* Princeton, N.J.: Princeton, 1978.(c)

Roberton, M.A.: "Movement Quality Not Quantity," *Motor Development Academy Newsletter,* 2, 2–3, 1981.

Roberton, M.A.: "Describing Stages Within and Across Motor Tasks," in J.A.S. Kelso and J. Clark (eds.), *The Development of Movement Control and Coordination,* New York: Wiley, 1982.

Roberts, J.A., and W.P. Morgan: "Effect of Type and Frequency of Participation in Physical Activity upon Physical Working Capacity," *American Corrective Therapy Journal,* 25, 99–104, 1971.

Robson, K.: "The Role of Eye-To-Eye Contact in Maternal-Infant Attachment," Journal of Child Psychology and Psychiatry and Allied Disciplines, 8, 13–25, 1967.

Rogers, D.R.: *Child Psychology,* Monterey, Calif.: Brooks/Cole, 1977.

Rossett, H.L., and L.W. Sander: "Effects of Maternal Drinking on Neonatal Morphology and State," in J. Osofsky (ed.), *The Handbook of Infant Development,* New York: Wiley, 1979.

Rothenberg, A.: "Understanding the Anorectic Student," *Today's Education,* 65, 48–49, 1976.

Rudel, R.G., and H.L. Teuber: "Discrimination of Direction of Line in Children," *Journal of Comparative Physiological Psychology*, 56, 892–899, 1963.

Sage, G.H.: *Introduction to Motor Behavior: A Neuropsychological Approach*, Reading, Mass.: Addison-Wesley, 1977.

Sapp, M.: "Developmental Sequence of Galloping," Unpublished materials, Michigan State University, 1980.

Saunders, J.B., et al.: "The Major Determinants in Normal and Pathological Gait," *Journal of Bone and Joint Surgery*, 35, 543–558, 1953.

Schaie, K.W., and P.B. Baltes: "On Sequential Strategies in Developmental Research: Description or Explanation," *Human Development*, 18, 384–390, 1975.

Schmidt, R.A.: "Schema Theory: Implications for Movement Education," *Motor Skills Theory into Practice*, 2, 36–48, 1977.

Scrimshaw, N.S.: "Malnutrition, Learning and Behavior," *American Journal of Clinical Nutrition*, 20, 493–502, 1967.

Seashore, H.G.: "The Development of a Beam Walking Test and Its Use in Measuring Development of Balance in Children," *Research Quarterly*, 18, 246–259, 1949.

Seefeldt, V.: "A Discussion of Walking and Running," unpublished research, Michigan State University, 1972.

Seefeldt, V.: "Critical Learning Periods and Programs of Intervention," Paper presented at the AAHPER Conference, Atlantic City, N.J., 1975.

Seefeldt, V.: "Physical Fitness Guidelines for Preschool Children," in *Proceedings of the National Conference on Physical Fitness and Sports for All*, Washington, D.C.: President's Council on Physical Fitness and Sports, 5–19, February, 1980.

Seefeldt, V., et al.: "Sequencing Motor Skills Within the Physical Education Curriculum," Paper presented at the AAHPER Conference, Houston, Texas, 1972.

Seefeldt, V., and D. Gould: *Physical and Psychological Effects of Athletic Competition on Children and Youth*, Washington, D.C.: ERIC Clearinghouse on Teacher Education, 1980.

Seefeldt, V., and J. Haubenstricker: "Developmental Sequences of Fundamental Motor Skills," Unpublished research, Michigan State University, 1972–1976.

Seefeldt, V., and J. Haubenstricker: "Developmental Sequence of Kicking: Second Revision," Paper presented at the Midwest AAHPERD Conference, Chicago, March 19, 1981.

Self, P.A., and Horwitz, F.D.: "The Behavioral Assessment of the Neonate: An Overview," in J.D. Osofsky, (ed.), *The Handbook of Infant Development*, New York: Wiley, 1979.

Sheldon, W.H., et al.: *The Varieties of Human Physique*, New York: Harper, 1940.

Sheldon, W.H., et al.: *Atlas of Man*, New York: Harper, 1954.

Shirley, M.: *The First Two Years: A Study of Twenty-Five Babies, I. Postural and Locomotor Development*, Minneapolis: University of Minnesota Press, 1931.

Sinclair, C.: *Movement of the Young Child*, Columbus, Ohio: Merrill, 1973.

Singer, R.N.: *Motor Learning and Human Performance*, New York: Macmillan, 1980.

Sloan, W.: *Manual for the Lincoln-Oseretsky Motor Development Scale*, Chicago: C.H. Stolting, 1954.

Smart, M.S., and R.C. Smart: *Preschool Children: Development and Relationships*, New York: Macmillan, 1973.(a)

Smart, M.S., and R.C. Smart: *School Age Children: Development and Relationships*, New York: Macmillan, 1973.(b)

Smith, D.W., and A.A. Wilson: *The Child with Down's Syndrome (Mongolism)*. Philadelphia: W.B. Saunders, 1973.

Smith, H.: "Implications for Movement Education Experiences Drawn from Perceptual Motor Research," *Journal of Health, Physical Education and Recreation*, 4, 30−33, 1970.

Smith, K.V., and W.M. Smith: *Perception and Motion: An Analysis of Space-Structured Behavior*, Philadelphia: W.B. Saunders, 1972.

Smith, O.W.: "Spatial Perceptions and Play Activities of Nursery School Children," *Perceptual Motor Skills*, 21, 160, 1965.

Smith, O.W., and P.C. Smith: "Developmental Studies of Spatial Judgements By Children and Adults," *Perceptual Motor Skills* (Monograph supplement), 22, 3−73, 1966.

Solkoff, N., et al.: "Effects of Handling on the Subsequent Developments of Premature Infants," *Developmental Psychology*, 1, 765−768, 1969.

Spears, W.C.: "Assessment of Visual Preference and Discrimination in the 4-Month Old Infant," *Journal of Comparative Physiological Psychology*, 57, 381−386, 1964.

Spitz, R.: "Hospitalism: An Inquiry into the Genesis of Psychiatric Conditions in Early Childhood," *Psychoanalytic Study of the Child*, 1, 53−74, 1945.

Stallones, R.A.: "The Rise and Fall of Ischemic Heart Disease," *Scientific American*, 243, 53−59, 1980.

Standley, K., et al.: "Local-Regional Anesthesia, During Childbirth and Newborn Behavior," *Science*, 18, 634−635, 1974.

Stanley, S.: *Physical Education: A Movement Orientation*, Toronto: McGraw-Hill, 1969.

Stein, E.A., et al.: "Coronary Risk Factors in the Young," *Annual Reviews of Medicine*, 52, 601−613, 1981.

Stewart, K.J., and B. Gutin: "Effects of Physical Training on Cardiorespiratory Fitness in Children," *Research Quarterly*, 47, 110−120, 1976.

Strauss, M.E., et al.: "Behavior of Nicotine Addicted Newborns," *Child Development*, 46, 887−893, 1975.

Sundberg, A.I., and C. Wirsén: *A Child Is Born*, New York: Delacorte, 1977.

Susser, M., et al.: "Birth Weight, Fetal Age and Perinatal Mortality," *American Journal of Epidemiology*, 96, 197−204, 1972.

Swartz, D., and M. Allen: "Residual Reflex Patterns as a Basis for Diagnosing Stroke Faults," in J.P. Clarys and L. Levillie (eds.), *Swimming II, Baltimore: University Park Press, 1975*.

Tanner, J.M.: *Fetus into Man*, Cambridge Mass.: Harvard University Press, 1978.

Tanner, P.: "Movement Education: A Total Program of Elementary School Physical Education, *Proceedings of the Contemporary Elementary School Physical Education Conference*, Georgia State University, Atlanta, Ga., 1979.

Taylor, B.J.: "Pathways To a Healthy Self-Concept," in T.D. Yarokey (ed.), *The Self Concept of the Young Child*, Salt Lake City, Utah: Brigham Young Press, 1980.

Thelen, E.: "Determinants of Amounts of Stereotyped Behavior in Normal Human Infants," *Ethology and Sociobiology*, 1, 141−150, 1980.

Thompson, H., and A. Gesell: "Learning and Growth in Identical Twins: An Experimental Study by the Method of Co-Twin Control," *Journal of Genetic Psychology Monographs*, 6, 1−24, 1929.

Thompson, J.D., and M.W. Thompson: *Genetics in Medicine*, Philadelphia: W.B. Saunders, 1973.

Tipton, C., and T.K. Tcheng: "Iowa Wrestling Study," *Journal of the American Medical Association*, 214, 1269–1274, 1970.

Travers, J.F.: *The Growing Child*, New York: Wiley, 1977.

Titchner, E.B.: *A Textbook of Psychology*, New York: Macmillan, 1909.

Tronick, E., and T.B. Brazelton: "Clinical Uses of the Brazelton Neonatal Behavioral Assessment," in B.Z. Friedlander and L. Rosenblum (eds.), *Exceptional Infant* (Vol. III), New York: Brunner/Mazel, 1975.

Tuddenham, R.S.: "Studies in Reputation III, Correlates of Popularity Among Elementary School Children," *The Journal of Educational Psychology*, 42, May 1951.

Twitchell, T.E.: "Attitudinal Reflexes," *Physical Therapy*, 45, 411–418, 1965.

U.S. Bureau of the Census, *Statistical Abstract of the United States*, Washington, D.C.: U.S. Department of Commerce, 1980.

Van Slooten, P.H.: "Performance of Selected Motor-Coordination Tasks by Young Boys and Girls in Six Socio-Economic Groups," Unpublished doctoral dissertation, Indiana University, 1973.

von Bermuth, H.G.L., and H.R.R. Prechtl: "Reflexes and Their Relationship to Behavioral State in the Newborn," *Acta, Pediatric Scandanavia*, 57, 177–185, 1969.

Vrijens, J.: "The Influence of Interval Circuit Exercise on Physical Fitness in Adolescents," *Research Quarterly*, 40, 595–599, 1969.

Vrijens, J.: "Muscle Strength Development in the Pre- and Post-Pubescent Age," in J. Borms and M. Hebbelinck (eds.), *Medicine, Pediatric Work Psychology and Sports Series, Vol. II*, Basel, Belgium: S. Karger, 1978.

Wade, M.: "A Plea for Process Oriented Tests," *Motor Development Academy Newsletter*, 2, 1, 1–2, 1981.

Wallace, R.N., and J. Stuff: "A Perceptual Program for Classroom Teachers, Some Results," *Genetic Psychology Monographs*, 87, 253–288, 1983.

Wapner, S., and H. Werner: *Perceptual Development: An Investigation Within the Sensory Tonic Field Theory*, Worcester, Mass.: Clark University Press, 1957.

Ward, D., and P. Werner: "Analysis of Two Curricular Approaches in Physical Education," *Journal of Physical Education and Recreation*, 52, 60–63, 1981.

Warkany, J., et al.: "Intrauterine Growth Retardation," *American Journal of Diseases of Children*, 102, 462–476, 1961.

Warren, K., and H. Rosett: "Fetal Alcohol Syndrome," *Alcohol Health and Research World*, HEW, 2, 2–12, Summer 1978.

Watson, E.H., and G.H. Lowrey: *Growth and Development of Children*, Chicago: Year Book, 1967.

Watson, R.I., and H.C. Lindgreen: *Psychology of the Child and the Adolescent*, New York: Macmillan, 1979.

Wattenberg, W., and C. Clifford: *Relationship of Self Concept to Beginning Achievement in Reading*, U.S. Office of Education, No. 377, Detroit: Wayne State University, 1962.

Wellman, B.: "Motor Achievements of Preschool," *Childhood Education*, 13, 311–316, 1937.

Werner, E.E., and N. Bayley: "The Reliability of Bayley's Revised Scale of Mental and Motor Development During the First Year of Life," *Child Development*, 37, 39–50, 1966.

Wertheimer, M.: "Psychomotor Coordination of Auditory-Visual Space at Birth," *Science,*
    134, 1692, 1961.
Westman, J.C. (ed.): *Individual Differences in Children,* New York: Wiley, 1973.
White, B.: *The First Three Years of Life,* Englewood Cliffs, N.J.: Prentice-Hall, 1975.
White, B., and R. Held: "Plasticity of Sensorimotor Development in the Human Infant," in
    J.F. Rosenblith and W. Allinsmith (eds.), *The Causes of Behavior: Readings in Child
    Development and Educational Psychology,* Boston: Allyn and Bacon, 1966.
*White House Conference on Children and Youth,* Conference Proceedings, Washington,
    D.C.: Superintendent of Documents, U.S. Government Printing Office, 1970.
Whithurst, G.J., and R. Varta: *Child Behavior,* Boston: Houghton Mifflin, 1977.
Whiting, H.T.A.: *Acquiring Ball Skill,* London: G. Bell and Sons, 1969.
Whiting, H.T.A.: *Concepts In Skill Learning,* London: Lepus Books, 1975.
Wickstrom, R.: *Fundamental Motor Patterns,* Philadelphia: Lea and Febiger, 1977.
Wild, M.: "The Behavioral Pattern of Throwing and Some Observations Concerning Its
    Course of Development in Children," *Research Quarterly,* 3, 20, 1938.
Williams, H.: "A Study of Perceptual-Motor Characteristics of Children in Kindergarten
    Through Sixth Grade," Unpublished paper, University of Toledo, 1970.
Williams, H.: "Perceptual-Motor Development in Children," in C. Corbin (ed.), *A
    Textbook of Motor Development,* Dubuque, Iowa: W.C. Brown, 1980.
Wilmore, J.H.: "The Role of the Health and Physical Educator," Symposium on
    Overweight and Obesity, AAHPER Conference, Anaheim, Calif., March 30, 1974.
Winchester, A.M.: *Human Genetics,* Columbus, Ohio: Merrill, 1979.
Winters, M.: "The Relationship of Time of Initial Feeding to Success of Breastfeeding,"
    Unpublished paper, University of Washington, 1973.
Witti, F.P.: "Alcohol and Birth Defects," *FDA Consumer,* 22, 20−23, 1978.
Wyke, B.: "The Neurological Basis of Movement: A Developmental Review," in K.S.
    Holt (ed.), *Movement and Child Development,* London: William Heinemann Medical
    Books, 1975.
Wylie, R.: *The Self Concept,* Lincoln: University of Nebraska Press, 1961.
Wylie, R.: *The Self Concept: A Critical Survey of Pertinent Research Literature,* Lincoln:
    University of Nebraska Press, 1974.
Yakacs, R.F.: "Heart Rate Response of Children to Four Separate Bouts of Training,"
    Unpublished doctoral dissertation, Texas A & M University, 1971.
Yamamoto, K.: *The Child and His Image,* Boston: Houghton Mifflin, 1972.
Yang, R.K.: "Early Infant Assessment: An Overview," in J.D. Osofsky (ed.), *The
    Handbook of Infant Development,* New York: Wiley, 1979.
Yang, R.K., et al.: "Successive Relationships Between Maternal Attitudes During Preg-
    nancy, Analgesic Medication During Labor and Delivery, and Newborn Behavior,"
    *Developmental Psychology,* 12, 6−15, 1976.
Yawkey, T.D. (ed.): *The Self-Concept of the Young Child,* Salt Lake City, Utah: Brigham
    Young Press, 1980.
Zaichkowsky, L.B., et al.: "Self-Concept and Attitudinal Differences in Elementary Age
    Children After Participation in a Physical Activity Program," *Movement,* 243−245,
    October 1975.

Zaichkowsky, L.D., et al.: *Growth and Development: The Child and Physical Activity,* St. Louis, Mo.: C.V. Mosby, 1980.

Zelazo, P.: "From Reflexive to Instrumental Behavior," in L.P. Lipsitt (ed.), *Developmental Psychology: The Significance of Infancy,* Hillsdale, N.J.: Lawrence Erlbaum, 1976.

Zelazo, P., et al.: "Walking in the Newborn," *Science,* 176, 314–315, 1972.

Zubek, J.P., and P. Solberg: *Human Development,* New York: McGraw-Hill, 1954.

# Appendix A

## Equivalent Measures

### English-Metric

1 inch = 2.54 centimeter
1 foot = 0.3048 meter
1 yard = 0.9144 meter
1 mile = 1.6093 kilometers

1 ounce = 28.349 grams
1 pound = 0.53 kilograms
1 short ton = 0.907 metric ton

1 fluid ounce = 29.573 millileters
1 pint = 0.473 liter
1 quart = 0.946 liter
1 gallon = 3.785 liters

### Metric-English

1 centimeter = 0.3937 inch
1 meter = 3.281 feet
1 meter = 1.0936 yards
1 kilometer = 0.6214 mile

1 gram = 0.35 ounce
1 kilogram = 2.2046 pounds
1 metric ton = 1.1 short ton

1 milliliter = .06 cubic inch
1 liter = 61.02 cubic inch
1 liter = 0.908 dry quart
1 liter = 1.057 liquid quart

# Appendix B

## Inches-Centimeters: Conversion Table

| IN | CM | IN | CM | IN | CM |
|----|-----|----|-------|----|-------|
| 1/32 | .08 | 24 | 61.0 | 52 | 132.1 |
| 1/16 | .16 | 25 | 63.5 | 53 | 134.6 |
| 1/8 | .32 | 26 | 66.0 | 54 | 137.2 |
| 1/4 | .64 | 27 | 68.6 | 55 | 139.7 |
| 1/2 | 1.27 | 28 | 71.1 | 56 | 142.2 |
| 1 | 2.5 | 29 | 73.7 | 57 | 144.8 |
| 2 | 5.1 | 30 | 76.2 | 58 | 147.3 |
| 3 | 7.6 | 31 | 78.7 | 59 | 149.9 |
| 4 | 10.2 | 32 | 81.3 | 60 | 152.4 |
| 5 | 12.7 | 33 | 83.8 | 61 | 154.9 |
| 6 | 15.2 | 34 | 86.4 | 62 | 157.5 |
| 7 | 17.8 | 35 | 88.9 | 63 | 160.0 |
| 8 | 20.3 | 36 | 91.4 | 64 | 162.6 |
| 9 | 22.9 | 37 | 93.8 | 65 | 165.1 |
| 10 | 25.4 | 38 | 96.5 | 66 | 167.6 |
| 11 | 28.0 | 39 | 99.1 | 67 | 170.2 |
| 12 | 30.5 | 40 | 101.6 | 68 | 172.7 |
| 13 | 33.0 | 41 | 104.1 | 69 | 175.3 |
| 14 | 25.5 | 42 | 106.7 | 70 | 177.8 |
| 15 | 38.1 | 43 | 109.2 | 71 | 180.3 |
| 16 | 40.6 | 44 | 111.8 | 72 | 182.9 |
| 17 | 43.2 | 45 | 114.3 | 73 | 185.4 |
| 18 | 45.1 | 46 | 116.8 | 74 | 188.0 |
| 19 | 48.2 | 47 | 119.4 | 75 | 190.5 |
| 20 | 50.8 | 48 | 121.9 | | |
| 21 | 53.3 | 49 | 124.5 | | |
| 22 | 55.9 | 50 | 127.0 | | |
| 23 | 58.4 | 51 | 129.5 | | |

# Appendix C

## Pounds-Kilograms: Conversion Table

| LB | Kg | LB | Kg | LB | Kg | LB | Kg |
|----|------|----|-------|----|-------|-----|-------|
| 1  | 0.54 | 26 | 11.77 | 51 | 23.10 | 80  | 36.24 |
| 2  | 0.90 | 27 | 12.23 | 52 | 23.55 | 81  | 36.69 |
| 3  | 1.35 | 28 | 12.68 | 53 | 24.00 | 82  | 37.14 |
| 4  | 1.81 | 29 | 13.13 | 54 | 24.46 | 83  | 37.59 |
| 5  | 2.26 | 30 | 13.59 | 55 | 24.91 | 84  | 38.05 |
| 6  | 2.71 | 31 | 14.04 | 56 | 25.36 | 85  | 38.50 |
| 7  | 3.17 | 32 | 14.49 | 57 | 25.82 | 86  | 38.95 |
| 8  | 3.62 | 33 | 14.94 | 58 | 26.27 | 87  | 39.41 |
| 9  | 4.07 | 34 | 15.40 | 59 | 26.72 | 88  | 39.86 |
| 10 | 4.50 | 35 | 15.85 | 60 | 27.18 | 89  | 40.31 |
| 11 | 4.98 | 36 | 16.30 | 61 | 27.63 | 90  | 40.77 |
| 12 | 5.43 | 37 | 16.76 | 62 | 28.08 | 91  | 41.22 |
| 13 | 5.88 | 38 | 17.21 | 63 | 28.53 | 92  | 41.67 |
| 14 | 6.34 | 39 | 17.66 | 64 | 28.99 | 93  | 42.12 |
| 15 | 6.79 | 40 | 18.12 | 65 | 29.44 | 94  | 42.58 |
| 16 | 7.24 | 41 | 18.57 | 66 | 29.89 | 95  | 43.03 |
| 17 | 7.70 | 42 | 19.02 | 67 | 30.35 | 96  | 43.48 |
| 18 | 8.15 | 43 | 19.47 | 68 | 30.80 | 97  | 43.94 |
| 19 | 8.60 | 44 | 19.93 | 69 | 31.25 | 98  | 44.39 |
| 20 | 9.06 | 45 | 20.38 | 70 | 31.71 | 99  | 44.84 |
| 21 | 9.51 | 46 | 20.83 | 71 | 32.16 | 100 | 45.30 |
| 22 | 9.96 | 47 | 21.29 | 72 | 32.61 |     |       |
| 23 | 10.41 | 48 | 21.74 | 73 | 33.06 |    |       |
| 24 | 10.87 | 49 | 22.19 | 74 | 33.52 |    |       |
| 25 | 11.32 | 50 | 22.65 | 75 | 33.97 |    |       |

# AUTHOR INDEX

# SUBJECT INDEX

Abilities: motor fitness, 49, 51; physical fitness, 49, 51; fundamental movement, 251, 332; sport skill, 258; performance, 326; reasonable expectations of, 335; free-play, 366; lead-up, 391

Adaptation, definition, 13

Adventure, activities, 332, 333

Aerobic capacity, 270, 271, 289

Affective development: term use, 14; of children, 337

Age periods, as time ranges, 7

Agility, definition, 283

Alcoholism, maternal, 69, 70

American Alliance for Health, Physical Education, Recreation, and Dance (AAHPERD), 8, 268, 283, 292, 327

Anorectic children, family of, 288

Anorexia nervosa: incidence of, 287; mentioned, 289

Apgar screening test, 401, 412, 413

Assessment instruments: process-oriented, 412; product-oriented, 412

Axial movements: definition, 230; developmental sequence, 230-231; visual description, 231-232

Balance: concerns of, 52-53; and vision, 279; types, 279, 280, 282; and kinesthetic abilities, 280; and tactile abilities, 280; concept of, 380

Ball rolling: developmental sequence

of, 222; visual description of, 222-223

Bayley Scales of Infant Development, 406, 408, 412, 413

Beam walk: developmental sequence of, 244; visual description of, 244-246

Behavior, goal-directed, 389

Behavioral assessment instruments, purposes of, 401

Birth: process, 75-76; risk factors of, 77; preterm, 82; home, 89

Body awareness: term use, 301; components of, 302

Body rolling: developmental sequence of, 236; visual description of, 237-238

Body weight, maintenance of, 284

Bonding, 88, 89

Brazelton Neonatal Behavioral Assessment Scale (BNBAS), 406, 412, 413

Bruininks-Oseretsky Test of Motor Proficiency (BOT), 408, 410, 412, 413

Bureau of Product Safety, 351, 353

Cardiovascular: endurance, 270, 289; health, 271

Catching: definition, 210; developmental sequence of, 210-211; visual description of, 211

Census: data (1980), 367; report (1970), 367

Challengers, program, 329, 330